Research Methods in
Communication Disorders

Dedication

For Joan and Archie
and Ellie and Ben

Research Methods in Communication Disorders

TIM PRING PhD

City University, London

W

WHURR PUBLISHERS

LONDON AND PHILADELPHIA

© 2005 Tim Pring

First Published 2005
Whurr Publishers Ltd
19b Compton Terrace, London N1 2UN, England and
325 Chestnut Street, Philadelphia PA19106, USA

British Library Cataloguing in Publication Data

A catalogue record for this book is available from the
British Library.

ISBN 1 86156 097 4

Printed and bound in the UK by Athenaeum Press Limited,
Gateshead, Tyne & Wear.

Contents

Foreword

This book is a delight. I've spent longer than I intended reviewing it because it is such a joy to read! It is witty, modest, authoritative, committed, serious, light hearted and above all reveals and conveys a love of its subject matter. It will be the only statistics textbook of which all this can be said.

Many aspects are impressive. First, the range of content is massive. From the simplest introductory material through to complex issues of power, effect, size, transformation, the author manages to maintain a kind of intimate almost chatty style which distinguishes this from any comparable book. I enjoyed particularly the references to King Lear in the castle, the 'double entendre' of Howell's quip about fatal abnormality, and perhaps most of all the opening of Chapter 14, the great dragons of the past! I can't imagine a reader who will fail to be seduced and drawn into a depth of understanding which they had never dreamt of reaching.

There is erudition here. The way in which each new concept and technique is grounded in the literature of SLT research shows a massive breadth of reading, but more to the point it supports the novice reader and builds a knowledge of the literature by proxy. The final chapters are mandatory reading not just for students in training but for each and every researcher in the field. And they will enjoy themselves!

Coverage of diverse areas and techniques within the remit of SLT studies is virtually complete, impressing the reader with the author's ability to apply the same rigour and conviction to observational studies as to analyses of simple main effects, to focus groups and transformations.

People will probably carp at this or that. Why no computer outputs? Why is stepwise regression thought respectable? Why no structural modelling? and so on. They will be missing the point. This is a lovingly crafted and immensely readable gift from an expert to all who are committed to working and researching within the field of communication disorders. It will provide interest, delight and even salvation to many others in related disciplines e.g. Special Education, Educational Psychology, Clinical Psychology, and of course the other therapy professions.

Chris Donlan
University College London

Preface

Books on research methods are commonplace. Look in your local university bookshop and you will find that almost every subject has research methods textbooks explaining the mysteries of experimental design and of statistical tests as they apply in their area. Psychology takes first prize. Whole shelves are filled with research methods books. Psychologists are obsessed with research methods. I should know; I am one and have many of these books at home on my own shelves. The other behavioural sciences, medicine, nursing and other health sciences are not far behind. Even quite esoteric subjects have them. Recently I found not one but two books on research methods for archaeology. The contents of these books (the odd hole in the ground apart) were quite familiar and included old friends like the t test. Research methods and statistical tests appear to be a necessary part of all scientific enquiry.

You may have guessed where this is leading. Given the ubiquitous nature of research methods, it is curious, to say the least that there are so few books on research methods in speech and language therapy. While lecturing in this area, I have been forced to recommend books written for students in other areas. Some are good, but I cannot help wondering what students make of the need to borrow research methods texts from other disciplines or whether they might feel happier with a book designed for their own needs. During the several years it has taken me to write this book (and lets acknowledge the patience of Whurr publishers at this point!) I have expected other authors to beat me to it. However, few other books have appeared. This only adds to the mystery. It cannot be that therapists are uninterested in research. Most that I meet are very aware of the need for it and anxious, not to say neurotic, about their lack of time and, perhaps, perceived lack of knowledge to contribute to it. The Royal College of Speech and Language Therapists has eleven thousand members. This adds up to a lot of anxiety and suggests that it cannot be lack of sales that is putting potential authors off.

There is a serious side to all this. Speech and language therapy, like all health interventions, progresses in a series of stages. Early interventions are haphazard. Those that appear to work acquire the status of superstitions. Superstitions that endure over time acquire a more respectable name. They become clinical experience. Therapists are not short of clinical experience; they also have plenty of energy and imagination. They have come up with lots of ideas about how to do therapy. What we lack is evidence that they work. Research methods are our means of discovering whether, why and with whom they work. In other words they are our means of making clinical practice more scientific.

Although not a therapist myself, I have tried to make this book as relevant to the needs of speech and language therapy as I can. It has been a great help to me in doing so that I have been able to hang around with therapists for many years and pick their brains. As a result I am much indebted to many colleagues (both stable and neurotic) with whom I have done research over the years and to the many students whose research projects I have supervised.

Chapter 1
Introduction

Why should speech and language therapists study research methods?

People train to become speech and language therapists (SLTs) for many commendable reasons. That they want to study research methods appears not to be one of them. So let's begin with some reasons why they should know how to do research.

First, they must be able to assess research critically. You might be familiar with the way research is reported in academic journals. Articles have:

- an introduction that summarizes existing knowledge and describes the aims of the research
- a methods section that describes the research design and the procedure used
- a results section in which the data is analysed
- a discussion of the results and their implications.

Journals look impressive and live in libraries. Reading them is hard work. The methods section is a bit dull (but with good reason as it must give the information readers need to repeat the research), and the results section can be hard going. It is tempting to skip these sections. This is a mistake. There is a lot of bad research in journals and to spot it you must assess the research design, the way the data are analysed and whether appropriate conclusions are drawn from this analysis.

A second reason is that therapists need to design research to investigate the effects of their therapy. We will be particularly interested in how to do this. It is not easy, and studies conducted in the past have led to controversy and misunderstanding.

A third reason is to be more involved in theoretical research. Research may be divided into applied and theoretical forms. In SLT applied research is about therapy and its outcome; theoretical research is about the nature and causes of communication disorders. Clinicians are often sceptical about theoretical research. It does have a habit of taking its time and researchers like nothing better than disagreeing with one another. However, its findings improve our knowledge of communication disorders and help us develop therapies. Therapists, with their experience of clinical practice, can bring a much-needed sense of urgency to this process.

Is research working?

Research on people's behaviour faces two big problems. The first is that many behaviours are hard to define and difficult to measure. Consider measuring the severity of a child's dysfluency. We could count the stammers. Unfortunately therapists can argue all day about what constitutes a stammer. Moreover, a count only tells us how many there are, not how severe they are. We might tape the child and have listeners rate the severity of the dysfluency. This has the advantage of assessing the impact a child's speech has on actual listeners, but it's hard work persuading people to listen to the tapes! These measures tell us about the child's speech but not about the effect that stammering has on them personally. This is even more difficult to measure. Many behaviours are like stammering — they are hard to define, don't come in fixed quantities and observers may disagree whether they have occurred or not.

Exercise 1.1

Think about how we might measure the following:

1. Children's conversational skills.
2. The effects of being dysfluent on people's personal life and well-being.
3. Depression in people with dysphasia.
4. The effects of language impairment on children's social behaviours.

A second problem is that many 'things' affect behaviour. Consider the causes of language delay in children or the factors that aid recovery after stroke. In each case a large variety of 'things' may be involved. In research 'things' are called variables. Often we want to study one variable but others are in the way. Research design tries to isolate the effects of interesting variables by controlling the ones that are in the way.

The difficulties of studying behaviour are frustrating for researchers and the public alike. The public may have two complaints. The first is 'I could have told you that for free, mate!' Such 'common sense' findings are often reported in the press. For instance, it was recently reported that babies prefer tuneful music to dissonant music. They were more content listening to Mozart than Schoenberg. No surprise there, then. Even dogs howl when they hear Schoenberg. In another recent experiment, subjects answered a self-esteem questionnaire and then waited in a room with well-dressed models. Later, when they repeated the questionnaire, their self-esteem was as dishevelled as their clothing. Not a finding designed to raise the public's regard for science!

In fairness it should be said that, although research and common sense may reach similar conclusions, they use very different methods. Common-sense judgements are based on our subjective observation of a limited range of people. Researchers are more systematic. They test a variety of people and try to measure their behaviour objectively. Then they analyse the data statistically to assess the importance of the findings and whether they can be generalized to other people.

Exercise 1.2

The speech of people with cerebral palsy is often dysarthric. Common sense might suggest that listeners with experience of such speakers are better able to understand them. What advantages are offered by an experimental demonstration of this?

A second complaint is that when researchers look at things that concern us they often can't agree on an explanation. Health research is a good example here. It is difficult to study the causes of many illnesses directly (we can't make some people smoke or not smoke to see if it affects their health) so we observe what happens naturally. Unfortunately potential causes of a disease and the illness itself are often widely separated in time and other possible causes intervene. Regular alarming newspaper stories have turned the world into a hazardous place full of threats to our health: pollution and toxic waste abound, eating is a perilous process and smoking is reported to increase the risk of Alzheimer's disease and impotence (as if lung cancer were not bad enough). Many of these reports are convincing and may be correct; however, these studies do not allow us (for reasons we discuss later) to link cause and effect with certainty.

How should we do research?

Research is done in different ways. We will divide it into three different approaches. The first approach is to do experiments. Most people think that all research is about doing experiments. However, researchers have a stricter definition of what an experiment is than the rest of us. Suppose we examine the effect of therapy on children who stammer. We put the children randomly into two groups: one receives therapy, the other does not. Here we 'manipulate' the variable we are interested in (therapy). Other variables are free to vary, but by putting people randomly into groups we hope that their average effect on the two groups is the same. This is a 'true' experiment and is the only type of research that lets us show that a variable directly causes a change in behaviour.

Unfortunately the experimental approach has problems when it is used to study people's behaviour. Real life is reluctant to stand still while we control the variables and so, as in the self-esteem example above, we may have to simulate it in laboratories. This lets us do experiments but is often criticized for being unnatural and producing atypical behaviour.

Another problem is that many variables can't be manipulated. Suppose we compare children with and without language delay to find the cause of their delay. This looks like an experiment, but the presence or absence of delay is not manipulated. Just as we can't force people to smoke or not to smoke, so they either have language delay or they do not. As a result we can't be sure that any difference we find between the groups of children is the cause of the delay. This sort of research is often called quasi-experimental — it resembles an experiment but we cannot draw cause-and-effect conclusions from it. The distinction between experimental and quasi-experimental research is important. Nevertheless, these approaches use broadly similar methods and are considered together in this book. It is up to you to be alert and spot quasi-experiments so that you avoid drawing inappropriate conclusions from them.

Sometimes researchers abandon any attempt to control or manipulate variables. Suppose we want to know the factors that aid recovery of language after a stroke. Variables like age, the severity of the stroke, the client's motivation and personality, help from carers and therapy may all aid recovery. Rather than trying to control these variables we might collect information on all of them and look for relationships between them. This is a correlational approach to research. It lets us discover relationships between variables, but we have to be careful about claiming that one causes another (a client's motivation may be a result of recovery not vice versa). Nevertheless, this approach to research is useful in complex situations where it is difficult to do experiments.

The third approach is the broadest of the three. It takes the sensible view that we might learn a lot about people's behaviour by asking them about it or watching them do it. This lets us study real behaviour without the need for experiments and sounds like more fun as well. We can do this in a variety of ways. Methods of asking people about their behaviour vary from having them fill in questionnaires to conducting in-depth interviews with them. Methods of observing behaviour also vary. We may observe people covertly or participate in the behaviour we want to observe. We may define types of behaviour in advance and record how often they occur or freely interpret the behaviour we observe.

Researchers are unlikely to restrict themselves to just one way of doing research. Our example above of treating children who stammer used an experimental approach. We assessed the children's fluency before and after therapy to see if it had improved. Combining this with other approaches might give a much better picture of the effects of therapy. We will probably find that some children respond better to therapy than others, and we might try to understand this by using a correlational approach to look at relationships between the amount of improvement made and other variables. We could observe them in school or playing with other children to see if they are fluent in situations outside the clinic, and we might interview their parents to find out more about the effects of dysfluency on the children and whether these had also changed with therapy.

Dividing up research methods in this way cuts across a traditional distinction between quantitative and qualitative approaches to research. The first two of the above approaches are quantitative; much, but not all, of the third is qualitative. Quantitative research, as its name suggests, likes to measure behaviour and collect numbers for analysis. Qualitative research is more concerned with interpreting behaviour than measuring it and uses interviews and observation to study it in real situations.

It's fair to say that many of the problems mentioned above are associated with quantitative methods. The problem of measuring variables arises because we want numbers to analyse, and our inability to get to grips with 'real' problems stems from the difficulty of doing experiments in real-life situations. In some instances these problems are so great that using a quantitative approach seems pigheaded. On the other hand, the apparent desire of some qualitative researchers to exclude all numbers from their research as though they are something nasty and probably catching is also shortsighted.

Many textbooks deal only with quantitative or with qualitative research, and researchers using one approach are sometimes suspicious of the other. This is silly. Qualitative methods are good for finding out about people's experiences or examining complex behaviours. We won't find out much about the problems faced by carers of people with communication disorders in a laboratory. Interviews or observation of real life will serve us better. In contrast, quantitative methods may be preferred to test theories about the nature of language disorders. Here the advantage of testing specific language-processing skills outweighs the disadvantage of being in a laboratory.

Theories and research

In the real world we accept theories if they seem to be true. In research their role is rather different. They summarize existing knowledge and stimulate research by suggesting which hypotheses should be tested (see Figure 1.1). This is especially true of experimental research, where it is normal to state, and then test, a particular hypothesis. Testing may support or disprove the theory. Disproof is important here: theories that cannot be disproved are not useful and become objects of faith – we believe them or not according to our prejudices.

This means that theories are temporary things. They help us to develop knowledge but are rejected when they fail to explain new results. Unfortunately, people have a tendency to strengthen rather than reject their beliefs when confronted with contrary evidence. Researchers are no exception. They are reluctant to dump their theories and often find ways to amend them so that they struggle on after their sell-by date. Sometimes this leads to a sudden exciting change or paradigm shift when a new approach finally replaces a worn-out theory. A classic example was the shift from a behaviourist to an information-processing approach when it became clear that cognition generally and language-learning in particular could not be explained by behaviourism.

One silly objection to experimental research is that its objectivity is inconsistent with new or creative ideas. The reverse is true. Experiments should be objective; theories need not be. They may come from clinical observations, intuitions or wild ideas on a sleepless night. This creative freedom illustrates why it is important that theories can be disproved. In return for letting you test your ideas (which may be completely potty), the experimental method asks that you at least expose them to the possibility of disproof.

Qualitative research is less dependent on theories and is often used in areas where theories are clearly inadequate or non-existent. Consequently it has an important role in developing new theories. These theories may make predictions that can be tested by quantitative methods. Here the two methods complement rather than compete with one another.

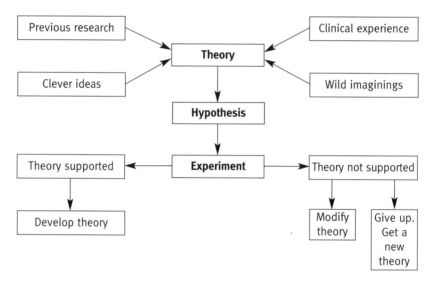

Figure 1.1 Theories and their role in research.

Exercise 1.3

Three of the biggest 'psychological' theories of the last century are Freud's psychoanalytic theory, Skinner's theory of operant conditioning and Piaget's theory of cognitive development. Assess them as theories in the light of what you have just read.

How does this book work?

There are many books on research methods, but few appeal directly to SLTs. They explain research methods without reference to the problems that interest therapists. In this book examples are drawn from the SLT literature with the hope that, if the examples are meaningful, the methods will be more comprehensible. (In some cases I have simplified the examples. You can go to the original sources to find out more. There are also a few non-SLT examples to add variety.)

Books on research methods face a problem. Sooner or later they have to show readers how to do statistical tests. Traditionally textbooks have devoted many fierce-looking pages to this and have made poor bedtime reading. Although difficult, these books do give an insight into how statistical tests work. The general availability of statistics programs on computers has provided a less tearful way of doing the calculations and has led to a new kind of textbook that explains how to do tests on computers. These bypass the arithmetic, often filling their pages with computer printouts that look just as fierce. Although useful, these books don't give you much help with designing experiments or understanding their results. In fact, the uncritical way in which computers gobble up numbers may even encourage unnecessarily complex and poorly designed research. The objective in this book is to help you to design research and understand statistical tests. Along the way we will work out some simple tests to see how they work. When this becomes too complicated, I will give you the results and try to explain what they mean. Generally the more advanced tests are beyond the level of this book, but I will describe a few of them in a non-mathematical way. A few sections of the book and one whole chapter are marked with an asterisk (*) to indicate that you may want to skip them on a first reading.

As you progress in research you will want to use one of the major statistical programs. People behave quite oddly about these, becoming very attached to their favourite program and having irrational grudges against alternatives. The dominant statistical package is currently SPSS, and this is likely to be the most readily available. It also has the advantage that several textbooks are available to take you through it (see, for example, Howitt and Cramer, 1999; Field, 2000; Dancey and Reidy, 2002).

Statistical analysis of research data is a less precise business than you might expect. Statisticians often disagree about how to proceed. In this sense applied statistics is more like law than mathematics. Opinions differ, precedents are set, fashions change and experts write heavy books on it (I will call these the 'big books'). Mere mortals need not become involved; however, it is surprising (and amusing) to find that such disagreements exist.

This book works its way through the approaches to research described above. Then it looks at research on the efficacy of therapy. You have to work hard. As you have already seen, there are exercises to do. These are mainly, but not entirely, used to give you some practice at some of the easier calculations needed to carry out statistical tests. They are compulsory – you are forbidden to look at the answers before at least working up a sweat. Before starting Chapter 2 you should do Exercise 1.4, which is about designing experiments. People know more about this than they think (or perhaps they don't know that what they do know is about designing experiments). Experimental design is a bit like riding a bicycle: things go pretty well until you start thinking about it (or having lectures on it). This exercise was designed to convince you that you already know more than you thought. We will refer back to it later on.

Exercise 1.4

This exercise takes a preliminary look at experimental design. It will give you an idea of some of the difficulties we often have when doing research. We look at some ways in which they may be overcome later in the book.

1. Does providing a sentence context assist children with word-finding difficulties?
2. Compare the progress made by treated and untreated children who stammer.
3. Compare the auditory reaction times of children with language impairment and children with normal language development.
4. Compare the 'naturalness' of people who stammer before and after therapy.
5. Assess the value of giving counselling/support on the psychological well-being of the carers of people with dysphasia.

Chapter 2
Designing experiments

Research methods and statistics

This chapter looks at experimental design and introduces some of the terminology used to discuss it. Then it explains why we need statistical tests and what they do for us.

Research methods and statistics are related skills that are learned in different ways. The former is about designing research and is a craft learned through experience. Each research project has its own design problems. Projects often go wrong. Don't be discouraged – it's part of the learning process. This book aims to help you to make a start; your own experience will finish the job. In contrast, statistical analysis is manual labour and not very popular as a result.

The first example in Exercise 1.4 was about cueing children who have word-finding difficulties. It illustrates two basic experimental designs. We can either put children randomly into two groups and compare naming by one with cued naming by the other or we can compare the performance of the same children doing both. These are the between-subjects designs (or independent-groups designs) and within-subjects designs (or related- or repeated-measures designs).

The between-subjects design

We will use the second example from Exercise 1.4 to illustrate the between-subjects design. It compared progress by treated and untreated children who stammer. In this example we will assume that we can randomly assign clients to treated and untreated groups. We will use the percentage of syllables stammered to measure dysfluency. To avoid upsetting any of the ideological factions that exist in stammering research, we won't say what the therapy is!

Stammering varies from person to person, in the same person over time, at different times in a person's life and in different situations.

In other words, it is affected by many variables. We need to control these variables.

In experiments we manipulate an independent variable (IV) and measure its effect on a dependent variable (DV). In our experiment the IV is therapy and it has two levels: clients are either treated or not. The DVs in experiments are the data we collect, but I have managed to choose an example where it's slightly more complicated than this. We want a measure of the children's change in fluency over time; so we must assess them before and after therapy, and our DV will be the difference between the assessments. We assess untreated clients at the same times to measure how much they change without therapy.

The IV has two levels; so the experiment has two conditions. These are the experimental and control conditions. The experimental condition measures change with therapy. If this is greater than in the control (untreated) condition, therapy has had an effect. Here it is obvious which are the experimental and control conditions. This is not always the case. For example, we may compare two different therapies. Here each acts as a control for the other.

Exercise 2.1

In the following experiments would a between- or a within-subjects design be used? Identify the IV and DV and the experimental and control conditions.

1. People with chronic aphasia (more than 6 months since onset) have computer-assisted treatment and their progress is assessed (see Aftonomos et al., 1997).
2. Children with specific speech and language difficulties (SSLD) and typically developing children complete a self-esteem assessment and their scores are compared. In a second experiment the scores of children with SSLD are compared with the scores given to them by teachers on the same assessment (see Lindsay et al., 2002a).
3. Clients with aphasia who are receiving SLT are tested to see if the use of amphetamines improves their language recovery (see Walker–Batson et al., 2001).

Experimental design is about controlling the variables in which we are not interested. We can divide these into subject and situational variables. People bring their subject variables with them. Among the more obvious ones are differences in their skills, attitudes and background. We control these by random assignment. In our experiment the severity of stammering is a subject variable. We can't control it directly and so we randomly assign clients to the treated and untreated groups. As a result the average severity should be equal in the groups (but individual children in each group will vary).

Situational variables arise within the experiment. People may react to the novelty of the situation, be suspicious or anxious to please and respond in unexpected ways to the experimenter or the experimental task. We can't control these reactions, but we can minimize their effects by using a standard procedure. We give everybody the same instructions about the experiment and test them under the same conditions. Sometimes this is taken to extremes. Must we really test everyone in the same room or at the same time of day? It all depends on whether these things affect their performance. If you think they will (or if you don't know that they won't), you should control them. If tiredness is a factor, test people when they are unlikely to be tired. If you want them to do a complex task or listen to tapes of people's speech, use the same quiet room. Ideally we want good conditions so people perform well, and consistent conditions to reduce the variability in their performance.

The experimenter is a major situational variable. It's easy to influence (deliberately or not) the way people behave in experiments. To reduce this we try to interact with each subject in the same way. One way to do this is to interact as little as possible! However, this produces a formal atmosphere and poor rapport with clients and gives the impression that experiments (and experimenters) are not much fun. It's a particular problem with children, who respond rather badly to serious strangers who ask them to do odd things and then sit frowning at them. On the other hand, we must be careful about giving encouragement or help during experiments. This affects performance and opens the door to the temptation to help children in the experimental group selectively (see below). It's a good idea to establish rapport with children before testing them and to have a procedure that lets you be equally friendly and encouraging with all the children.

One of the beauties of adhering to the above is that it controls all of the variables that might affect the outcome of an experiment. Some variables will be obvious, but there will always be others we have not considered. Random assignment and a standard experimental procedure will control both known and unknown variables.

If subjects are not randomly assigned, other variables may inadvertently be manipulated along with the IV. These are confounding variables. They may affect the DV, and their effect may be mistaken for that of the IV. They often occur in therapy studies. One sure way to get confounding variables is to cheat on the random assignment. If we have a hunch about which clients respond to therapy, why not put them in the treated group? Sounds sensible enough! Notice that it doesn't matter if the hunch was right or not; the problem is that the groups are now different. Concern about withholding treatment may persuade you to use clients who cannot be treated as a control group. For instance, some people with aphasia have transport or mobility problems and can't come to the clinic. This is just well-intentioned cheating. These problems are more likely in the elderly or people with severe aphasias; so any difference we find between the groups may be due to age or severity and not to therapy. A similar situation occurs in Exercise 1.4, Example 5.

This is a good moment to introduce the randomized control trial (RCT), which is widely used in medical research – particularly in drug trials. A lot of mystique and confusion has grown up around RCTs. As a research design they are no big deal. Typically they are like our experiment with children who stammer. They use a between-subjects design to compare treated and untreated people. Their attention to detail makes them special. Care is taken to ensure random allocation and to avoid the effects of variables – such as receiving attention from a doctor – which are confounded with treatment. In drug trials, assignment to the drug or control (placebo) condition is random so that neither doctors nor patients know who gets the drug. This is referred to as a double-blind study. It's difficult to do therapy studies like this. The contact is more personal and we can't easily disguise who is having treatment; nor is it clear what the placebo should be. We return to the use of RCTs in therapy research later on.

So far we have discussed doing experiments as if the subjects we need are just lining up at the door full of enthusiasm to start. Sadly this is rarely the case. In fact, a most irritating aspect of research is that the clients who were in your caseload only last year can't be found for love nor money when you want to do research on them (see Hodgson and Rollnick, 1996, for this and other cautionary tales about doing research). This often means that research is done over a period of time as new clients enter a caseload. It's a misperception that all subjects must do an experiment at the same time. Normally it is unnecessary and undesirable to keep some waiting until others appear. No problem arises as long as we use a common procedure throughout (but the chances of its changing increase with time).

In clinical research we often want to compare different clinical groups or clinical with non-clinical groups. Here we need a clear definition of the membership of the clinical groups to use as an entry criterion for the experiment. Unfortunately clinical diagnoses that sound fine in textbooks may be more difficult to make on the factory

Exercise 2.2

Confounding variables are often present in research on communication disorders. What confounding variables might exist in the
following studies?

1. Studies have found that children with specific language
   impairment (SLI) are more likely to have had parents who
   smoke (see Tomblin et al., 1998).
2. Children attending language units at 7 years of age were
   followed up at 11. Some had moved to mainstream schools, and
   the progress of these children was compared with children
   who remained in language units (see Conti-Ramsden et al.,
   2002).
3. Research has shown that measures of short-term phonological
   memory (usually non-word repetition) are related to measures
   of language development in both children with normal
   development (Adams and Gathercole, 1995, 1996) and
   children with SLI (Gathercole and Baddeley, 1990).

Exercise 2.3

People think that the study of art and literature is important because
they reveal profound truths about humanity. Actually, studying
research methods changes lives and knowing about confounding
variables plays a big part in this. Open the newspaper most days and
you will find reporters failing to detect confounding variables. Here
are some examples. Can you spot the possible confounding variables?

1. The increasing anarchy in the nation's schools has led to differences of opinion about what to do with disruptive children. One
   view is that they should be excluded from school; another argues
   that they should not be, on the grounds that excluded children go
   on to participate in a variety of anti-social activities in later life.
2. Research has shown that regular users of Ecstasy are more
   prone to psychiatric problems in later life. More than 1 in 4
   have psychiatric illnesses, whereas fewer than 1 in 5 non-users
   do (which sounds alarmingly high anyway).
3. The government has argued that students can afford to pay top-
   up fees to attend university on the grounds that graduates will
   earn £400,000 more than non-graduates over their working life.
   What's wrong with the reasoning here?

floor. Conflicting findings may result because researchers include different types of people within the same clinical diagnosis. Entry criteria should be set before an experiment and maintained throughout. A dilemma may arise because they restrict the number of clients available for the experiment. As subjects fail to appear and the completion date for the research recedes, the temptation to change the entry criteria can become very strong. Objective entry criteria, such as performance on standardized tests, may hold this in check. Research on children with SLI, for example, may require that they be below a specified score on a language test but not on a test of non-verbal ability. This approach has two advantages. It makes the research more disciplined by excluding doubtful subjects and it makes it clearer to whom the results apply. In cases where we are forced to rely on more subjective criteria it may be a good idea to have two or more clinicians see the clients and agree that they are suitable for the research.

Random assignment is fairly easy when we know the clients we need. A first step is to decide if all of them can do the experiment. In the example above it is probably better to exclude the people with mobility problems. Even if we allocate them randomly, their potential non-attendance will be a nuisance. We then randomly assign the rest. How you do this may depend upon your liking for drama. Drawing names from a hat (but a hat is not essential) and assigning them alternately to treated and untreated groups is usually fine, although the temptation to cheat is surprisingly strong. If you don't trust yourself, you can give the clients numbers and draw and assign the numbers to groups or have someone who doesn't know the clients randomly assign them.

Random assignment is trickier when clients enter the experiment over time and/or must meet strict entry criteria. Having to assess clients to see if they meet the entry criteria may influence assignment ('This one looks like a good subject. I'll put him in the experimental group' or 'I'm not catching this kid's cold, he can be a control'). Changing the entry criteria because of a shortage of subjects is one thing; much worse (and, yes, it happens) is when clients who satisfy the criteria are assigned to the experimental group and the dodgy ones are put in the control group. This is a really smart way of producing confounding variables. A good approach in these circumstances is to have a list that randomly assigns subjects to conditions by their order of entry into the experiment. This is entrusted to another person who is only consulted when the researcher has decided that a client meets the entry criteria.

Unfortunately random assignment alone can't control all confounding variables. They can occur within the experiment if researchers behave differently with the experimental and control groups. The more contact there is between subjects and researchers, the more likely this is (which is why RCTs keep group membership a secret) and the more likely that confounding variables will be present.

Unfortunately therapy studies are a prime example here. In language therapy, therapists do many 'nice' and encouraging things. These may be confounding variables. If we want to know specifically about therapy (and since we are unlikely to persuade SLTs not to be 'nice') we may need a control group that they can be nice to without giving therapy (and I'll volunteer for that one).

Further problems arise when we assess clients. Researchers may influence the outcome of experiments by influencing the way subjects respond at assessments. Some assessments (like reaction times – see Example 3 of Exercise 1.4) offer little scope for this. However, assessments in SLT usually involve personal contact. If assessors know which group a client has been in, they may (deliberately or otherwise) allow this to influence their performance (such assessments are called 'reactive'). The usual (but inconvenient) way around this is to have the clients assessed by someone who does not know them or whether they have been treated or not.

Why we need statistical tests

Random assignment makes the *average* effect of subject variables the same in each condition of an experiment. But individual differences between subjects remain. In our experiment the changes in fluency will vary among clients in both the treated and untreated groups. Treatment will not help all the treated group equally, and some of the untreated group will improve for reasons of their own. Table 2.1 gives some possible data. Although overall improvement is greater in the treated group, individual clients vary. Despite our best efforts designing the experiment, it is difficult to tell if the IV has had an effect. (To simplify the example, all the scores are positive – no one became worse.)

Table 2.1 Data from the experiment – the scores are the differences in percentage of syllables stammered before and after therapy

Control group (no therapy)		Experimental group (therapy)	
Subject 1	14	Subject 7	19
Subject 2	0	Subject 8	11
Subject 3	12	Subject 9	15
Subject 4	9	Subject 10	17
Subject 5	3	Subject 11	13
Subject 6	10	Subject 12	3
Mean (average) score	8	Mean (average) score	13

Data like these are common in behavioural research and show why we need statistical tests. Individuals vary so much that it is hard to tell if the treated group made more improvement. Clients vary in their fluency over time, and perhaps the treated group has done better because, by chance, it includes more clients who improved during the experiment. Now do Exercise 2.4.

Exercise 2.4

Here are three more sets of results from our experiment. Compare each with the data in Table 2.1. Would you be more or less confident that the groups are different in these examples?

1. **Control group (no therapy)**   **Experimental group (therapy)**

Subject 1	14	Subject 7	22
Subject 2	0	Subject 8	14
Subject 3	12	Subject 9	18
Subject 4	9	Subject 10	20
Subject 5	3	Subject 11	16
Subject 6	10	Subject 12	6
Mean (average) score	8	Mean (average) score	16

2. **Control group (no therapy)**   **Experimental group (therapy)**

Subject 1	16	Subject 7	25
Subject 2	0	Subject 8	4
Subject 3	10	Subject 9	17
Subject 4	12	Subject 10	22
Subject 5	2	Subject 11	9
Subject 6	8	Subject 12	1
Mean (average) score	8	Mean (average) score	13

3. **Control group (no therapy)**   **Experimental group (therapy)**

Subject 1	14	Subject 13	19
Subject 2	0	Subject 14	11
Subject 3	12	Subject 15	15
Subject 4	9	Subject 16	17
Subject 5	3	Subject 17	13
Subject 6	10	Subject 18	3
Subject 7	14	Subject 19	19
Subject 8	0	Subject 20	11
Subject 9	12	Subject 21	15
Subject 10	9	Subject 22	17
Subject 11	3	Subject 23	13
Subject 12	10	Subject 24	3
Mean (average) score	8	Mean (average) score	13

It is important to understand what statistical tests do. We must decide if a difference between the conditions in our experiment is real (due to the IV) or due to chance (the treated group happens to have more clients who changed positively). Any difference can occur by chance. However large it is there is a possibility (but, in statistics, we call it a probability) that it is, due to random variation by the subjects. Statistical tests calculate the probability of a chance result. If it is small, we say the test is significant. We set the level of significance. The widely accepted level is 5%. If a test tells us there is less than a 5% probability (written $p < 0.05$) that a result is due to chance, we call it 'significant'. This means there is a 5% probability that we have made an error (but we won't know this) and that the result is due to chance. These are called type-one errors. They play a big part in the lives of statisticians, and we will meet them again frequently. The reverse, where we fail to get a significant result that does exist, is called a type-two error.

The significance level is the probability of a type-one error. Normally it is 5%. However, if we want a *lower* level of risk, we can use a *higher* level of significance (for example $p < 0.01$). Now a type-one error is less likely, but a type-two error more likely.

Exercise 2.5

When we use the 0.05 level of significance:

1. What probability is there that a significant result is a type-one error?
2. How do we know we have made a type-one error?
3. How many researchers must do an experiment before one finds a type-one error?
4. What might happen when the researchers in 3 submit their work for publication?

Exercise 2.6

People often become mixed-up when talking about the significance of results. Sometimes a result is said to be significant even though it is not statistically significant. Sometimes results are statistically significant but are said to be not clinically significant. Do these statements make sense?

When we do research, we must state the hypothesis we are going to test. Our hypothesis seems simple enough – that therapy improves fluency – so it may surprise you that we are expected to state two hypotheses and in a rather odd way. They are the null and experimental (or alternative) hypotheses. Our null hypothesis is that:

> Any difference in the change in fluency between subjects who have and have not been treated can be accounted for by chance.

and the experimental hypothesis is that:

> Any difference in the change in fluency between subjects who have and have not been treated is unlikely to be accounted for by chance.

If the statistical test is significant, we 'reject' the null hypothesis.

You may think that someone is taking the Mickey here. You might also have noticed that authors in journals state their hypotheses in a more straightforward way or even get away without stating them clearly at all. This is one of many instances where beginners must follow the rules while club members get away with murder. There is a reason for stating hypotheses like this, however. It reminds us that we never prove a hypothesis. We only show that a result is (fairly) unlikely to be due to chance. So we reject the null hypothesis; we don't prove the experimental hypothesis.

The need to reject the null hypotheses affects how we design experiments. In experiments we want subjects to behave as consistently as possible. Bad design increases subject variability and decreases the chance of finding a significant result. Consequently we should avoid doing experiments to show that no difference exists between groups of subjects (to prove the null hypothesis). This would just reward poor research design.

Suppose we know a therapy is effective but want to show that another therapy, which is more economical to deliver, is equally good. Here we are trying to prove the null hypothesis, and consequently there is no incentive to conduct the experiment rigorously. An alternative might be to use three groups, a control group and groups receiving each of the therapies. If each therapy is better than the control, we have at least shown that the new therapy works and that our experiment can detect a difference. As a result we can be more confident about the lack of a difference between the two therapy groups.

Sometimes there is no way around this problem, and theory demands that we show that no difference exists between groups of people. An example concerns parental speech to children who stammer. Starkweather and Gottwald (1990) suggested that parental speech may make demands that exceed the child's capacity for fluency, and therapies to change parental input are often used (see Matthews et al., 1997). Contrary evidence comes from failures to demonstrate that differences exist in parental speech to fluent and dysfluent children close to the onset of stammering (see Miles and Bernstein Ratner, 2001).

The within-subjects design

Example 1 in Exercise 1.4 compared picture naming with and without cues by children with word-finding problems. Here a between- or a within-subjects design might be used. In the former the problems described above arise. Children in each group will vary in performance making it difficult to see if cueing has had an effect. In a within-subjects design differences between children do not matter. Here we have the advantage that we can directly compare each child's performance with and without cues. And we don't need as many subjects either.

Table 2.2 shows the data from this experiment as a between- and a within-subjects design. It should be clear why we are more confident about the outcome in the latter. Here we ignore differences between the children and compare their performance in the two conditions. As a result we stand a much better chance of getting a significant result. Unfortunately there are many occasions where we can't use a within-subjects design. Clinical research often compares groups of subjects defined by a clinical diagnosis (see Example 3 of Exercise 1.4), and most therapy research compares treated and untreated groups. Both require between subject designs.

When subjects do both conditions of an experiment, the first may influence the second. There may be practice or fatigue effects or changes in performance as subjects learn stimuli or gain insight about the experiment. These order effects are the equivalent of the confounding variables in between-subjects designs. To overcome them we counterbalance the subjects across conditions. With two conditions half the subjects do one first while half do the other first; so order effects should affect the two conditions equally.

Counterbalancing alone may not solve the problem. Sometimes order effects are asymmetric. When one condition is first, it affects the other, but little effect is seen in the reverse order. In our experiment cueing is expected to help naming. Children in the cued condition first may learn the words and perform well in the uncued condition. The reverse effect will be much weaker. Children who do

Table 2.2 Possible outcomes of our naming experiment using a between-subjects or a within-subjects design (scores are numbers of pictures named out of 20)

Between-subjects design

	Naming		Naming with cue
S1	6	S7	18
S2	17	S8	14
S3	7	S9	6
S4	2	S10	10
S5	12	S11	16
S6	9	S12	12
Mean (average) score	8.8		12.7

Within-subjects design

	Naming	Naming with cue
S1	6	10
S2	17	14
S3	7	12
S4	2	6
S5	12	18
S6	9	16
Mean (average) score	8.8	12.7

the former will show small differences between the conditions, while those who do the latter show much larger differences. This inconsistency makes it more difficult to obtain a significant result.

Within-subjects designs can be modified in two ways to deal with this. In our experiment we could separate the conditions over time or use different words. Spreading conditions over time helps remove order effects and is a good idea where tiredness (or boredom) might affect performance, but it is inconvenient and subjects (especially those who get bored) may fail to reappear to complete the experiment. It is also difficult to judge the interval needed; it must be long enough to avoid subjects recalling their responses but not so long that they have changed for other reasons. As a precaution we still counterbalance the conditions even when they are separated in time.

Having different words eliminates learning effects but has other disadvantages. We need twice as many words, and the sets of words must be equally difficult (otherwise the words become a confounding variable). There are two ways around this. If we know what makes words difficult (for example their frequency of use), we can match pairs of words and place one of each pair in each set.

However, we may not know what makes them difficult and, anyway, matching is no fun. A better approach is to assign a pool of suitable words randomly to two sets. The objective, like randomly assigning subjects, is to ensure that, on average, the sets are equally difficulty. It's still a good idea to counterbalance sets across conditions (so half the subjects get cues for set A but not set B and vice versa), and, of course, we still counterbalance order of conditions across subjects. At which point you may feel the between-subjects design is not such a bad idea after all.

With different sets of items no interval is required between testing. We might even present all the items together in a random order, giving cues when needed. Here we do not need to counterbalance conditions across subjects (but must counterbalance sets of words across conditions). It also controls for practice or fatigue as each condition is spread across the experiment and will be equally affected. A problem is that the changes in the experimental task may be puzzling for the subject and stressful for the experimenter, who, sooner or later, will get her cues in a twist. Figure 2.1 summarizes these designs.

One final problem is that adjacent items may have unpredictable and idiosyncratic effects on each other (for example items in our naming test might prime one another so the second one is unexpectedly easy). If everyone has the same order, this will affect the results; so we should vary the order across subjects. The thorough approach is to have different random orders for each; the simpler approach is to have alternate subjects do the items in reverse order.

Counterbalancing is also important when we ask subjects to do a series of assessments. The reason is similar to that for items. One assessment may affect performance on another, and we don't want everyone to be affected in the same way. Assessments take a long time; so we should also think carefully about both subject and experimenter fatigue.

It is not always possible to counterbalance conditions in within-subjects designs. In Example 4 of Exercise 1.4 the naturalness of clients' speech was compared before and after therapy. Here the effect of therapy is confounded with the order of assessments. The design is weak because it cannot rule out other explanations. We can strengthen it in two ways. Ideally we need a control group to assess changes in naturalness over time without therapy. This, of course, is a between-subjects design. An alternative is to assess the clients, first during a period without treatment then over a period of treatment and finally over a further period of no treatment. This lets us see whether improvement only occurs with treatment and whether it is maintained afterwards.

1. Simple counterbalancing

	Order of testing	
Subject 1	naming	cued naming
Subject 2	cued naming	naming
Subject 3	naming	cued naming
Subject 4	cued naming	naming
Subject 5	and so on.	

2. Counterbalancing and an interval between tests

	Test 1	Interval	Test 2
Subject 1	naming		cued naming
Subject 2	cued naming		naming
Subject 3	naming		cued naming
Subject 4	cued naming		naming
Subject 5	and so on.		

3. Conditions and sets of items counterbalanced across subjects

Select items: place in set A and set B by (1) random assignment or (2) matching items

	Order of testing	
Subject 1	naming (set A)	cued naming (set B)
Subject 2	cued naming (set B)	naming (set A)
Subject 3	naming (set B)	cued naming (set A)
Subject 4	cued naming (set A)	naming (set B)
Subject 5	and so on.	

4. Random order of items and sets counterbalanced across conditions

Subject 1 (set A naming, set B cued naming), e.g. A1 A2 B1 A3 B2 B3 A4 B4 B5 B6 A6 etc.

Subject 2 (set B naming, set A cued naming), e.g. A1 A2 B1 A3 B2 B3 A4 B4 B5 B6 A6 etc.

Order may be reversed for half the subjects or a new random order created for each subject.

Figure 2.1 Possible within-subjects designs for our naming experiment.

Exercise 2.7

1. Consider how we might design an experiment to examine the effect of word length on the naming ability of clients with dysphasia.
2. How could we compare naming by people with dysphasia of items presented either as line drawings or as colour photographs?

Exercise 2.8

You might be wondering about our experiment on therapy for stammering. Why did we not treat that as two related designs? We could have compared the before and after scores of the treated group to see if they had changed and the scores of the untreated group to show that they had not. Why didn't we do this?

Counterbalancing is obviously a complicated business. Fortunately it's usually easier in your own experiment where you are more aware of the possible problems and of the need to counterbalance to overcome them. On the other hand, things could be worse. We might want to test the children's response to more than one type of cue. Just think what fun counterbalancing will be with three (or more) conditions. We will come back to this.

Matched-subjects designs

The matched-subjects design is a compromise between the between- and within-subjects designs. We use two groups of subjects but match pairs of subjects, one from each group, on one or more variables. In effect, the design converts situations where subjects can't do both conditions of an experiment (where a between-subjects design is required) into one where pairs of scores may be compared (as in a within-subjects design). The pairs may occur naturally. We may compare siblings or twins or children's language with that of their parents. More often we have to 'create' the pairs ourselves. We may match pairs of treated and untreated clients for the severity of their communication disorder or compare clinical and non-clinical groups matching them on relevant variables. Owen and McKinlay (1997), for example, compared motor skills in children with language disorders and normally developing children matching the children on non-verbal intelligence.

The design is not easy to use. Subjects must be assessed on the variables on which they are matched. We may have to test many more subjects than we need to get matched pairs, and, once you start down this road, it's easy to think of other variables that subjects might be matched on. Matching on one variable is irritating; matching on several may be impossible. As a result the design is mainly used when a variable has a large effect on the DV. A common example in SLT research is age. Suppose we compare a clinical group with a control group of normally developing children. The clinical group is hard to find; so it is difficult to find children of the same age. The children's performance on the DV will vary with their age, and we end up with data like those in Table 2.1. Differences between the clinical and control groups are now obscured by differences due to age, and we may fail to obtain a significant result. A better approach is to pair each member of the clinical group with a normally developing child of the same age. Our data now look like that in a within-subjects design (see Table 2.2). Owen and McKinlay (1997) matched pairs of subjects for age and gender (as well as non-verbal IQ). As a result each child with a language disorder was compared directly with a normally developing child of the same age, and the effect of age on performance was eliminated.

Experiments, quasi-experiments and causal relationships

Example 3 of Exercise 1.4 compared the reaction times of children with language impairment and with normal language development. This is a between-subjects design but without random assignment. It is a quasi-experiment, and we cannot draw cause-and-effect conclusions from it. The reason for this should be clear. Without random assignment, confounding variables may cause a change in the DV. Quasi-experiments tell us that a relationship exists between an IV and a DV, not that it is causal. Suppose we are interested in interactions between parents and children with normal and delayed language. We can compare their interactions but cannot manipulate the IV (type of child/parent); so this is not a true experiment. If interactions differ, we may conclude that this is related to the children's speech but not that one is causing the other. Clearly it's plausible that parents can affect their children's language, but it's also plausible that children's delayed language may affect the parents' language. No doubt causal factors exist in each direction. This is a rather extreme example of a quasi-experiment. Others are less obvious; so you have to be alert to spot them.

The term 'quasi-experiment' suggests there is something wrong with this research. This is not so. Quasi-experiments are widely used in clinical research. In fact, they are so familiar that researchers often fail to warn us to be cautious about the conclusions we draw. Readers are expected to sort this out for themselves.

Choosing a control group

So far we have said very little about control groups. In our therapy experiment controls were assessed then shunted off to 'no therapy' before returning to be reassessed. They deserve more attention than this. Our choice of control group can help to control confounding variables and eliminate alternative explanations for our experimental findings.

We saw above that a difficulty in assessing therapy is that other things accompany it. These may include increased attention and encouragement, increased confidence and self-esteem, having time off school and getting a chocolate biscuit at the clinic (some nasty things might happen as well). If we just compare therapy and no therapy, all these things become part of the IV and make it unclear whether any improvement was specifically due to the therapy.

Speech and language therapy has been a bit sloppy in its approach to this problem. Admittedly it is difficult to control for the non-specific effects of therapy, but the reluctance of therapists to be specific about what therapy is hasn't improved matters. The clearer we are about what therapy is, the easier it is to control for non-specific effects. An example is Katz and Wertz (1997), who assessed the effects of computer therapy on the reading of people with aphasia. Use of a computer may also improve concentration, interest and motivation; so treated clients were compared with a control group who had equal time on a computer doing non-verbal tasks that were not expected to benefit reading. This controlled for the non-specific benefits of the intervention. In other cases this is more difficult. One possibility is to use some form of group activity that offers extra stimulation and attention, but not the specific benefits of a therapy. Alternatively we might compare different therapies. Here both groups might gain from any non-specific benefits that are on offer with the therapies.

The choice of a control group is also important in quasi-experimental designs. Here it may help us to eliminate some confounding variables and draw clearer conclusions. A good example occurs in research comparing children who have language disorders with children who have normal development. Here we may use controls that are the same chronological age (with more advanced language) or the same language age (but younger). This approach is often used in research on dyslexia, where both reading-age (RA) and chronological-age (CA) controls are used. Suppose we want to show that phonological working memory capacity is related to reading. This is confirmed if children with dyslexia are worse than CA controls and similar to RA controls (but we still can't tell if one causes the other). If they are as good as CA controls and better than RA controls, it's unlikely to be the cause of their problems.

A good example of this occurs in a study of theory of mind by Miller (2001). Theory-of-mind tasks are not thought to require verbal skills; so they should not be impaired in children with SLI. However, explanation of the tasks themselves may require complex language.

Miller (2001) compared children with SLI same-age and language-age normally developing controls. She used tasks that varied in their linguistic complexity. When linguistic demands were low, children with SLI performed like same-age controls (so they can do theory of mind), but, when they were high, they were like language age controls.

Samples and populations

Statistical tests do more than tell us that a difference exists between groups in an experiment. They let us generalize from our samples to the populations from which they were drawn. The term 'population' is a confusing one. Sometimes it means everybody; more frequently it means a particular type of person. In our experiment we had two samples of people with dysfluent speech. If the treated sample improved more than the untreated one, we infer that therapy is effective for the population of dysfluent people (although statisticians would probably say there are two populations – dysfluent people receiving and not receiving therapy – and that we infer that these populations differ).

A distinction is made between statistical generalization to the population sampled and non-statistical generalization to a wider population. Researchers often do the latter, sometimes plausibly, usually not. For a start, experiments often take place in universities and use non-random groups of subjects. Many are undergraduates; others are members of the public who, suspiciously, have nothing better to do with their time. Undergraduate behaviour is not typical, and there is a rumour going about that they are smarter than other people. The researcher then generalizes the results to a wider population than that sampled (actually they rarely admit to doing this – they just forget to warn the reader not to do it). For this to be legitimate they need a random sample of undergraduates who are, in turn, a random sample of people. Neither is very likely. Generalization to all people may or may not be reasonable; it is not statistical.

In clinical research we only want to generalize our findings to other members of the client group we are studying. Here, the problem is identifying the clients. Researchers may use different definitions of client groups and draw their samples from different populations. Although researchers receive a big share of the blame for the confusion that results, they have had some help along the way. The whole business of putting clients into categories is an emotive issue and subject to social and educational pressures too. Clinicians are, quite reasonably, more impressed by clients' individual needs than similarities between them and don't like classification systems. In contrast, parents like names (especially fashionable ones) that 'explain' children, and education authorities that must plan provision are quite keen on them too. Early research on, for example, developmental dyslexia and autism tried hard to exclude children who did not meet certain criteria. Subsequently these diagnoses have become public property and have been casually extended to other children. This may have helped the children (although I'm not sure about that), but it has not helped research. As you can see, it's easy to become hot under the collar and rant about this. Nevertheless, it is a big problem. The most fundamental lesson you will learn about research is that you don't find significant results when subjects respond inconsistently. So it's a good idea to be careful about who they are in the first place.

In our dysfluency experiment we were not very fussy about who the clients were. Suppose we sample the whole population of dysfluent people (different severity, ages and so on). This seems like a good move. It's easy to find subjects, and we can generalize the result to all people who stammer, but, if the clients respond inconsistently to therapy we will produce a non-significant result. An alternative is to have a more closely defined sample that responds more consistently. Here we can only generalize to people like those in our sample. Of course, it's tempting to generalize further and, even if we resist temptation, readers of our research may do it for us. This is why research reports should give full details of the subjects. Then readers know to whom the results apply.

Exercise 2.9

Suppose we do the experiment above in which a wide range of people who stammer are treated and we fail to get a significant result. We notice that some subjects improved and that they have something in common; so we disregard the others and claim that therapy is effective with this type of client. What is wrong with this? What should we do instead?

Conclusion

In this chapter we have looked at some basic issues about experimental design. The problems of design vary from experiment to experiment, and it's difficult to make general rules about how it should be done. You will learn through experience; so don't expect to do wonderful experiments immediately.

When we read other people's research, two questions often spring to mind. The first is what might happen if we tried to repeat the experiment ourselves; the second is whether we believe the results. These are questions about the reliability and validity of the research (reliability and validity are discussed in Chapter 11). Repeating the research assesses the reliability of its findings. Researchers often report a series of experiments in which they substantiate and expand their findings. This is not entirely convincing, however. They may continue to make the same mistakes, and, anyway, they have a vested interest in not undermining their own work. A more convincing test is for other researchers to repeat the research and produce similar findings. This is called replication. They might attempt to recreate the original experiment exactly. More frequently they vary some aspects of the procedure, the experimental task or use different types of subjects. These are sometimes called 'literal' and 'constructive' replications respectively. The latter are valuable because they broaden the findings and extend the population to whom they apply. They can cause problems, however. Failures to replicate the findings may mean either that the result does not apply in the new circumstances or that the original result was unreliable. It's common for this to lead to prolonged quarrelling between researchers about exactly how and with which subjects an experimental result may be demonstrated.

In reporting experiments, researchers claim that their manipulation of the IV has caused a change in the DV. They will also say (or imply) that this result is true of the populations from which their samples came. These are claims about the experiment's internal and external validity. It has internal validity if it convincingly demonstrates that the IV affects the DV. It has external validity if the results extend to the population from which the samples were drawn and to behaviours outside the experimental setting. Many of the issues discussed in this chapter affect validity. A major threat to internal validity comes from confounding variables. Random assignment and a standard experimental procedure help to protect us against these. When random assignment can't be used, we must be alert to other explanations for our findings. The major threats to external validity are that researchers generalize their results to a wider population than that sampled and that subjects behave one way in research studies and quite differently in real life. The term 'ecological validity' is used for research findings that apply in real life. As we have seen, the need to measure behaviour and control variables in experimental research may create artificial situations and atypical behaviour. As a result we should maintain a healthy scepticism about the ecological validity of many experimental findings.

Chapter 3
Describing data

Descriptive and inferential statistics

Chapter 2 explained the need for statistical tests and described how they work. Statistical tests decide for us whether we have a significant result in our data. They also allow us to infer that the result applies to the population that we sampled. This part of statistics is called inferential statistics. We return to these tests in Chapter 5. In this chapter we look at some methods used to describe data. This area is called descriptive statistics.

Measures of central tendency

Descriptive statistics provide some simple measures for describing data to other people. Suppose we test 20 4-year-old children with specific language impairment (SLI) on the British Picture Vocabulary Test (BPVS). The scores are:

17, 20, 21, 23, 25, 25, 26, 26, 26, 26, 27,
28, 28, 29, 29, 30, 31, 33, 35, 38.

Suppose we want to tell someone what a typical score in this sample is. We would probably use the average score. Everybody is familiar with averages and knows how to work them out. So naturally statisticians try to confuse matters by calling them 'means' and by disguising a simple calculation with a mathematical formula. It is:

$$\bar{x} = \frac{\Sigma x}{n}$$

where $\bar{x}$ is the mean. Individual scores are represented by x, and Σx (sigma x) is their sum. n is the number of children. In our example $n = 20$ and $\Sigma x = 543$; so the mean is 27.15.

The mean is a measure of central tendency. It is the best measure but not the only one. Alternatives are the mode and the median. The mode is the most frequently occurring score. In our data it is 26. The median is the middle score. As we have an even number of scores, the point midway between the two middle scores is the median (the mean of the two middle scores). It is 26.5. The three measures are very similar. This will often be the case.

Figure 3.1 is a histogram of the scores. It shows that most scores are in the middle (25–29) with a few above and below them. This shows why our mean, mode and median are similar. The mode and median are likely to be in this middle group, and the large number of scores in this area strongly affects the mean.

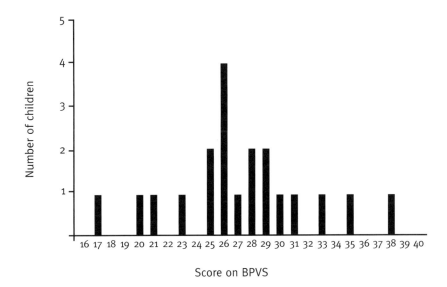

Figure 3.1 Histogram of our sample of BPVS scores.

Suppose we persuade other therapists to collect similar data until we have scores for 1,000 children. Figure 3.2 is a histogram of the scores. The mode is still 26. So is the median. The mean is 26.26 (take my word for it). These values are similar to our original ones. This sample is so large that we would probably get the same results if we tested the whole population of 4-year-olds with SLI. So our original sample is a pretty good estimate of the population mean.

Statisticians don't like histograms. They prefer frequency distributions. We can get a frequency distribution by joining up the tops of the bars in the histogram. This distribution would be fairly smooth and nearly symmetrical. The frequency distribution of our 20 subjects is anything but. Nevertheless, data like ours (with the mean

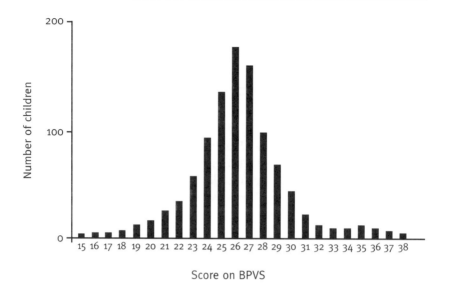

Figure 3.2 Histogram of our sample of 1,000 BPVS scores.

and median about equal and scores clustered in the middle) suggest that the population is symmetrically distributed. Consequently, and because they look better, we will draw smooth frequency distributions from now on. In fact, we (and other researchers) will often claim that our data come from a normally distributed population. The normal distribution is a symmetrical distribution with special mathematical properties and is important in inferential statistics. We meet it again later on.

The distributions in Figure 3.3 show the relationship between a distribution and its mean and median. In (i) the mean and median (and mode) are identical. This occurs when the distribution is symmetrical. The others are skewed. In (ii) the skew is negative and in (iii) positive. We can detect skew by comparing the mean and median. The mean is the most sensitive measure of central tendency as it takes each score into account. Consequently extreme scores affect the mean more than the median. So if the mean is > (greater than) the median, a distribution is positively skewed. If it is < (less than) the median, it is negatively skewed.

Distributions that are very skewed tell us something about the samples and the populations that they came from. Their means will be pulled a long way from the central peak of scores, and the median may be a better measure of central tendency as it is a more 'typical' score. In practice nearly all distributions are likely to be at least a little skewed. Ours is, but the skew is so slight that we can ignore it.

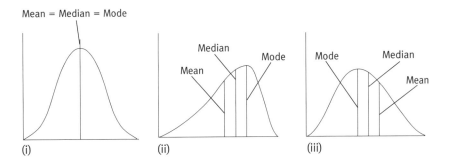

Figure 3.3 In (i) mean = median, distribution symmetrical. In (ii) mean < median, distribution negatively skewed. In (iii) mean > median, distribution positively skewed.

Measures of dispersion

The mean (or mode or median) tells us what a typical score from our data is. But how typical is it? In other words, how spread out around the mean are the rest of the scores? Measures of this 'spread outness' are called measures of dispersion and are important both for describing data and, later, in inferential statistics.

The simplest measure of dispersion is the range. It is the distance from the lowest to the highest score. For our data it is 17–38. The range is easily understood but is misleading when there are extreme scores ('outliers'). A way round this is to use the interquartile range (also called the midspread). Its calculation is similar to the median. We put the scores in ascending order. The middle score is the median, and the scores a quarter of the way up and three-quarters of the way up show the interquartile range. It is often used as a measure of dispersion when the median is used as the measure of central tendency. But working it out is a messy business. With large numbers of scores it takes a while and doesn't even reward us by making us feel much like mathematicians. We will avoid it.

A better measure of dispersion would be one that takes each score into account giving them all equal influence. We could add up the differences between each score and the mean. This is indicated by:

$$\sum (x - \bar{x})$$

However, this is made up of positive and negative differences (scores above and below the mean); in fact, the differences add to zero (do you know why?); so it won't be much use to us. Statisticians have a

Exercise 3.1

1. The diagrams below are the distributions of scores on the BPVS of 4-year-olds with SLI and of 4-year-olds with normal language development. What does each diagram tell you about the children?

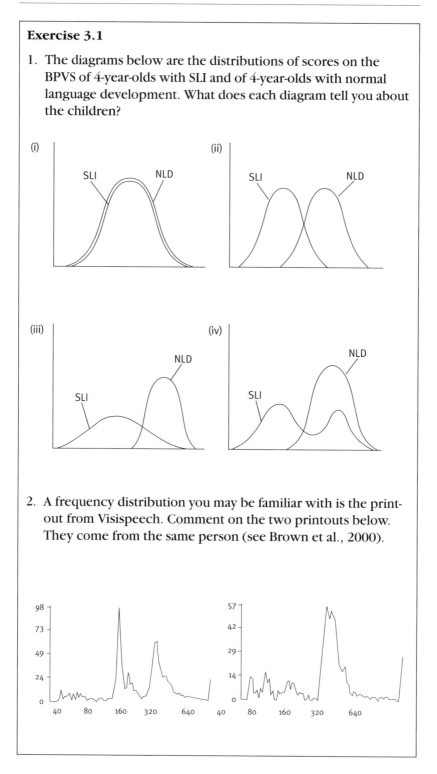

2. A frequency distribution you may be familiar with is the print-out from Visispeech. Comment on the two printouts below. They come from the same person (see Brown et al., 2000).

solution to this problem: they square the differences between the scores and the mean. As it happens statisticians are never happier than when they are squaring things and here they have the perfect excuse. Squaring the positive and negative differences makes all the differences positive. Adding them up we get:

$$\sum(x - \bar{x})^2$$

This is called the sum of squares. If we divide it by n, we get the variance.

$$\frac{\sum(x - \bar{x})^2}{n}$$

The variance is an important statistical quantity and is used in many formulae, but it is not a good descriptive statistic because, after all that squaring, its relationship to the original data is less than clear. So we use its square root. This is the standard deviation.

$$\sqrt{\frac{\sum(x - \bar{x})^2}{n}}$$

The variance and standard deviation are the most used measures of dispersion. In Chapter 2 when we were trying to guess whether two sets of scores were different we found that our confidence was influenced by how spread out they were around their means. You may have wondered how we were going to measure this 'spread outness' – now you know.

Research reports rarely give the scores of individual subjects, but they should give the means and standard deviations of groups of subjects. A lot can be learned from these. For reasons we discuss in the next chapter, most scores are within two standard deviations above and below the mean (if the mean is 10 and the standard deviation 2, most scores will be between 6 and 14). You should use this rule of thumb in Exercise 3.2.

The defining and computational formulae and a lot of fuss about n and $n - 1$

The formulae above for variance and standard deviation have the advantage that you can see what you are doing as you do it (not always the case in statistics). They are called 'defining formulae'. It's

---

Exercise 3.2

Researchers should report the means and standard deviations of their data. You can discover quite a lot from this information. What do the following examples tell you?

1. In an experiment comparing the progress of treated and untreated clients with aphasia, the mean improvement of each group is:
   (a) Treated group – mean change 16, standard deviation 5.7.
       Untreated group – mean change 5, standard deviation 5.1.
   (b) Treated group – mean change 18, standard deviation 12.7.
       Untreated group – mean change 7, standard deviation 5.8.
   (c) Treated group – mean change 22, standard deviation 10.8.
       Untreated group – mean change 17, standard deviation 9.4.

2. Children with normal language development and children with SLI are asked to name pictures of 20 objects. The mean number that each group names correctly is:
   (a) Normal language development – mean number correct: 14.5, standard deviation 2.1.
       SLI – mean number correct: 10.9, standard deviation 1.7.
   (b) Normal language development – mean number correct: 19.3, standard deviation 0.3.
       SLI – mean number correct: 13.1, standard deviation 3.9.
   (c) Normal language development – mean number correct: 19.1: standard deviation 0.8.
       SLI – mean number correct: 17.6, standard deviation 4.6.

---

a shame, therefore, that we have to change the formulae in a way that makes them less sensible and causes a lot of confusion. So pay attention!

The first change is to divide by $n - 1$ instead of n. As a result the formulae become:

$$\text{Standard deviation} = \sqrt{\frac{\Sigma(x - \bar{x})^2}{n - 1}}$$

$$\text{Variance} = \frac{\Sigma(x - \bar{x})^2}{n - 1}$$

Exercise 3.3

In Exercise 2.4 we compared sets of data from our dysfluency experiment to test our confidence that a difference existed. Below are the means and standard deviations of the original data and the data from part 2. We concluded that the first was more likely to give a significant result. Do the standard deviations confirm that judgement?

Original data	Control group	mean = 8	std dev = 5.40
	Experimental group	mean = 13	std dev = 5.66
Data from part (ii)	Control group	mean = 8	std dev = 6.07
	Experimental group	mean = 13	std dev = 9.82

This is an odd thing to do. If we are going to divide by anything, n seems like a good choice! The reason for the change may surprise you. It's that we don't want the standard deviation and variance of our sample after all; we want them of the population (all 4-year-olds with SLI). This problem did not arise with the mean, because the sample mean is a good estimate of the population mean. However, the sample variance and standard deviation are inaccurate ('biased') estimates. The best ('unbiased') estimate is obtained by dividing by n – 1 not n. Of course, the two values are not very different and the difference becomes smaller as n increases.

You might feel that this is just a statistical storm in a teacup. Nevertheless, you should understand what the storm is about. It is confusing for three reasons. The first is that some books use the n formula and so calculate the actual standard deviation and variance of the sample not estimates for the population. We will use the n – 1 formula and obtain population values. This will make us feel like real (if confused) statisticians. It also makes sense in the real world. It's unlikely that other people will want to know about our specific children. They want an indication of how all children with SLI perform.

The fact that we can estimate things about populations at all is another source of confusion. That samples represent populations is one thing, but estimating their variance seems to be pushing our luck. As we go on we shall find that statisticians flit back and forward between the here-and-now world of samples and the Never Never Land of populations with alarming ease. The rest of us find the transition a bit trickier. To clarify things they use a notation that distinguishes between actual population values and estimates of those values from samples. Estimates are called statistics and are designated by Roman letters. The mean is $\bar{x}$, the standard deviation s and the variance s^2. The actual values are called parameters and are designated by Greek letters. The mean is μ (mew), the standard deviation σ (sigma) and the variance σ^2. Meanwhile, back in English, we refer to s and s^2 as the sample standard deviation and variance (but use them to estimate the population values) and σ and σ^2 as the population standard deviation and variance.

A third confusion is that calculators (which have special routines for working out standard deviations) offer us a sample (σ_{n-1}) and a population (σ_n) standard deviation. The first estimates the population value from a sample and is the one we want but, having just learned that we want the population value, you may be misled and use the second. Calculators work like statisticians – they always aim at population values. Consequently they use σ_{n-1} to estimate the population value and σ_n in the unlikely event that the whole population has been tested. Then we are not estimating its value so we don't need the $n - 1$ formula!

Having established that the $n - 1$ formula estimates population values, we now change the formulae a second time. In the defining formulae we could see what we were doing, but the calculations are tedious, especially with lots of subjects. The computational formulae below are not clear at all (in fact, they look rather fierce), but the calculations turn out to be easier.

$$\text{Standard deviation} = \sqrt{\frac{\sum x^2 - \frac{\left(\sum x\right)^2}{n}}{n - 1}}$$

$$\text{Variance} = \frac{\sum x^2 - \frac{\left(\sum x\right)^2}{n}}{n - 1}$$

The formulae $\sum x^2$ and $\left(\sum x\right)^2$ need an explanation. In English they are homophones! Mathematically they are different, however. In the first we square each x then add them; in the second we add first and then square the total. Table 3.1 gives the notation and formulae for the standard deviation and variance.

The standard error

Suppose we take several samples from the same population. It might worry you that these samples have different means and that, as a

Table 3.1 Sample statistics and population parameters

	Mean	Variance	Standard deviation
Sample values for estimating population values (statistics)	$\bar{x}$	$s^2 = \dfrac{\sum x^2 - \dfrac{(\sum x)^2}{n}}{n-1}$	$s = \sqrt{\dfrac{\sum x^2 - \dfrac{(\sum x)^2}{n}}{n-1}}$
True population values (parameters)	μ	σ^2	σ

Exercise 3.4

Work out the variance and standard deviation of our BPVS scores. You can do this with your calculator or by using the defining or computational formula. If you do either of the latter, it's a good idea to be methodical and set out the calculations in a table like the one below. From the table you can get $\sum x$, $\sum(x-\bar{x})^2$ and $\sum x^2$ which allows you to work out the mean, standard deviation and variance.

Subject	Score	$(x - \bar{x})$	$(x - \bar{x})^2$	x^2
1	17			
2	20			
3	21			
4	23			
5	25			
6	25			
7	26			
8	26			
9	26			
10	26			
11	27			
12	28			
13	28			
14	29			
15	29			
16	30			
17	31			
18	33			
19	35			
20	38			

$\sum x =$ $\bar{x} =$ $(\sum x)^2 =$ $\sum x^2 =$ $\sum(x-\bar{x})^2 =$

result, estimates of the population mean vary. This reminds us that $\bar{x}$ is only an estimate of s, the population mean. It would be useful to know how good an estimate it is. Clearly, if the means of different samples vary a lot, any one mean may not be a good estimate. If we take lots of samples and calculate their means (unlikely, I know, but it disguises the fact that another statistical flight of fancy is coming up), we can obtain a frequency distribution of these means. This distribution is called the sampling distribution of the mean and its standard deviation is the standard error.

The standard error tells us how good an estimate the sample mean ($\bar{x}$) is of the population mean (μ). You might have guessed that we don't need repeated samples to find it out. We can do this by dividing the population standard deviation by the square root of our sample size.

$$\sigma / \sqrt{n}$$

The origin of this formula is going to have to remain a mystery. However, it may reassure you to see that it is consistent with common sense. The standard error is small (and our estimate good) if σ is small (so scores in the population – and our sample – don't vary much) and the sample is large.

To use this formula we need the population standard deviation σ, which we can estimate from the sample standard deviation s. You might think that something a bit fishy is going on here. First, we estimate the population variance from the sample, and then we use this estimate to find out how good an estimate the sample mean is of the population mean. This won't be the last time that you may feel that statisticians can stand on a ladder and move it at the same time! Despite this conjuring trick, the standard error is an important statistical concept that plays a big part in statistical tests.

If you have done Exercise 3.4, you know that s, the standard deviation of our BPVS scores, is 4.96; so the standard error of the scores is:

$$\sigma / \sqrt{n} = 4.96 / \sqrt{20} = 1.11$$

We can now use the standard error to determine how good an estimate the sample mean is of the population mean. We can define a range of scores around the mean of our sample within which the true population mean is likely to fall. This is called a confidence interval.

We usually use a 95% confidence interval, which is a range of scores that is 95% likely to contain the population mean.

This is similar to the procedure we used in Exercise 3.3. There we used a rough rule that most of the scores in a set of data would lie in a range from 2 standard deviations below to 2 standard deviations above the mean. Here we are defining a range of scores that are likely to contain the population mean. As we shall see in Chapter 4, 95% of the scores making up a normal distribution fall within 1.96 standard deviations of the mean (2 standard deviations was a rough rule). So a 95% confidence interval for a mean extends from 1.96 standard errors below the estimated mean to 1.96 standard errors above it. Our estimate of the population mean was 27.15; so the 95% confidence interval is:

$$27.15 \pm 1.96 \times 1.11$$

Which is from 24.97 to 29.33.

Box-and-whisker plots

In research reports means and standard deviations are used to describe data. Exercise 3.2 showed that we could tell quite a lot about data from their standard deviations. Researchers normally plot means on graphs. Figure 3.4 shows the improvement scores for the groups in our dysfluency study (see above) as a bar chart and as a graph. We can add information to these by using box-and-whisker plots. 'Boxes' and 'whiskers' can be used to indicate the standard deviation, the standard error or both. The commonest arrangement is 'whiskers only' to indicate one standard deviation about the mean. These are shown in the diagrams (i) and (ii). In (iii) the box indicates the standard error; the whiskers, the standard deviation.

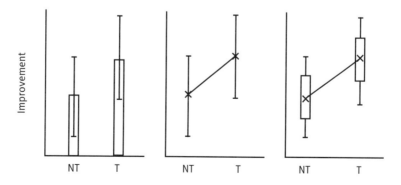

Figure 3.4 Box-and-whisker plots of the data from the dysfluency experiment: NT = no treatment, T = treatment.

Chapter 4
The normal distribution and standardized tests

The normal distribution

The distribution of children with SLI in the last chapter seemed sensible enough. It was nearly symmetrical (mean = median = mode). Most scores were close to the mean, and there were fewer and fewer as we moved away from it. Such distributions are described as 'normal'. The normal distribution plays a large role in statistics because many naturally occurring variables are assumed to be normally distributed. I say 'assumed' because we can't be sure unless we have a very large sample. Even then, the distribution may not be perfectly normal but will look like it is trying to be.

The normal distribution is important because many statistical tests assume that variables are normally distributed in the population. We discuss this later. For the moment our interest in the normal distribution is that it allows us to design and use standardized tests.

Exercise 4.1

We conduct a survey of a large number of SLTs. In it we collect information on their:

1. heights
2. ages
3. IQs
4. shoe sizes
5. marks on a research methods exam.

Which of these variables would you expect to be normally distributed?

Z-scores

You have probably used the British Picture Vocabulary Scale (BPVS) (Dunn et al., 1997) to assess whether a child's receptive vocabulary is at the level expected for their age. We can do this because it is a standardized test. We know how other children perform on it and can compare our child with others of his or her age.

Suppose we test a child (never mind, for the moment, what the test is) and find that his score is 93. We know that the mean score for children of the same age is 100; so he is 7 below the mean. This tells us that he is below average but not how poor his score is or whether we should worry about his language. However, the test also gives us the standard deviation of the scores of children who are his age. So we can measure how many standard deviations he is below the mean. This gives us a z- or standard score where z is the number of standard deviations a score is from the mean.

$$z = \frac{(x - \bar{x})}{s}$$

Where x = the individual's score, and $\bar{x}$ and s are the mean and standard deviation of children of a similar age taken from the test. Notice that I have used the sample mean and standard deviation. You will see this formula using μ and σ, the population values. The samples on which tests are based are usually large so there is little difference between them and the population.

If the standard deviation of the children's scores is 15, our child has a z-score of:

$$z = \frac{(x - \bar{x})}{s} = \frac{-7}{15} = -0.467$$

You may think that this has not taken us very far. Being 7 below the mean may not tell us much, but having a z-score of –0.467 (being 0.467 standard deviations below the mean) is even more puzzling. Things would obviously improve if we knew how many standard deviations cover the range of scores on the test.

This is where the normal distribution comes in. If a variable is normally distributed, we know how subjects are distributed around the mean. Figure 4.1 shows the percentage of subjects we expect to find 1, 2 or 3 standard deviations from the mean. Most scores (99.74%) are within 3 standard deviations of the mean. Two standard deviations cover a little over 95% of the population (recall that in

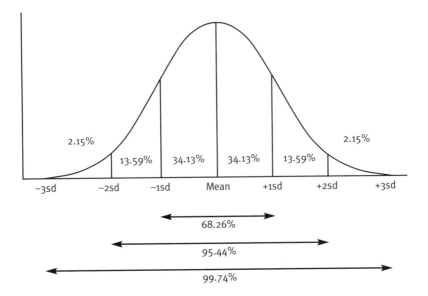

Figure 4.1 The percentage of subjects with scores 1, 2 and 3 standard deviations from the mean.

Exercise 3.2 we assumed that most scores were within 2 standard deviations of the mean).

Intelligence quotient (IQ) scores are an example of normally distributed scores. Although there is controversy about what IQ tests measure, there is no dispute about their status as standardized tests. Vast efforts have been made to standardize them. The mean IQ on tests such as the WISC and the WAIS is 100, and the standard deviation is 15 (as in the example above). So a little over two-thirds (68.26%) of people have IQs between 85 and 115 and a little over 95% have IQs between 70 and 130.

We now have a way to convert z-scores into percentages or percentile scores that are easily understood. A person's percentile score is the percentage of people who score lower than they do. So, if children receive a z-score of −2 on the BPVS, their percentile score is 2.28% (we would probably say they are in the bottom 3% of the population). This is because 50% are above the mean and 47.72% between the mean and 2 standard deviations below it; so the percentile score is 100 − (50 + 47.72).

The z-tables (Appendix 1) allow us to convert any z-score to a percentile score. If a subject scores 125 on an IQ test with mean 100 and standard deviation 15, then:

$$z = \frac{125 - 100}{15} = 1.66$$

The z-tables give the proportion of people between a score and the mean. For 1.66 the table value is 0.4515. So 0.4515 or 45.15% of people are between this score and the mean. The tables are for half the normal distribution. So the calculation of a percentile score differs if someone is above or below the mean. For $z = 1.66$ we add the 50% below the mean so the percentile score is 95.15%. If a subject is below the mean, the z-tables give the percentage between that score and the mean. So the percentile score is 50% minus the table value. So $z = -1.66$ converts to a percentile score of 4.85.

Use of the z-tables requires a little practice (see Exercise 4.2). They can be used with any variable that is normally distributed. If you have used standardized tests, you know they have tables to convert raw scores (the actual score on the test) into z, percentile or age-equivalent scores (the age for which a raw score is the mean).

Exercise 4.2

1. The mean score of 6-year-old children on an assessment is 50 and their standard deviation is 10. What is the standard (z) score of children who have a raw score of (a) 40, (b) 70, (c) 37 and (d) 61?
2. What is the percentile score of children whose standard scores are (a) 0.5, (b) -0.5, (c) 1.24, (d) -1.37, (e) 1.96 and (f) -1.96?
3. What z-score divides the half of the population who are close to the mean from the half that is further away?

Standardized tests allow us to do three things:

- Compare a client's score with the population. A difference here indicates that a person is performing poorly and may be used as an indication that therapy is appropriate.
- Assess change over time. We will want to monitor progress with therapy. Children's performance improves with age; so it is difficult to know if they have improved as a result of therapy or as a result of growing older. Developmental tests are standardized for different ages (usually every 3 months); so we can convert scores to z- or percentile scores and compare performance at different ages.
- Compare test performances. We can't compare raw scores from different tests. However, if each is standardized, we can compare z- or percentile scores. The profile of a child's performance across tests tells us whether they have a general or a specific problem.

Points 2 and 3 show that z-scores are not used only to compare people with their age group. They convert scores at different ages and on different scales to a common unit for comparison.

Standardizing a test

Standardizing a test is a serious business. The procedures are usually described in the test manual. We can look briefly at how it's done using the CELF-3 (Semel et al., 1995). The first step is to obtain a large number of items that may be suitable for the test. Usually we involve as many other clinicians and experts as possible so that a wide range of items are found. Existing tests are a useful guide to the range of items needed. A large sample of people is tested, and their responses are used to select the best items. These items must vary in difficulty so that the test covers a range of ages and ability levels. Items must be sensitive – there is no point having items that everybody gets right or wrong. They must also be consistent. This is tested by looking at responses to different items. Subjects should not answer harder items correctly and easier ones incorrectly, and subjects with similar scores should show similar profiles of correct and incorrect responses to items.

The CELF-3 (Semel et al., 1995) was developed from the CELF-R (Semel et al., 1987) so the general philosophy of the test and the types of items were already known. Nevertheless, the test was amended in the light of comments from users of the earlier version. To make sure that the views of users were taken into account, discussions and focus groups were held to get their opinions. Two parallel forms of the test were developed, and 'tryout' testing began. Eight hundred children without a language disorder and 143 with such a disorder were tested by 225 SLTs, who submitted notes and answered questionnaires giving their opinions on the test. A committee of SLTs then examined the data and amended the scoring system, and a special panel considered all the test items to determine whether any were biased in favour or against any group of children. Items from the two versions of the test were then chosen to make up the final test.

Once a definitive version of the test has been selected, the test can be standardized. The standardization sample must represent the population on which the test is to be used. When we test subjects, we compare them with the data from this standardization sample. These samples are large, and care is taken to make them representative so it is reasonable to claim that we are comparing the subject with the population. The standardization sample for the CELF-3 consisted of 2,450 children selected to match the US population for age, gender, race, geographical region and parental education.

Testing was carried out by 384 SLTs. All the children were scored by two clinicians, and discrepancies in their scores resolved by a third.

Next comes the mathematical part. The raw scores and standard deviations for children of different ages must be calculated. If the raw scores are normally distributed, it is easy to convert them to z- or percentile scores. They are unlikely to be normally distributed, however (see below). The common way around this is to convert the raw scores to a scaled score (the CELF calls this a standard score equivalent) that is normally distributed. Many tests do this but conceal from users what is actually going on by providing tables which convert directly from raw scores to z-, percentile or age-equivalent scores (see below). A final stage in developing a test is to get data on its reliability and validity. We will look at this in Chapter 11.

Speech and language therapists and their troubles with standardized tests

Standardized tests are clearly useful; so it is surprising that therapists complain so much about them. One problem is that, once a test has been standardized, we are stuck with it. We want to compare our subject with the test norms, and so we must follow the same procedure as that used to standardize the test. This usually means observing time limits, not giving encouragement and generally behaving in a less-than-friendly way. My guess is that when children struggle with tests, those conducting them feel uncomfortable and find it difficult to stick to the rules. Unfortunately these are exactly the children who we want to compare with the test norms. Bending the rules a little may help them perform better but may not do them any favours if, as a result, they are deemed not to need therapy. (Note, though, that a departure from the standardized procedure is advocated in dynamic assessment – see Gutierrez and Pena, (2001). Here standard and non-standard procedures are compared to discover if some children – such as those from diverse cultural backgrounds – are being penalized by the formal test procedure.)

Standardizing a test is a dreadful job; so we can't expect authors to revise them at anything less than lengthy intervals. Tests become dated or go out of fashion either because test items are less appealing or, more fundamentally, because our view of what needs to be tested alters with changes in theoretical thinking and/or clinical practice. We should nevertheless maintain a balanced view of the merits of standardized tests. We may have more modern or attractive test materials, but we are unlikely to want to standardize them, and so they will not have the advantages of standardized tests.

A further complaint is that each test comes with its own tables to convert raw scores into z- or percentile scores. The procedure varies from test to test, and the differences between tests are confusing. This is partly due to tests making well-meaning but different attempts to simplify the process of conversion for us. In each case it is based on the z-tables, and, if you have understood how they work, you should be able to follow what any given test is doing.

Figure 4.2 summarizes the various scores into which a raw score may be converted. The easiest step is to find an age-equivalent score. This can usually be obtained directly from a table giving the mean raw scores of children of different ages. The age-equivalent score is the age of the children whose mean score is equal to the raw score obtained.

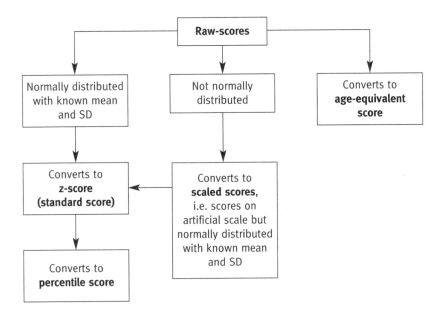

Figure 4.2 From raw scores to age-equivalent, z- and percentile scores.

Obtaining z- and percentile scores is rather more tricky, and different tests use their own tables to ease the process of conversion. If raw scores on the test were normally distributed, we could use the z-formula above. In fact, raw scores are seldom, if ever, normally distributed. One reason for this is that developmental tests must cater for a wide range of ages. Even if one age had normally distributed raw scores, another would not. In particular the youngest and oldest children for whom the test is intended will have scores near the bottom and top of the range of scores on the test. Their distributions will be squeezed up against the floor and ceiling scores on the test and will be skewed as a result. To avoid this, tests often convert raw scores to what I am calling a scaled score (but which they often call a standard score). This is an artificial but normally distributed score that can be converted to z- or percentile scores. All this may become a little clearer in the examples below.

Some tests and how they go about it

A very popular and apparently simple test is the 'bus story' (Renfrew, 1997). The test is standardized on children aged from 3.9 to 8.5 and a mean score (for amount of information) given for each month. This allows an age-equivalent score to be obtained easily by finding the age of child who ought to get the raw score obtained. The test also gives the overall mean and standard deviation for children in 6-month bands. These could be used to obtain z- or percentile scores, but the test has no table to do so. It's likely that this is because the standard deviations are large. A 5.8 child is expected to score 26 but the standard deviation is 6.48. Applying our 2-standard-deviation rule gives a range from 13 to 39, which covers almost the whole test. Even one standard deviation covers an age range from 4.7 to 7.2. This is not really surprising. The test appears simple, but storytelling uses a wide range of language skills. As a result children vary considerably and the test is a poor guide to whether they are at an age-appropriate level. Its popularity probably stems from its ability to give an overall, if subjective, view of a child's language and because children like doing it.

The Symbolic Play Test (Lowe and Costello, 1988) is for children from 12 months to 36 months. A problem with developmental tests is that they are less accurate at the extremes of their age range. It is difficult to standardize tests for very young children, because the children vary and change very rapidly and, at the upper end of the age range, ceiling effects make tests less useful. There are ceiling effects in the Symbolic Play Test, and the manual suggests that it is most useful for children between 15 months and 24 months. A table converts raw scores into z-scores directly, and a second table converts them to age-equivalent scores.

The more trouble that test designers take standardizing a test, the longer (and less readable) the test manuals tend to be. The tables are more complicated and the tests become fussier about the procedure to be used. This is fair enough for the reasons discussed above. The BPVS looks like a serious test, has lots of tables and quite an elaborate procedure. It converts raw scores (Table A) into what it calls a standard score (or, in the older version, a standardized score equivalent). In my terminology this is a scaled score. It is an artificial but normally distributed score with mean 100 and standard deviation 15, which is easily converted to a z- or percentile score. This scaled score is similar to that used in many IQ tests. This makes it familiar to some users, but it should not be confused with IQ. Suppose we test a 6-year-old, who scores 76. This converts to a standard score (a scaled score) of 115. We can easily convert this to a z- or percentile score. Table B (on the score sheet) converts it to a percentile score. In this case the z-score is +1 and the percentile score is 84. Table C converts raw scores directly to age-equivalent scores and gives a 68% confidence interval for them. For our child the age-equivalent score is 7.5.

The CELF-R has 10 subtests. Of these, three add together to give a receptive language score and three to give an expressive language score. The receptive and expressive scores add to give a total language score. The three latter scores are referred to as composite scores, and tables (Appendix E and Appendix F of the test) convert the raw scores on these to standard score equivalents (a scaled score) with a mean of 100 and a standard deviation of 15, as in the BPVS. The individual subtests also convert into standard score equivalents but with mean 10 and standard deviation 3. These tables also provide confidence intervals at the 68% and 95% levels for the standard score equivalents. A strength of the test is that receptive and expressive scores or scores on different subtests may be compared to find relative strengths and weaknesses in a child's language. The confidence intervals provide a way to determine whether a difference exists. Further tables convert the standard score equivalents into percentile scores (Appendix G of the test) and convert the sum of the raw scores on the six subtests to an age-equivalent score (Appendix H).

The Reynell Developmental Language Scales III (Edwards et al., 1997) is divided into a comprehension and an expressive subscale. Tables convert raw scores to age-equivalent and percentile scores. The latter are handy as they bypass the scaled scores on which they are based. A further table converts raw scores to a scaled score (again called a standard score) with a mean of 50 and standard deviation of 10.

As you can see from the above, many tests convert raw scores to what they call a standard or standardized score. I have insisted on calling this a scaled score to avoid confusing it with a true standard or z-score. My preference would be to go directly to a true standard score, which tells us how many standard deviations children are above or below the mean. This score is common to all standardized tests and allows comparisons across tests. The procedure of many tests seems to assume that users can't understand z-scores. I would rather be optimistic and assume that they can!

Language tests used with adults usually avoid the need for standardization and all the scores and tables that follow from this. They can do so by assuming that adults with no language impairment would score at or very near ceiling on the test. Anyone who scores much below this has a problem. Suppose we want to test the naming of a person with dysphasia. If we use items that people without dysphasia can name easily, any failure should be apparent. The Boston Naming Test (Goodglass et al., 1983) takes this approach. Norms for people aged 20 to 60 show that they score about 55 (out of 60). The standard deviation of their scores is low, and a range is given so we can determine whether a client is scoring abnormally. Other tests use a similar approach. The Pyramids and Palm Trees test (Howard and Patterson, 1992) tells us that people without dysphasia made no more than three errors. The Psycholinguistic Assessment of Language Processing in Aphasia (PALPA; Kay et al., 1992) takes this approach to the extreme providing 60 tests that appear to be easy for people without dysphasia (some, but not all, have norms to prove this). Here any failure is obvious. Nor is PALPA very concerned about the degree of failure. The tests are designed to isolate particular deficits by showing that clients fail some but do well on others.

Chapter 5
Some statistical tests

Introduction to inferential statistics

Chapter 2 looked at why we need statistical tests and the nature of the decisions they make for us. Now we look at the tests themselves. In this chapter we look at tests that compare two sets of data from between- and within-subjects designs.

In choosing a test we must make two decisions. First, which design did we use? Second, what sort of data do we have? The first decision should be easy if you have designed your own experiment. The second is more complicated. Tests are of two kinds – parametric and non-parametric (or distribution free). Normally we want to use parametric tests because they are more powerful (more likely to get a significant result). However, they make assumptions about the data; so you may not be allowed to use them. Non-parametric tests are more flexible; they make few assumptions about the data, and, as applied research often produces data that are unsuitable for parametric tests, this is an important consideration. Table 5.1 summarizes the two decisions and the tests we can use.

Table 5.1 Deciding which tests to use

	Is the design?	
Are the data	Between-subjects	Within-subjects
Parametric?	Independent t-test	Related t-test
Non-parametric?	Mann-Whitney test	Wilcoxon test or Sign test

Parametric tests may be used when:

- the data are drawn from normally distributed populations.
- the data are drawn from populations with approximately equal variances. This assumption is called homogeneity of variance.
- the data are measured on an equal-interval scale.

The first two assumptions are about the populations we have sampled. Usually our only guide to whether they are normally distributed or have homogeneous variances is to look at the samples. These may not be very helpful. We saw in Chapter 3 that small samples are a poor guide to the population distribution, and, although we can estimate the population variances from the samples, it's unclear what 'approximately equal' means. Of course, it's unlikely that the populations will be perfectly normally distributed or have identical variances. So strict adherence to the rules is not possible. For the moment we will follow common practice of using parametric tests unless there is clear evidence that we should not. If we feel guilty about this, we can say (along with many other researchers) that the tests are 'robust'. When data do not meet the assumptions, parametric tests may give wrong answers. Saying they are 'robust' amounts to saying that this isn't very likely.

The third assumption concerns the scale on which the data are measured. The traditional view, in most statistics texts, is that parametric tests require equal interval data. Here the units of measurement are equal, as in physical measures (lengths, times, temperatures and so on). Our data are more likely to count behaviours (such as the number of dysfluencies made by a child telling a story or the number of pictures a person with dysphasia can name) rather than being physical measures. Strictly these are not equal-interval scales as the instances of the behaviours may not be equal in magnitude. However, such measures are treated as equal-interval and qualify for parametric tests.

In Chapter 1 we discussed the difficulties in measuring behaviour. There are occasions where we cannot directly measure a behaviour and have observers rate it instead. Example 4 of Exercise 1.4 used listeners' ratings as a measure of the naturalness of dysfluent speech. Use of ratings is quite straightforward, if a bit inconvenient, and it produces numerical data by converting opinions into numbers. These are not equal-interval data. They are measured on an ordinal scale. Many statistics texts say that parametric tests should not be used with such data. We will stick with this view for now, but we will look at it again in Chapter 8.

Nominal scales of measurement are quite different from the others. Suppose we test children in their first year at school to see if they have delayed language. We can put the children into one of four categories (boys or girls with or without language delay). Here the subjects do not give us data – they are the data. Each is a score in a category (we also call this categorical data), and a test can be used to see if the categories are associated (if boys are more likely to have language delay than girls). Such data have their own tests. We look at them in Chapter 9.

Exercise 5.1

On what scales of measurement are the data in the following research?

1. The time taken to name pictures is compared in children with SLI and children with no language impairment (see Lahey and Edwards, 1996).
2. The number and type of errors made naming pictures is compared in children with SLI and children with no language impairment (see Lahey and Edwards, 1999).
3. Singers and non-singers indicate which symptoms of vocal attrition they experience. They are then divided into those who have no symptoms, those who have one or two and those who have three or more (see Sapir et al., 1996).
4. Carers of elderly people with stroke or dementia are compared on the General Health Questionnaire (GHQ) (Goldberg and Williams, 1988). This has a series of questions with a four-point scale on which the subject responds (see Draper et al., 1992).

Exercise 5.2

What statistical tests would you use in the following?

1. The fundamental frequency of the speech of people with and without chronic sinusitis is compared (see Cecil et al., 2001).
2. Clients with aphasia attend communication groups. Their psychological well-being is assessed by having them complete a rating scale before and after 6 months of attendance at the groups (see Hoen et al., 1997).

Exercise 5.2 (cont)

3. The number of errors made by children with phonological impairments is compared in a picture-naming task and a conversational task (see Wolk and Meisler, 1998).
4. People with and without dysphonia complete a self-rated assessment (the SF-36) of their quality of life (see Wilson et al., 2002).
5. The early language development (< 36 months of age) of children with HIV and children exposed to but uninfected by the virus is compared. The two groups are divided into those who score more than or less than 2 standard deviations below the mean on the test (see Coplan et al., 1998).

The independent t-test

We start with the independent t-test. We will use the made-up data on therapy for dysfluency from Chapter 2 (see Table 2.1). There we assessed the subjects before and after the treated group had therapy and subtracted the number of dysfluencies after therapy from the number before to get a measure of change. The scores are shown below.

Table 5.2 Scores (in ascending order) and means and standard deviations from our experiment on therapy for people who stammer

	Subjects' scores (decrease in number of dysfluencies)										x	s
Treated group	2	3	4	5	6	10	11	12	12	14	7.90	4.36
Control group	0	1	3	4	4	4	5	7	8	9	4.50	2.88

First we should consider whether the data allow us to use a parametric test. There is no clear evidence that the scores are not normally distributed. Squaring the standard deviations to obtain the variances shows that they are not very equal. It could also be argued that the data are not equal-interval data, as not all dysfluencies are the same. This shows how difficult it is to be confident about this decision. Each assumption is questionable. Now look at journal articles where similar data are analysed. You will find that parametric tests are almost always used. In other words, researchers are quite pragmatic when it comes to assumptions.

Looking at the data before analysing them may help you to understand the result of the statistical test. There is a lot of overlap between the groups. Five of the treated group scored lower than at least one person in the untreated group. Other treated subjects received high scores – five were higher than any of the control groups. So it is no surprise that the treated group had a higher mean. It also had a higher standard deviation because some clients responded better than others.

Will this data give us a significant result? The overlap in the two groups of scores and the variability in the treated group suggest that it may not. If we fail to get a significant result (or even if we do), we are likely to look to see which clients improved and which did not. You must be cautious here. You don't receive much credit for saying 'the result was not significant but some clients improved a lot' – even if they did. Some clients always improve more than others, and we can't tell whether this is because therapy helped them or whether they changed for reasons of their own. Nevertheless, it would be silly not to look for reasons why some improved and some did not. Perhaps the therapy does help certain types of clients, and we can make our hypothesis more specific and test it with this sort of client in a new experiment. But this is jumping too far ahead. Let's do the t-test.

The formula for the independent t-test is: $t = \dfrac{(\bar{x}_1 - \bar{x}_2)}{\sqrt{\left(\dfrac{1}{n_1} - \dfrac{1}{n_2}\right) s_p^2}}$

where: $\quad s_p^2 = \dfrac{(n_1 - 1)s_1^2 + (n_2 - 1)s_2^2}{n_1 + n_2 - 2}$

In these formulae $\bar{x}_1$ and $\bar{x}_2$ are the means of the two groups and n_1 and n_2 are the numbers of subjects in the groups. s_p^2 is called the pooled variance. Essentially it is the mean of the two group variances s_1^2 and s_2^2 (weighted for sample size – but ours are the same size).

This formula doesn't look very friendly. However, we can see what it is doing. It compares the difference in the means (numerator) with the variances (denominator). We want it to be as large as possible; so we want a big difference between the means and small variances. You will recall that in Chapter 2 these things affected our confidence about whether the means of the groups differed. This may reassure you that there is nothing in the formula that you would not expect to be there.

To work out the formula we need the sample means and standard deviations and the number of subjects. From Table 5.2 (with the treated group as group 1 and the untreated as group 2) these are:

$$x_1 = 7.9 \quad x_2 = 4.5 \quad s_1 = 4.36 \quad s_2 = 2.88 \text{ and } n_1 = 10 \text{ and } n_2 = 10$$

We then obtain a pooled estimate of the population variance from:

$$s_p^2 = \frac{(n_1 - 1) s_1^2 + (n_2 - 1) s_2^2}{n_1 + n_2 - 2} = \frac{9 \times 4.36^2 + 9 \times 2.88^2}{18} = 13.65$$

and calculate the value of t from:

$$t = \frac{(\bar{x}_1 - \bar{x}_2)}{\sqrt{\left(\frac{1}{n_1} - \frac{1}{n_2}\right) s_p^2}} = \frac{7.9 - 4.5}{\sqrt{\left(\frac{2}{10}\right) \times 13.65}} = \frac{3.4}{1.65} = 2.06$$

We now look up this result in the t-tables (Appendix 2). If our result (2.06) is bigger than the table value, it is significant. To find the appropriate table entry we must decide what the degrees of freedom are, what significance level we are using and whether we are using a one- or a two-tail test.

The degrees of freedom for the independent t-test are $(n_1 - 1)$ + $(n_2 - 1)$ (the total number of subjects minus 2). Few statistical mysteries are more puzzling than degrees of freedom (d.f.). Let's just say that they are the number of subjects minus 2 because we used the data to estimate the *two* population means. In the t-tables you use the row corresponding to the d.f. of your test.

We discussed the significance level in Chapter 2. It is the probability that a result is due to chance. Alternatively it is the risk of a type-one error. Conventionally 5% is used; so, if a result has less than a 5% probability of being due to chance, it is significant. The columns in the t-tables correspond to different levels of significance. If our value is higher than the table value, then the result is significant. If we find that it is significant at a higher level than $p < 0.05$ ($p < 0.01$), we report this because it increases confidence that the result is not a type-one error.

Experimental hypotheses may be directional or non-directional. In our experiment we predicted that treated clients would improve more than untreated ones; so we used a one-tail test. In other experiments we might not predict the direction of the result. For instance, we might compare two different treatments and have an open mind as to which is better. Here we have a non-directional hypothesis and use a two-tail test.

A statistical test is significant when a difference in our experiment is unlikely to be due to chance. The 5% level of significance lets us call significant the 5% of results that are least likely to have occurred by chance. If an experiment has two possible outcomes, we must divide this 5% between them. A result in either direction is only significant if it can be accounted for by chance less than 2.5% of the time. The total of significant outcomes remains at 5%, but the chance of either outcome being significant is now only 2.5%. A directional hypothesis rules out one outcome and allows 5% of results in the predicted direction to be significant.

If we make a directional prediction in advance, we use a one-tail test; if we are in doubt about the outcome, we must use a two-tail test. Sometimes a result is significant for a one- but not for a two-tail test. However, the prediction must be made before the results are known. Claiming that you had a directional hypothesis after the results are known is not only cheating but rarely carries conviction. If we had no reason to predict the result beforehand, we are unlikely to find a good one afterwards. So, if we start with a two-tail test, we must stick with it. On the other hand, it is noticeable that researchers in communication disorders often use two-tail tests when a one-tail test appears to be justified. This is unduly cautious. When we make a directional prediction, we should use a one-tail test.

We can now, at last, look up our t-value in the tables. The first column is the d.f.; so we look in the '18' row. Choose the column for $p < 0.05$ for a one-tail test. You will find the value 1.73. Our t-value is higher than this; so the result is significant. We reject the null hypothesis that any difference in the improvement of treated and untreated clients who stammer is due to chance. We write the result as $t(18) = 2.06$, $p < 0.05$. This gives the value of t, the d.f. used and the level of significance obtained.

There are two things to notice about this result. First, the table value for $p < 0.025$ is 2.10, which is slightly higher than our value. Therefore, our result is not significant at this higher level. Had it been significant at a higher level we would report this; that it isn't shouldn't surprise you in view of our initial doubts about the data. Second, the value 2.10 is the table value for a two-tail test at $p < 0.05$. If we had used a two-tail test, our result would not have been significant.

Exercise 5.3

1. Look up the critical value in the t-tables for the following
   (a) a one-tail test with 10 d.f. at the 0.05 level of significance.
   (b) a two-tail test with 10 d.f. at the 0.05 level of significance.
   (c) a one-tail test with 10 d.f. at the 0.025 level of significance.
   (d) a one-tail test with 20 d.f. at the 0.01 level of significance.
   (e) a two-tail test with 30 d.f. at the 0.01 level of significance.

2. Suppose we compare the BPVT scores of the 20 children with SLI from Chapter 3 with the scores of 10 normally developing children.
   (a) What are the degrees of freedom in this experiment?
   (b) An independent t-test is used giving $t = 1.87$. Is the result significant? What do you make of this result?

Exercise 5.4

In Exercise 2.4, we compared different sets of data from our experiment on treating dysfluency. The aim was to convince you that our confidence about getting a significant result depends upon the difference in the means of the groups, how big the standard deviations of the groups are and how many subjects take part. Now we are in a position to check our judgements against the results of t-tests on the data. You will have noticed that the formulae above allow us to calculate t if we know the means and standard deviations (we don't need the individual subject scores). Reports of research normally give means and standard deviations so you may find this useful. The means and standard deviations; for the treated and untreated groups are given below. Work out the t values and check their significance in the tables.

	n	Treated group Mean	Treated group Standard deviation	Untreated group Mean	Untreated group Standard deviation
Original data	6	13	5.40	8	5.66
Exercise 2.4 (1)	6	16	5.40	8	5.66
Exercise 2.4 (2)	6	13	9.82	8	6.07
Exercise 2.4 (3)	12	13	5.39	8	5.15

The related t-test

The advantage of the within-subjects design is that each subject does each condition and we can compare their performance directly. Subject variability, which was such a headache in the between-subjects design, is no longer a problem. This advantage is seen in the related t-test. We reduce each subject's performance to the difference between his or her scores in the two conditions of the experiment. We do so by subtracting the scores to get a difference or d-score for each subject. Common sense suggests that we should find a significant result if the difference scores are:

- mainly in one direction
- reasonably consistent
- large.

These expectations are fulfilled in the formula:

$$t = \frac{\bar{d}}{s_d / \sqrt{n}} \qquad \text{where} \qquad s_d = \sqrt{\frac{\sum d^2 - \frac{(\sum d)^2}{n}}{n - 1}}$$

Large values of t will result if the mean difference (numerator) is large and the standard deviation of d (denominator) is small. The difference between the conditions is measured by $\bar{d}$ but does not tell us about individual subjects. A particular value of $\bar{d}$ might occur because subjects have consistent difference scores or because some have large scores while others show no difference. The latter situation is not one we would expect to give us a significant result because the value of s_d will be large.

In other respects the related and independent t-tests are similar. We again use the t-tables to look up the significance of the result, this time with $n - 1$ degrees of freedom, and must decide in advance whether to use a one- or two-tail test.

Our example on the cueing of children with word-finding problems used a within-subjects design and can be analysed with a related t-test. Children named pictures with or without a sentence completion task as a cue. Below are data from 10 children doing the experiment. Scores are out of 20.

Table 5.3 Scores of 10 children naming pictures with and without a sentence cue

	Naming pictures	Naming pictures with a sentence completion cue	difference (d)	d^2
Subject 1	6	10	4	16
Subject 2	17	14	-3	9
Subject 3	7	12	5	25
Subject 4	2	6	4	16
Subject 5	12	18	6	36
Subject 6	9	16	7	49
Subject 7	0	3	3	9
Subject 8	18	20	2	4
Subject 9	10	10	0	0
Subject 10	5	11	6	36
Mean	8.6	12.0	$\Sigma d = 34$ $\bar{d} = 3.4$	$\Sigma d^2 = 200$
s	5.89	5.23		

$$S_d = \sqrt{\frac{\Sigma d^2 - \frac{(\Sigma d)^2}{n}}{n-1}} = \sqrt{\frac{200 - \frac{1156}{10}}{9}} = 3.06$$

$$\text{and} \quad t = \frac{\bar{d}}{S_d / \sqrt{n}} = \frac{3.4}{3.06 / \sqrt{10}} = 3.51$$

There are a few points to note about these data and calculations. Eight of the subjects improved their naming when cued. One showed no effect, and one did worse. As a result one d score is negative. We expected the cued naming to be better; so it made sense to subtract the naming scores from the cued naming scores so that positive values of d are consistent with our directional hypothesis. This doesn't matter, but positive numbers are less disconcerting. Had we subtracted in the opposite direction, t would be the same but negative. We ignore this when looking in the tables; the sign just reminds us of the direction of the result.

Notice how variable the subjects are. One only makes two errors in the whole experiment; another only names three items. This variation would be troublesome in a between-subjects design. Here it has little effect because the d scores are very similar.

When we look up the table value of t; we do so for 9 d.f. using the 5% significance level and a one-tail test. The table value is 1.83; so our result is easily significant. If we continue across the d.f. = 9 row, we find that our value is higher than the table values up to 0.005 for a one-tail test. So we report the result as $t(9) = 3.52$, p < 0.005.

Exercise 5.5

1. The experiment above might be done as a within-subjects design or as a between-subjects design. In Chapter 2 we decided that we should use a within-subjects design both here and elsewhere if it was possible to do so. To reassure yourself that we made the right decision analyse the data in Table 5.3 as if they had come from a between-subjects design (do an independent t-test on the data).
2. Goberman et al. (2002) compared fundamental frequencies of the speech of clients with Parkinson's disease before and after taking medication. Data from 10 clients are shown below. Does medication affect their fundamental frequency? Work out the values of d and d^2 in the table and then use a related t-test to find out.

	Before	After	Difference (d)	d^2
Subject 1	92	104		
Subject 2	124	123		
Subject 3	203	186		
Subject 4	156	162		
Subject 5	132	140		
Subject 6	86	91		
Subject 7	141	139		
Subject 8	167	160		
Subject 9	101	115		
Subject 10	97	101		

*The one-sample z- and one-sample t-tests

In Exercise 5.3 we compared the performance of 20 SLI children with a group of children with normal language development. You might have felt this was an odd thing to do, and you would have been right. Why should we get scores for children with normal language when the BPVS has done it for us? Can't we compare our sample with the data from the test?

The one-sample z- and t-tests let us compare a sample with the performance of a population. In effect they ask whether the sample came from the population. If this is unlikely, we reject the null hypothesis. Standardized tests give us an opportunity to use the one-sample z- and t-tests. We can compare a sample from some clinical group with the scores from the test using these as the performance of the population. This is cheating slightly as the tests' scores are also based on a sample; however, it is usually a very large one, which has been carefully selected to represent the population.

Standardized tests will normally give us both the mean and the standard deviation of the population. Here we use the one sample z test. Its formula is given below.

$$z = \frac{\bar{x} - \mu}{\sigma / \sqrt{n}}$$

where $\bar{x}$ is the sample mean, μ the population mean, σ the population SD and n the size of the sample.

We look up this value of z in the z-tables. Previously we did this to get a percentile score. Here we do the same thing but with the aim of showing that the sample mean is within the 5% (for a one-tail test) or 2.5% (for a two-tail test) of the most extreme scores found when standardizing the test. If it is, then the result is significant and the sample differs from the population by an amount that is unlikely to occur by chance.

Exercise 5.6

We have a sample of 16 children with a history of petit mal attacks. At 5 years we test their comprehension on the BPVS (mean 100, SD 15) to see if they have any difficulty. Their mean raw score is 43.2. This converts to a standardized (scaled) score of 92. Has epilepsy affected the children's comprehension?

Sometimes we know the population mean but not its standard deviation. Here we can't use the one-sample z-test. In such cases statisticians have resorted to another of their conjuring tricks. They use the sample standard deviation *s* to estimate the population standard deviation σ (even though they are planning to show that the sample is different from the population). However, this underestimates the value of σ; so when *n* is small we need to use the one-sample t-test. The formula is:

$$t = \frac{\bar{x} - \mu}{s / \sqrt{n}} \quad \text{with } n - 1 \text{ d.f.}$$

and we look the resulting value up in the t-tables as before. As sample size increases the estimation of σ improves and we can use *z* again. Thirty is the usual cut-off point for using *z*.

Non-parametric tests

We have seen that parametric tests may only be used if our data shapes up. There are many occasions when it does not and we need non-parametric tests. This is particularly the case when we use observers to rate behaviours that cannot easily be measured.

Non-parametric tests do not use the actual data. Instead they rank them and use the ranks in their formulae to assess significance. The underlying philosophy of the tests is the same, however. We still set a level of significance (p < 0.05), reject the null hypothesis and use one- or two-tail tests, and we can still make type-one and -two errors.

The Mann-Whitney test

The Mann-Whitney test is used for between-subjects designs where the data are non-parametric. Like other non-parametric tests, it requires very little arithmetic but has a convoluted procedure that makes it easy to go wrong. Here we use the data from our dysfluency experiment again but analyse it with a Mann-Whitney test. The scores are given in Table 5.4.

First, we rank the scores. We give the lowest score (in either group) the rank 1 and continue until all the scores have a rank. In the above the score 0 receives the rank 1, the score 1 is ranked 2 and so on. If a tie occurs, each tied score is given the mean of the ranks that would have been used. In the above, two subjects score 3. They would have been ranked 4 and 5; so each is ranked 4.5. This can

Table 5.4 Ranks of the scores from our experiment on therapy for people who stammer

Subject	Score	Rank	Subject	Score	Rank
1	0	1	11	2	3
2	1	2	12	3	4.5
3	3	4.5	13	4	7.5
4	4	7.5	14	5	10.5
5	4	7.5	15	6	12
6	4	7.5	16	10	16
7	5	10.5	17	11	17
8	7	13	18	12	18.5
9	8	14	19	12	18.5
10	9	15	20	14	20
		$R_1 = 82.5$			$R_2 = 127.5$

become complicated when there are a lot of ties. Four subjects scored 4 and so receive the rank 7.5 (the mean of 6, 7, 8 and 9).

We add the ranks in the first group and call the total R_1. In the example the ranks of both groups have been added, but we will call the untreated subjects group one; so $R_1 = 82.5$. We now use R_1 and n_1 and n_2 (the numbers of subjects in the groups) to get U.

$$U = n_1 n_2 + \frac{n_1(n_1 + 1)}{2} - R_1 = 10 \times 10 + \frac{10 \times 11}{2} - 82.5 = 72.5$$

and then work out U' where $U' = n_1 n_2 - U = 10 \times 10 - 72.5 = 27.5$

To look up the table value (see Appendix 3) we must decide if we are using a one- or two-tail test and the significance level we want. No degrees of freedom are involved – we look up the table entry for the numbers of subjects in the groups. If either U or U' is less than or equal to the table value, the result is significant. Here we use a one-tail test as we expect greater improvement by the treated group. For the 5% level of significance and 10 subjects in each group the critical value is 27. As neither U nor U' is less than the table value, the result is not (quite) significant.

The logic of the Mann-Whitney test is quite simple. If a difference exists between the groups, one should have mainly low scores and the other mainly high ones. The rankings will reflect this giving low ranks to one group and high ones to the other. The formula assesses whether one group has sufficient low rankings for the result to be significant.

Some people prefer non-parametric tests because the maths is easier. Although the Mann-Whitney test does not offer the mathematical thrills of the independent t-test, it is quite easy to go wrong. The ranks are a problem, particularly when there are ties. There are two quick checks you can use. First, the highest rank should be equal to the number of subjects. Second, the sum of the ranks should equal the sum of the numbers 1 to n where n is the number of subjects (1 to 20 sum to 210 as do $R_1 + R_2$).

Confusion may also arise when getting R_1. It doesn't matter which group is group 1 (and R_1), but we must label n_1 and n_2 accordingly (if the numbers in the groups are not the same). If the treated group had been made group 1 in our example, the values of U and U' would have been reversed.

You may find it disconcerting that we found a significant result with a t-test but not with a Mann-Whitney test. This is because the t-test is more powerful, which shows that we should use it if we can.

A final point is that the test does not use the actual scores. Suppose subjects 16 to 20 all reduced their dysfluencies by 10 more than at present. This would have caused all sorts of problems for the t-test. The population would not be normally distributed, the variances would not be homogeneous and the t-value would change. Here the outcome is unaffected. This illustrates the value of the non-parametric approach, which is unaffected by extreme scores, non-normal distributions and unequal variances.

The Wilcoxon test

Our table has two tests for within-subjects designs with non-parametric data. The Wilcoxon test is the stronger test. We can illustrate its use by again analysing the data from our picture-naming experiment (see Table 5.5).

The procedure is simple. Subtract the pairs of scores. It doesn't matter which way we do this, but, as with the related t-test, it makes sense for scores favouring our hypothesis to be positive (if we are using a one-tail test). One child shows no difference. The Wilcoxon test has no patience with subjects like this. It drops them from the experiment and reduces n.

We now rank the differences ignoring their signs. The lowest difference is ranked as 1. Again ties receive the mean of the ranks that would have been used. Now we add the ranks of the differences with the least occurring sign and call it W. In our case only one difference score is negative, and it receives the rank 2.5. Hence $W = 2.5$.

Look up the table value (Appendix 4) for 9 subjects (the number after ties are dropped). If W is less than or equal to the table value,

Exercise 5.7

Kunkel et al. (1997) described a non-invasive method of measuring velopharyngeal muscle function, which may be used to monitor progress during therapy with children with cleft palate. To assess the measure they compared children with and without cleft palate. They used a Mann-Whitney test to compare their epipharyngeal volumes (in cubic centimetres). Do a Mann-Whitney test on the made-up values below.

People with cleft palate			People without cleft palate		
Subject	Score	Rank	Subject	Score	Rank
1	6		9	8	
2	5		10	5	
3	4		11	6	
4	4.5		12	8.5	
5	6		13	9	
6	9		14	7.5	
7	7		15	10	
8	6.5		16	9.5	
			17	6.5	
		$R_1 =$			$R_2 =$

Table 5.5 Ranks of difference scores for children naming pictures with and without a sentence cue

	Naming pictures	Naming pictures with a sentence completion cue	Difference (d)	Rank
Subject 1	6	10	4	4.5
Subject 2	17	14	-3	2.5
Subject 3	7	12	5	6
Subject 4	2	6	4	4.5
Subject 5	12	18	6	7.5
Subject 6	9	16	7	9
Subject 7	0	3	3	2.5
Subject 8	18	20	2	1
Subject 9	10	10	0	–
Subject 10	5	11	6	7.5

the result is significant. In our case we use a one-tail test and the 5% level of significance. The table value is 8; so our result is easily significant; in fact, it is significant at $p < 0.01$ (table value = 3).

The logic of the test is simple. It finds how many scores go against the trend and uses their ranks to assess how seriously they do so. Again the actual scores are not used. In our example several of the subjects could have improved more strongly without changing the ranking of the sole subject who went against the trend.

Exercise 5.8

The Lidcombe program (see Chapter 15) is known to reduce dysfluency in children. One explanation for its effect is that it subtly alters speech timing. Onslow et al. (2002) investigated this by comparing acoustic variables from pre- and post-treatment speech of eight children who had successfully completed the programme. Data for mean vowel duration (in ms) are shown below and were analysed with a Wilcoxon test. What result do you find?

	Pre-treatment	Post-treatment	Difference (d)	Rank
Subject 1	0.116	0.122		
Subject 2	0.140	0.141		
Subject 3	0.114	0.124		
Subject 4	0.126	0.106		
Subject 5	0.114	0.136		
Subject 6	0.150	0.139		
Subject 7	0.127	0.129		
Subject 8	0.165	0.152		

The sign test

The sign test is an even simpler test for non-parametric data from within-subjects designs. It just assesses whether subjects change in the same direction. In our example above the test asks how likely it is that eight of nine subjects change in the same direction by chance alone (the tied score is eliminated). Give all the subjects a + or – sign to indicate their direction of change (use + for the right direction in a one-tail test). Call the number of scores that go against the trend S. Then look up the value in the tables (Appendix 5), and, if S is less than or equal to this value, reject the null hypothesis. In our example $S = 1$. For nine subjects, a one-tail test and the 5% level of significance the table value is 1; so our result is just significant.

You may be wondering why we bother with other more troublesome tests when the sign test does the job so easily. The answer is simple. The sign test is less powerful than the Wilcoxon test or the

---

Exercise 5.9

You may know that footballers are superstitious people. Having kicked balls every day for 20 years they still think that, on any given day, their ability will be affected by whether they put their left sock on before their right or wear their lucky suit to the match. Perhaps they have a case after all. When cup finals were moved to the Millennium Stadium in Cardiff, the first nine were won by teams using the north dressing room. A feng shui expert was called in to put things right. Is there a statistical case for avoiding the unlucky south dressing room?

---

related t-test. So why bother with it at all? One answer is that we can quickly discover if a result is significant. We can even do it without knowing the scores. If we are told, for example, that 16 subjects were given a therapy and that 13 improved, we can consult the sign test tables to see if this is significant.

*Using non-parametric tests with large *n*

You may have noticed that the tables for non-parametric tests do not allow you to test data from large groups of subjects. As n increases, the distributions of non-parametric test statistics approach the normal distribution. You can work out the tests in the normal way then substitute the values of U, W or S into formulae that give you a z-score and look this up in the z-tables (as with the one-sample z-test). The formulae are:

$$z = \frac{U - \dfrac{n_1 n_2}{2}}{\sqrt{\dfrac{n_1 n_2 (n_1 + n_2 + 1)}{12}}} \quad \text{for the Mann-Whitney test}$$

$$z = \frac{W - \dfrac{n(n+1)}{4}}{\sqrt{\dfrac{n(n+1)(2n+1)}{24}}} \quad \text{for the Wilcoxon test}$$

$$\text{and} \quad z = \frac{S - \dfrac{n}{2}}{\sqrt{\dfrac{n}{4}}} \quad \text{for the Sign test}$$

Chapter 6
Analysis of variance I

Introduction: variables and levels

You might have noticed that all our experiments to date have had only one IV with only two levels. Analysis of variance (ANOVA) is a set of experimental designs (and statistical tests) where IVs can have more than two levels and where more than one IV may be manipulated. This lets us do more exciting experiments. We can examine the effect of two or more IVs in the same experiment and look at their combined effects. As a result ANOVA is the most commonly used approach to experimental research, and you must know how it works. In fact, it is so important that we will give it two chapters.

The calculations needed to work out ANOVAs are no fun at all; so you won't be doing them. Computers are faster and don't make mistakes. Many books show you how to do the calculations (see, for example, Greene and D'Oliveira, 1982; Keppel, 1991; Hinton, 1995; Howell, 1997; Howitt and Cramer, 1999). One day you will want to know all about ANOVA and you might consult them. A word of warning is required, however. Books use different notations in the formulae; so it is important to find a book you like and get used to the system it uses.

Although computers can carry out ANOVAs for you, you won't get very far unless you can recognize the different types of ANOVA and know which to use in your research. You also need to understand and interpret the results. This may involve drawing graphs and carrying out further analyses.

One-factor designs

One-factor ANOVAs have one IV, which is manipulated, at more than two levels. The term 'factor' is confusing. It indicates that there is one IV; so two- or three-factor designs have two or three IVs. We use the terms 'one-factor design' and 'one-factor ANOVA' interchange-ably, but strictly one is the design and the other is the statistical test.

There are two one-factor designs. We may compare several groups of people doing a single experimental task (a step up from the independent t-test) or the same people doing several tasks or the same task at several different times (like a related t-test). We call these the 'one-factor between-subjects' and 'one-factor within-subjects' designs. (You might see them called the 'one-factor completely randomized' design and the 'one-factor repeated-measures' design.)

Yorkston and Beukelman (1980) were concerned that existing language assessments were insensitive to change in people with mild aphasia. They devised a measure (actually several, but one will do here) to detect high-level changes in language. To see if it worked, they tested five groups of people – adults and elderly adults with normal language development and three groups of people with aphasia classified as mild, high moderate and low moderate – to see if it could distinguish their performance. This is a one-factor between-subjects design. It has one IV with five levels. It is easy to become confused between IVs and their levels; so it helps to give them names. Here we might call the IV 'type of subject' and the levels are the five types of people listed above. Notice also that this is not a true experiment, as the subjects already belong to the levels of the IV and cannot be randomly assigned.

DuBois and Bernthal (1978) tested whether errors by children with articulation problems varied with the context in which they are tested. They tested the same children on three different tasks: a picture-naming task, retelling a story told by a therapist and telling a story from pictures (the same target words were in each). This is a one-factor, within-subjects design. Again there is one IV – the type of assessment – with three levels.

In these designs ANOVA does what the t-test did. It decides if differences between the levels of the IV are due to chance or whether this is unlikely. The procedure is so similar that you might wonder if we could do without ANOVA (especially as I have been so alarmist about its difficulty) and compare pairs of levels with t-tests. There are two reasons for not doing so. The first is that we would need many t-tests (10 in Yorkston and Beukelman) to compare each pair. One t-test may be easier than an ANOVA, but 10 can be rather tedious. You should already have realized the second reason. It is that 10 tests carry a much greater risk of a type-one error. In contrast, ANOVA has only the usual 5% chance of a type-one error.

An ANOVA gives us an F-value, which we look up in the tables of the F-distribution to see if the result is significant (computers do this for us). This tells us if there is a significant difference between any of the conditions in the experiment. It doesn't tell us which are different from which. We look at this problem later.

Exercise 6.1

Which ANOVA would you use in each of the following? What is the independent variable and how many levels does it have? What might the dependent variable be?

1. Children's dysfluencies are compared during interaction with a parent, play with a clinician, play under pressure, story retelling and picture description (Yaruss, 1997).
2. The performance on the Boston Naming Test of two groups of bilingual adults (French/English and Spanish/English) is compared with monolingual English speakers (Roberts et al., 2002).
3. Knowledge of the meaning of proverbs is tested at different ages. Young and older adolescents and people in their 20s. 30s, 40s, 50s, 60s and 70s are tested (Nippold et al., 1997).
4. Adults with profound and multiple-learning disabilities were taught to use objects of reference. A scoring system was devised and their performance at baseline and at four five-week intervals was assessed (Jones et al., 2002).
5. The educational achievement of children with language impairment is assessed when they are 16 years old. The children are divided into three groups: those whose problems had resolved by age 5.06, those whose problems persisted and those with general delay (poor-language and non-verbal ability) and compared with children with no history of language impairment (Snowling et al., 2001).

The one-factor between-subjects design: a closer look

We now take a closer look at the results of a one-factor between-subjects ANOVA. I have made up some data based on the experiment by Yorkston and Beukelman. One assessment asked subjects to describe pictures. The number of 'content units' (specified by the authors) in their descriptions was counted. Table 6.1 is the number of content units for three groups of subjects (simplified from the original five groups). You can see that we have our familiar problem:

the group means are different but there is a lot of variation within the groups. As usual, it's difficult to be confident that the groups differ.

Table 6.1 Numbers of content units for three groups of subjects

Group A. Elderly adults		Group B. People with mild aphasia		Group C. People with high moderate aphasia	
S1	12	S11	12	S21	9
S2	15	S12	8	S22	7
S3	13	S13	10	S23	10
S4	12	S14	11	S24	8
S5	11	S15	8	S25	6
S6	10	S16	9	S26	10
S7	12	S17	10	S27	12
S8	14	S18	9	S28	9
S9	15	S19	13	S29	12
S10	12	S20	10	S30	9
	Mean = 12.6		Mean = 10.0		Mean = 9.2
Mean of all scores = 10.6					

If we analyse this on a computer, we can produce a printout like Table 6.2 below. This is an ANOVA table. Columns 5 and 6 give the F-value from the calculations and the exact probability of the result occurring by chance. This probability is surprisingly low and the result highly significant. We normally round off significance levels (to 0.05, 0.01, 0.001 and so forth); here we would round it off to $p < 0.001$.

Table 6.2 ANOVA table for the data in Table 6.1

1	2	3	4	5	6
Source of variance	Sum of squares	d.f.	Mean square	F	p
Between-groups	63.20	2	31.61	10.43	0.0004
Within-groups (error)	82.00	27	3.03		
Total	145.20	29			

The F-value itself comes from dividing 31.6 by 3.03 from column 4. These numbers are the between-groups and within-groups mean squares. Actually they are variances (see column 1), but statisticians have decided to call them 'mean squares' just to make things even more confusing. We look at where they came from in the optional section below. So F is actually a ratio (it's often called the F-ratio) of the between-groups and within-groups variances. That's why it's called analysis of variance!

If we had worked the ANOVA out ourselves, we would have looked up its significance in the F-tables (Appendix 6). These tables need 2 degrees of freedom, 1 for the numerator and 1 for the denominator of the F-ratio (see column 3). These are 2 for the numerator (between-groups variance) and 27 for the denominator (within-groups variance). The F-tables give the values for the $p < 0.05$ and $p < 0.01$ levels of significance. They are 3.35 and 5.49. Notice that the F-tables do not have one-tail and two-tail versions. When we compare two levels of an IV, it is quite likely that we will have a directional hypothesis. When we compare several levels, as we often do in ANOVA, making predictions about the outcome is more difficult, and those we make may involve several levels of the IV. As a result there is normally no equivalent of a one-tail test in ANOVA. When we write up the results of our experiment, we normally give the F-value, the probability and the d.f. So this result would be written $F(2, 27) = 10.40$, $p < 0.001$.

*What does ANOVA do and why does it need a table to do it?

As promised, we won't work out any ANOVAs but we will do some arithmetic in this section to try to get a clearer idea of what an ANOVA does and how to understand its table. There are 30 scores in our data (3×10 subjects). We can calculate their variance. We will call this the total variance. As always, subjects vary for two reasons. One is because the IV is affecting them; the other is because individual people differ. We will call the effect of the IV the treatment effect and the effect of individual differences the error variance.

We must decide if there is a treatment effect. This should sound familiar – it's the problem we had with the t-test. We have to show that the treatment effect is large enough that it is unlikely to be due to chance (error variance). We can't measure it directly, but we can measure the between- and within-groups variances. The first measures the difference between the groups (it's the equivalent of the difference in the means in the independent t-test). The groups may differ for two reasons. First, because they are at different levels of the IV; second, because individuals in the groups differ from one another (error variance). The within-groups variance is only affected by differences between individuals in the same group (error variance). Here there is no effect of the IV. As:

$$F = \frac{\text{between-groups variance}}{\text{within-groups variance}}$$

$$F = \frac{\text{treatment effect} + \text{error variance}}{\text{error variance}}$$

You can see that, when there is no treatment effect, F should equal 1. It is unlikely that it will do so exactly, as our two measures of error variance are estimates and won't be the same. Nevertheless, F-values close to 1 indicate that there is little or no treatment effect. If there is a treatment effect, F will be greater than 1 and the F tables tell us how big it must be for the effect to be significant. Conversely researchers reporting non-significant results sometimes report that F < 1, as a way of emphasizing that there was no evidence of an effect.

The values in the above table can be obtained by using the usual formula for the variance.

Remember that this is $\dfrac{\Sigma(x - \bar{x})^2}{n - 1}$

and that $\Sigma(x - \bar{x})^2$ was called the sum of squares.

The mean of all 30 scores is 10.6. So, if we subtract 10.6 from each score and square and add the results, we find the total sums of squares. It may or may not surprise you that the answer is 145.2, the number in column 2 of the ANOVA table.

The difference between the groups is given by the variance of their means about the mean of all the scores. Its sum of squares will be:

$$(12.6 - 10.6)^2 + (10 - 10.6)^2 + (9.2 - 10.6)^2 = 6.32$$

If we multiply this by 10, the number of subjects, we get 63.2. This is the between-groups sum of squares.

The within-groups sum of squares is found by squaring the differences between each subject and the mean of his or her group. Subjects in each group are at the same level of the IV; so it has no effect on them and only individual differences are seen. This gives 82.

These calculations show that it is not difficult to find the sums of squares in the ANOVA table. To find the variance we normally divide the sum of squares by $n - 1$. Here we divide by the degrees of freedom for each sum of squares (column 3), which is just a more complicated version of the same thing. For the total, it is the number of subjects -1 (29) and for the between-groups sum of squares it is the number of groups -1 (2). For the within-groups sum of squares it is the number of subjects – the number of groups. Here one degree of freedom is lost when we estimate the population means from each group. When we divide the sums of squares by these degrees of freedom, we find the variances (mean squares), which are in column 4.

Once we have done all this, we don't need the sums of squares; so why are they in the ANOVA table? One reason is that the between- and within-groups sums of squares add to give the total sum of squares. If you have to do the calculations by hand, it is useful to have this as a check on your arithmetic.

Looking at these calculations might convince you that ANOVA is not quite the mystery you initially thought it was. You may even think these calculations are not too tricky and that you might, after all, do ANOVA without a computer (or maybe not). It's only fair to warn you that the calculations become much worse as the number of variables and levels in the ANOVA increase. Unequal numbers of subjects in the conditions also add to the problems.

The one-factor within-subjects design

Suppose we assess a group of children who stammer before and after therapy and 6 months later we assess the effect of therapy and if it is maintained. The data in Table 6.3 are the number of dysfluencies reading aloud a set passage. This is a one-factor within-subjects design; the IV is time, and it has three levels – before, after and 6 months after therapy.

Table 6.3 Number of dysfluencies before and after treatment and at follow-up

	Before therapy	After therapy	6 months post-therapy	Mean
S1	19	15	17	17.00
S2	8	7	6	7.00
S3	12	8	7	9.0
S4	21	15	13	16.33
S5	7	8	6	7.0
S6	14	10	15	13.0
S7	22	16	19	19.0
S8	18	12	10	13.33
Mean	15.12	11.37	11.62	

Subjects complete all the conditions; so we can now add across the rows to obtain a mean score for each subject. This measures their over-all severity. The ANOVA table for this analysis is given in Table 6.4.

This ANOVA table looks pretty much like the last one but has an extra source of variance. Again we need an F-ratio that compares 'treatment plus error' with 'error'. Now, however, there are two

Table 6.4 Analysis of variance table for a one-factor within-subjects ANOVA on the data in Table 6.3

Source of variance	Sum of S	d.f.	Mean square	F	p
Time	70.33	2	35.17	8.64	0.0036
Subjects (error)	451.62	7	64.52		
Subjects × time (error)	57.00	14	4.07		
Total	578.95	23			

sources of error. Subjects are one source of error variance. This is the equivalent of the within-groups variance in the one-factor between-subjects ANOVA, except that we measure it by looking at their mean performance across the levels of time (their mean severity across the experiment). The other is called 'subjects × time' and measures how much subjects' scores vary over time. We use the latter to measure error variance. You should be able to work out why. It doesn't matter if subjects vary in severity as long as they respond consistently to therapy. If they are not consistent, the 'subjects × time' variance will be large and the result non-significant. This is like the related t-test. There we subtracted pairs of scores to obtain d, and it was the consistency of d that decided whether we found a significant result.

This shows, once again, why it is an advantage to use the within-subjects design if we can. The significance of the result is not affected by differences between the subjects. If they all respond in a similar way, we obtain a significant result. Here the result is highly significant ($p < 0.01$); we would report it as $F(2, 14) = 8.64$, $p < 0.01$.

Exercise 6.2

The ANOVA table below is for our dysfluency data analysed as if they were from a between-subjects design. This is silly. However, comparing this table with the correct one given above reveals some interesting things about the two designs. What do you notice?

Source of variance	Sum of S	d.f.	Mean square	F	p
Time	70.33	2	35.17	8.64	0.0036
Within-groups (error)	508.62	21	24.22		
Total	578.95	23			

Planned and unplanned comparisons

Both of our one-factor ANOVAs found highly significant results. This tells us that a significant result exists somewhere in the data. It does not tell us which levels of the IV are different. This is not good enough. We didn't ask if there was a difference somewhere in the data. In the between-subjects example we wanted to know if the groups differed, particularly those with aphasia. In the within-subjects example we wanted to know whether subjects had improved after therapy and whether they maintained this at the follow-up assessment.

This shows that ANOVA is rarely the end of a data analysis. We often need to compare pairs of means (of different levels of the IV) to find which differ from one another. I can hear you stamping your foot at this point. If carrying out lots of t-tests was such a bad idea, how come we end up doing it anyway? The reason for not doing the t-tests was to avoid type-one errors. This remains the main consideration when we start comparing means.

There are two ways of comparing means after ANOVA. We use either planned (also called a-priori) or unplanned (also called post hoc or, even, a posteriori) comparisons. Planned comparisons are planned before the experiment and are part of our hypothesis. Unplanned comparisons are those we decide to do after we see the results! In both we need to avoid type-one errors. We are only allowed to do a few planned comparisons; so the chance of a type-one error is not high. With unplanned comparisons we can do as many as we like; however, an adjustment is made to avoid type-one errors, and we are less likely to obtain significant results.

Planned comparisons compare pairs or combinations of conditions in an experiment. In our between-subjects design we might want to compare:

1. people with and without aphasia (Group A versus Groups B and C) – if the assessment can't tell these apart, then it's not much good
2. groups of people with aphasia (Group B versus Group C) – this would detect a high-level change in aphasic language, the original objective of the experiment.

In our within-subjects ANOVA, we want to compare:

1. before therapy and after therapy
2. before therapy and 6 months after therapy.

This is to test whether therapy works and whether its benefits are still seen 6 months later.

To ensure that the risk of a type-one error is not too great, we must only do a few planned comparisons. So are we allowed to do the ones above? Books offer us two rules on this. One is quite strict; the other trusts our honesty. The strict rule says comparisons must be orthogonal (we will come back to what that means) and defines both how many we may do and which ones are permissible. The honesty rule says that we are allowed to do the comparisons predicted by our hypothesis. This sounds like an invitation to cheat; however, exponents of this approach say that a properly argued hypothesis would clearly justify some comparisons but not others, and so limit the number to be carried out.

*Carrying out planned comparisons

The procedure for planned comparisons is quite straightforward, if a little strange. Although it is easily done on a computer, it is useful to know about the calculations to understand what planned comparisons are and which ones we are allowed to do. We will do it for our data in the one-factor between-subjects design above. Remember that we wanted to compare:

- group A with groups B and C
- group B with group C.

To do this we need an F-ratio that compares the mean square of the comparison with the mean-square error:

$$F = \text{MS}_{\text{comp}} / \text{MS}_{\text{error}}$$

Hence we need MS_{comp} (MS_{error} comes from the main analysis).

The means for the three conditions were: elderly 12.6, mild aphasia 10.0, and high moderate aphasia 9.2. The first step is to select coefficients to define the comparisons we want to make. In the first case we want to compare the elderly with the performance of the two groups of people with dysphasia, and so we use the coefficients 1, -0.5 and -0.5 and obtain φ where:

$$\varphi = (1) \times 12.6 + (-0.5) \times 10.0 + (-0.5) \times 9.2 = 3$$

This might seem a very odd thing to do, but stick with it. Basically all we have done is to find the difference between the mean for the elderly group and the mean of the means of the other two groups! We can now use φ to find the SS comp that we need:

$$SS_{comp} = \frac{s(\varphi)^2}{\Sigma(c_i)^2} = \frac{10(3)^2}{1.5} = 60$$

where s = number of subjects per group and c_i = the coefficients used in the formula for φ. Since all comparisons have 1 degree of freedom this is also the MScomp.

$$\text{So } F = \frac{MS_{comp}}{MS_{error}} = \frac{60}{3.03} = 19.80 \text{ (d.f. 1, 27) } p < 0.001$$

We can repeat this process for comparison 2. Here we use 0, 1 and -1 as the coefficients:

$$\varphi = (0) \times 12.6 + (1) \times 10.0 + (-1) \times 9.2 = 0.8$$

$$SS_{comp} = \frac{s(\varphi)^2}{\Sigma(c_i)^2} = \frac{10(0.8)^2}{2} = 3.2$$

Again the comparison has 1 degree of freedom; so this is the MScomp:

$$F = \frac{MS_{comp}}{MS_{error}} = \frac{3.2}{3.03} = 1.06 \text{ (d.f. 1, 27) not significant}$$

So these comparisons show that the assessment can easily distinguish people with and without aphasia but not the two groups of people with different severities of aphasia (but remember these are only my made-up data!).

So we have carried out the comparisons that we planned; but were they orthogonal? And, by the way, what does 'orthogonal' mean? We can decide whether they were orthogonal (but, of course, we should have done this as part of our pre-planned strategy for analysing the data) by multiplying the coefficients in our comparison.

The sum of the products of the coefficients (see Table 6.5) is 0 $(-0.5 + 0.5)$; so these comparisons are orthogonal. Other sets of comparisons can be orthogonal; however, the number that make up an orthogonal set is given by the degrees of freedom of the variable

Table 6.5 Testing the coefficients to check for orthogonality

	Group A. Elderly adults	Group B. People with mild aphasia	Group C. People with high moderate aphasia
Comparison 1	1	-0.5	-0.5
Comparison 2	0	1	-1
Comparison 1 × Comparison 2	0	-0.5	0.5

being analysed. So in this example, orthogonal comparisons exist in pairs (d.f. = 2).

When we do the maximum number of planned comparisons allowed and they are orthogonal, their sums of squares will add to the sums of squares of the variable we are analysing. So in the example above:

$$SS_{comp1} + SS_{comp2} = 60 + 3.2 = 63.2$$

which is the between-groups sums of squares in the original ANOVA. This demonstrates that our comparisons account for all the variance in the means of the groups, and it helps to explain orthogonality. Orthogonal merely means that the comparisons are independent of one another. When they are, their sums of squares equal the sums of squares in the ANOVA. Had we made comparisons that were not independent, then each comparison would have included some common part of the original variance and the sums of squares would have been greater than that in the original analysis.

As stated above, some authors are more flexible than others on the issue of planned comparisons. The issue is not straightforward. In our within-subjects ANOVA we want to compare the pre- and post-scores and the pre- and follow-up scores. Only two comparisons are needed; so the risk of a type-one error is not very great. However, the rules tell us that these are not orthogonal comparisons. There is a clash between the clear intention of the experiment and orthogonality. Keppel (1991) took the sensible view that experimental interest is more important than following rules about orthogonality. Consider the original Yorkston and Beukleman experiment, however. It tested five groups of subjects and probably intended to show that the assessment could distinguish all of them. Were they, therefore, allowed to compare all the groups with one another claiming that they are planned comparisons? This sort of thing is too much, even for the free thinkers among statisticians, to tolerate. Keppel suggests that we interpret non-orthogonal comparisons carefully and that, when they greatly exceed the total allowed by the degrees of freedom (4 in the Yorkston and Beukleman experiment), we adjust the significance level required.

Unplanned comparisons

Suppose we don't plan our comparisons in advance. When we obtain the results, some means look different and some don't. What is to stop us saying that the former are the ones we planned to compare? Here we are only doing a few comparisons, so the risk of a type-one error is quite low. The problem, of course, is that doing only comparisons that look hopeful amounts to doing all the comparisons as far as type-one errors are concerned (we let them all have a go at being significant, then pick out the ones that look like they are going to make it). Unplanned comparisons allow for this by adjusting the significance level to protect against type-one errors. The adjustment will take into account all the comparisons that might have been done (not just those we fancy doing); so we normally use unplanned comparisons to evaluate the differences between all the pairs of means. Several tests are available to do unplanned comparisons. They include the Newman-Keuls test, the Tukey test – sometimes called the Tukey HSD (honestly significant difference!) test – and the Scheffé test. These tests differ in their formulae and in the adjustments they make to avoid type-one errors. Further details of the tests, their relative merits and their calculation can be found in the 'big books' (see, for example, Howell, 1997).

Exercise 6.3

Many people think that ANOVA is an obscure and complicated ritual. So here is an example of its use in everyday life. You drive a car to work each day varying the route you take. Each route seems quicker than the others on some days but on others there are hold-ups that delay you. Design an experiment to decide which route is quickest. How would you analyse the data?

Exercise 6.4

The examples in Exercise 6.1 would all require comparisons to be made between their different conditions. Would you expect these to be planned or unplanned?

Counterbalancing in the within-subjects ANOVA design

It is important to counterbalance the order in which subjects do the conditions of an experiment in within-subjects designs. In the example where DuBois and Bernthal (1978) compared articulation errors in three different situations the same words were used in each condition; so learning or practice may affect performance. Counterbalancing is more difficult with more than two conditions. Call the three conditions a, b and c. We might then assign subjects to orders as in Table 6.6.

Table 6.6 Simple counterbalancing with three conditions

	1st	2nd	3rd
Subject 1	a	b	c
Subject 2	b	c	a
Subject 3	c	a	b

Here each condition occurs in the first, second and third position once. Subject 4 restarts the cycle, in the same order as subject 1, and we need multiples of three subjects to maintain counterbalancing in the experiment. However, many books dislike this solution as the sequence is always the same (b only follows a and never c, and so forth). Table 6.7 gives a better solution for situations where there are three or four conditions in an experiment.

Table 6.7 Counterbalancing an IV with 3 and 4 levels.

	1st	2nd	3rd
Subject 1	a	b	c
Subject 2	b	c	a
Subject 3	c	a	b
Subject 4	c	b	a
Subject 5	a	c	b
Subject 6	b	a	c

	1st	2nd	3rd	4th
Subject 1	a	b	c	d
Subject 2	c	a	d	b
Subject 3	b	d	a	c
Subject 4	d	c	b	a

By using sets of six subjects we completely counterbalance the order of conditions with each occurring equally often in each position and after each other condition. We now need multiples of six subjects to maintain counterbalancing. Perversely the whole business is easier with 4 conditions. Here counterbalancing requires multiples of 4 subjects. In fact, counterbalancing an even number of conditions requires the same number of subjects, while counterbalancing an odd number requires twice that number of subjects.

In within-subjects designs it is tempting to add conditions by continuing testing the same people. In contrast, between-subjects designs restrain our enthusiasm by demanding more people every time we think it would be nice to have another condition! The above shows that when counterbalancing is important you may find you need more subjects than you bargained for in the within-subjects design as well.

Non-parametric analysis of variance

You may have guessed that ANOVA is only used with parametric data. Researchers often use it with data that look suspiciously non-parametric, saying, as usual, that it is a 'robust' test. The Kruskal-Wallis and Friedman tests are non-parametric versions of one-factor between- and within-subject ANOVAs. As someone who is a bit cavalier with assumptions myself, I confess that I almost never use them. You may not use them much either; but, just in case, this is how you work them out.

Suppose that three clinics have different approaches to helping children with language delay. Parents are asked to rate aspects of their child's language after treatment. The sum of these ratings (out of 30) for each child is shown in Table 6.8.

Table 6.8 Ratings of children after treatment

									n	R	R^2/n
Clinic 1	scores	23	21	15	22	19	13		6		
	ranks	15	13	7	14	1	5			65	704.16
Clinic 2	scores	14	12	9	11	20	8	17	7		
	ranks	6	4	2	3	12	1	9		37	195.57
Clinic 3	scores	27	25	24	18	16			5		
	ranks	18	17	16	10	8				69	952.20
										$\sum R^2/n = 1851.93$	

In the Kruskal-Wallis test we first rank all the scores in ascending order and sum the ranks to get R for each group. Square the values of

R and divide by n, the number of subjects in each group. Adding these gives us:

$$\sum \frac{R^2}{n} = 1851.93$$

Now find H where $H = \dfrac{12}{N(N+1)} \sum \dfrac{R^2}{n} - 3\,(N+1)$

and N = the total number of subjects.

$$H = \frac{12}{18 \times 19} \times 1851.93 - 3 \times 19 = 7.98$$

We look H up in the chi-square tables using k − 1 d.f.
where k = number of groups.

$$\text{d.f.} = k - 1 = 2,\ \text{p} < 0.025$$

So there is a significant difference in the ratings given by parents to children from different clinics. I hope you have noticed that this is a poor piece of research. Children were not randomly assigned to clinics; so confounding variables may be present. Clinics may differ in the children they treat, their catchment areas, their therapists and many other things.

Exercise 6.5

High-level language deficits may be present in multiple sclerosis and may be difficult to detect with language assessments designed for people with dysphasia. Laakso et al. (2000) designed a test to detect these and assessed its
ability to do so by testing people with MS who reported having language problems (MS+), people with MS who reported no problems (MS−) and similarly aged people without MS. They compared the scores from the three groups with a Kruskal-Wallis test. Is there a difference?

									n	R	
MS+	Scores	257	156	248	243				4		
	Ranks										
MS−	Scores	270	276	298	281	259			5		
	Ranks										
Controls	Scores	261	253	247	291	286	287	273	7		
	Rank										
									$\sum R^2/n =$		

Suppose that, in our experiment on therapy for dysfluency above, we videotaped the children at each of the assessment points and asked judges to rate their fluency (on a scale from 1 to 10). The data are given in Table 6.9.

Table 6.9 Ratings of children before and after therapy and at follow-up

	Before		After		6 months after	
	Rating	Rank	Rating	Rank	Rating	Rank
S1	4	1	8	3	7	2
S2	2	1	3	2	5	3
S3	5	2	9	3	4	1
S4	7	1	8	2	9	3
S5	2	1	9	2	10	3
S6	1	1	5	2	6	3
S7	3	1	10	3	8	2
S8	4	1	7	2	8	3
		$R_1 = 9$		$R_2 = 19$		$R_3 = 20$
		$R_1^2 = 81$		$R_2^2 = 361$		$R_3^2 = 400$

The Friedman test ranks the scores of each child across the conditions. We give the rank 1 to the lowest score; so the pre-therapy score of child 1 is ranked 1, their follow-up score ranked 2 and their post-therapy score ranked 3. This is probably the order we would expect as it reflects an improvement with therapy and then a decline, but not to the pre-therapy level, at follow-up.

Now add the ranks for each condition to find R_1, R_2 and R_3. If no differences exist between conditions, scores across them will be random and sums of ranks will be similar for each condition. If there are differences, the sums should differ. Square and sum the values of R to find $\sum R^2 = 842$. Now we find a value of chi square with the formula:

$$\chi^2 = \frac{12}{Nk(k+1)} \sum R^2 - 3N(k+1)$$

where N = the number of subjects and k = the number of conditions and chi square has $k - 1$ degrees of freedom.

$$\chi^2 = \frac{12}{8 \times 3 \times 4} \times 842 - 3 \times 8 \times 4 = 9.25 \quad \text{d.f.} = 2 \quad p < .01$$

In both of these examples I have cunningly avoided having any tied scores. In the Kruskal-Wallace test, the procedure is normally to give tied scores the mean of the ranks they would have received as in the Mann-Whitney test. Leach (1979) said this method is acceptable if less than a quarter of scores are tied but gives a modified formula for cases where more are tied. In the Friedman test, the mean rank is used to resolve tied scores. Again, Leach gave an alternative formula for cases where there are many ties.

With both tests there is the problem that a significant result does not identify which conditions are different from which others. The first rule is that we should only compare pairs of conditions if the overall test is significant. We do this for the Kruskal-Wallace test with the Mann-Whitney test and for the Friedman test with the Wilcoxon test. This takes us back to all the fuss about planned/unplanned comparisons after ANOVA. A safe procedure with both tests is to adjust the level of significance either by dividing it by the number of comparisons made (when these are planned) or by the total number that can be made (when not planned). The total number is $k(k - 1)/2$ where k is the number of conditions. So the significance level for unplanned comparisons should be $0.05/[k(k - 1)/2]$.

Chapter 7
Analysis of variance II

Two- (and three- and four-) factor designs

The real superiority of ANOVA over the other tests we have discussed is that it can analyse research designs that have more than one IV. This has two advantages:

- We can look at the effect of each IV in the same experiment. The ANOVA gives us an F-value for each IV allowing us to see if each has a significant effect.
- We can see whether two (or more) IVs interact with one another. Again the analysis gives us an F-value that tells us whether the interaction is significant.

The effects of individual variables are called 'main effects' and their combined effects are called 'interaction effects'. If we do a two-factor ANOVA, there are three results: the main effects of each IV and their interaction. With more IVs the number of results quickly escalates. With three there are three main effects and four interactions (between each pair of IVs and between all three).

It's important to understand interactions. Usually we design experiments specifically to look at them. Let's go back to the experiment on therapy for dysfluency in Chapter 5. You might have thought that measuring improvement by subtracting scores after therapy from those before was a bit naff. With ANOVA we can put both scores in the analysis. This is a two-factor ANOVA. The variables are type of subject (with two levels: treated and untreated) and time of assessment (with two levels: before and after therapy). Figure 7.1 shows a possible result of the experiment.

This design compares treated and untreated groups over time and is widely used to examine the effects of therapy. The ANOVA evaluates the main effects of time and type of subject. Both may be significant,

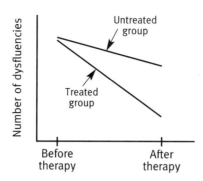

Figure 7.1 Graph of the results of our dysfluency experiment.

but neither of them is the result we want. Time compares all the subjects before and after therapy. Both groups show a decrease in dysfluency; so it is likely to be significant. The main effect of type of subject compares the overall performance of the two groups (before- and after-therapy scores). This may be significant, reflecting the overall better performance of the treated group. At first sight either result might suggest a positive treatment effect. In fact, neither does: we need to compare the change in performance of the treated group with the change in the untreated group. The interaction does this.

This is a two-factor ANOVA because there are two IVs. We have manipulated whether subjects are treated or not and the time of assessment. To describe it fully we must go further, however. Time is a within-subjects variable (subjects do both levels of it), while type of subject is a between-subjects variable. This is a two-factor mixed design (sometimes called a 'split-plot design'). We can also use a two-factor between-subjects design or a two-factor within-subjects design. It's important that you can recognize which design is which. The above does not exhaust the ANOVAs at our disposal. We can use three- and four- (and so on) factor designs of each of the above types, and mixed designs can vary in how they combine between- and within-subjects variables.

Working out the two-factor mixed design

We now look at the two-factor mixed design in a little more detail. It is the one you are likely to use if you want to compare the progress of groups of treated and untreated clients. In other words, it is the analysis used to assess randomized control trials. The data in Table 7.1 are from children with dysfluency randomly assigned to a treated or an untreated control group. They are similar to, but not the same

Exercise 7.1

Below are four further outcomes in our experiment on treating
dysfluency. Make sure you can identify which effects might be
significant and say what conclusion you would draw from each.
This is actually a silly exercise. You should not be guessing the
results of an ANOVA from a graph. Normally we do things the
other way round – obtain the ANOVA results then use a graph to
help us understand what they mean – but it might help you
understand how a two-factor ANOVA works.

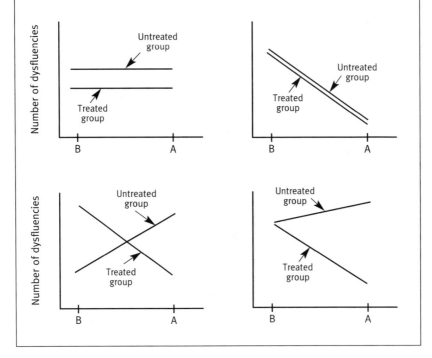

Exercise 7.2

What ANOVA would you use in the following? What are the
variables, how many levels have they and are they within- or
between-subjects variables?

1. A longitudinal study of child language is carried out. Mean
   lengths of utterance when talking to mothers and fathers are
   obtained at 1.5, 2.5 and 3.5 years of age (McLaughlin et al.,
   1983).

> **Exercise 7.2 (cont)**
>
> 2. A study looks at errors in picture naming. Three groups are tested – children, children with word-finding difficulties and adults. They are tested naming the pictures and naming them after a semantic cue is given to assist them (McGregor and Windsor, 1996).
> 3. A computer-reading scheme for people with aphasia is tested. Subjects are divided into three groups who either use the scheme or spend equal time doing non-verbal cognitive tasks on the computer or have no computer time. They are tested before and after 13 and 26 weeks of the trial (Katz and Wertz, 1997).
> 4. Intelligibility of a tracheo-oesophogeal speaker is studied. Single words, and five- and 10-word sentences were produced using either a tracheostoma valve or finger occlusion. Listeners either had experience of such speech or no experience (Fujimoto et al., 1991).
> 5 (i) A study examines the learning of names of Blissymbols by children and adults with normal cognitive abilities. Four groups of symbols are used which are high or low in complexity and high and low in translucency. (ii) The same study is carried out but tests of symbol recognition are conducted four times during the experiment (Fuller, 1997).

Table 7.1 Data from our experiment on therapy for dysfluency

	Untreated group			Treated group	
	Before	After		Before	After
S1	14	12	S11	16	17
S2	15	17	S12	23	12
S3	18	15	S13	9	6
S4	14	11	S14	10	4
S5	22	13	S15	18	12
S6	16	19	S16	21	12
S7	21	15	S17	12	5
S8	9	6	S18	14	2
S9	12	9	S19	20	11
S10	14	12	S20	15	7
Mean =	15.5	12.9	Mean =	15.8	8.8

as, the data we used for the independent t-test in Chapter 5 (to make it more realistic I have let a few clients deteriorate). Here we include both the before and after scores in the analysis instead of subtracting them as we did with the t-test. So we have a two-factor mixed design in which:

- group is a between-subjects variable (with two levels – treated versus untreated)
- time is a within-subjects variable (with two levels – before and after therapy).

As you can see from the graph of these data at the beginning of the chapter and from the means in the table, the dysfluency levels in the two groups were nearly equal before therapy. Both groups improved with time, but the treated group improved more. The control group did not receive therapy; so its change must be due to other factors such as increased familiarity with the assessment and the people conducting it. There is nothing in the rules to say that control groups can't change! The essential thing is that they show the change (or lack of it) that occurs without therapy. The ANOVA table for this data is shown in Table 7.2. As promised it has three F-values, one for each main effect and one for their interaction. The main effect of group (the overall difference between the groups taking both the pre- and post-therapy assessments into account) is not significant, but there is a significant effect of time of assessment. The latter reflects the fact that both groups improved. The most important result, however, is the interaction that shows that the improvement in the treated group is significantly greater than in the untreated group. There are two error terms in this ANOVA table. The between-subjects variable (group) is evaluated with the 'subjects' error term. The within-subjects variable (time) and the interaction are evaluated with the 'subjects × time (error)' term.

Table 7.2 ANOVA table for our dysfluency data

Source of variance	Sum of squares	d.f.	Mean square	F	p
Groups	36.10	1	36.10	1.18	0.2911
Time	230.40	1	230.40	34.79	0.0000
Groups × time	48.40	1	48.40	7.31	0.0145
Subjects (error)	549.40	18	30.52		
Subjects × time (error)	119.20	18	6.62		
Total	983.5	39			

Having looked at several graphs, you will have noticed that an interaction occurs when the lines are not parallel. To put it even more simply it occurs when they cross over (or would have done had they been slightly longer). Of course, as Exercise 7.1 showed, this is a very crude way of deciding if an interaction has occurred. Normally we do the analysis and then draw a graph to sort out what has happened. A more sophisticated definition is that the effects of one IV on the DV are different at different levels of the other IV. In our example the effect of time is different on one group (because it is treated) than it is on the other group.

When we find a significant interaction, we want to know why it is significant. In our example the source of the significant result is quite obvious, but it might not be in more complicated interactions. To do this we carry out further analyses on its component parts. The best way is to analyse the simple main effects. This tells us whether the effects of each IV are significant at the different levels of the other IV (as in our definition of an interaction above). Thus, while the main analysis tells us whether there is a significant difference between the groups over the whole experiment (there wasn't), simple main effects tell us whether there is a difference at the pre- and post-therapy assessments (at different levels of time). Likewise they tell us whether the effect of time is significant for each of the groups individually. Table 7.3 gives the simple main effects for our data.

Table 7.3 Simple main effects on our dysfluency data

		Sum of squares	d.f.	MS	F	p
Groups at	before	0.45	1	0.45	0.02	0.8772
	after	84.05	1	84.05	4.53	0.0403
	error	668.6	36	18.57		
Time at	untreated	33.8	1	33.8	5.10	0.0365
	treated	245.0	1	245.0	36.99	0.0000
	error	119.2	18	6.62		

The simple main effects show that:

1. The groups did not differ before therapy. We would have been worried if they had, as we randomly assigned the clients with the aim of making the groups the same.
2. The groups do differ significantly ($p < 0.05$) after therapy. This result is due to the greater improvement of the treated group.

3. The improvement in the untreated group is significant ($p < 0.05$).
4. The improvement in the treated group is highly significant ($p < 0.0001$).

Result 3 demonstrates the importance of the significant interaction. Suppose we had chickened out of doing an ANOVA and had just compared the before- and after-therapy scores of the treated group with a related t-test and then that we had done the same with the untreated group. We would be hoping to find a significant result for the first but not the second. We would not have found it here. Even if we had, it would have been potentially misleading. By doing two separate tests we have not compared the groups. If the difference in improvement is small, we may find a situation where the treated group is just significant and the untreated group just misses out.

In the experiment above we would want to follow up the clients some time later to see if the benefits of therapy are maintained. This may not be straightforward in practice. In all experiments that extend over time there is a danger of losing subjects. As a result, data from later assessments may be incomplete and are not easily compared with those obtained earlier in the experiment. This is a real pain statistically. The solution may be to analyse only those subjects with complete data. This is irritating and may be misleading. When subjects are lost from an experiment, we have to worry whether those who disappear are a random subset of the original sample or whether particular types of subjects are more likely to depart than others, changing the sample and affecting the interpretation of the results. Follow-up assessments, although desirable, increase the possibility that subjects will drop out. In our experiment it's possible that treated subjects who feel they have not improved will decide it's a waste of their time; alternatively those who have improved may feel they don't want to go back (in case they catch it again!). It's also possible that some subjects (particularly those we didn't treat) have had treatment elsewhere in the gap between post- and follow-up assessments.

Leaving all this aside, suppose we do have a follow-up assessment and the results look like Figure 7.2. The ANOVA tells us that there is a significant interaction of groups and time, but what is significant? The groups are the same before therapy and different after it, but at follow-up the treated group has deteriorated and it's unclear whether it is now better than the untreated group, which has shown gradual improvement over time. Here simple main effects are crucial. They tell us if there is a difference between the groups at each assessment. There is obviously no difference before therapy, and the difference after it is likely to be significant, but what of the follow-up assessment?

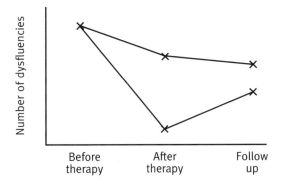

Figure 7.2 Graph of pre-, post- and follow-up assessments of children in our dysfluency experiment.

It's no exaggeration to say that the outcome of the whole experiment depends on this. If the difference is not significant then the effects of therapy are not maintained over time and we need to be much more cautious in claiming that it was effective.

How to obtain (and not obtain) a significant interaction

The example above is important because the design is widely used to examine therapy effects. The crucial result is the interaction of groups by time; so it is important to understand what may make this significant. Of course, the obvious way to not get a significant interaction is for the treated clients not to improve (or not to improve more than the controls). This result is unambiguous, and we have to conclude that therapy has not worked. However, there is a more irritating way of obtaining a non-significant result. As we have seen with other statistical tests, we only obtain significant results when subjects behave fairly consistently. In Table 7.4 I have adjusted the scores from our experiment, keeping the means the same but making the treated clients less consistent. The resulting ANOVA table is also shown.

The interaction is no longer significant. One message to take from this demonstration is that we can't judge whether an interaction is significant from a graph alone. The means and graph of these data have not changed, but the interaction is not significant because individual clients are less consistent. We can see in the ANOVA table why this has happened. The sums of squares and mean squares (variances) of the main effects and interaction remain as before because the scores are

Table 7.4 Data and ANOVA table on the rearranged data from the dysfluency experiment

Untreated group				Treated group	
	Before	After		Before	After
S1	14	12	S11	16	7
S2	15	17	S12	23	2
S3	18	15	S13	9	17
S4	14	11	S14	10	12
S5	22	13	S15	18	6
S6	16	19	S16	21	4
S7	21	15	S17	12	12
S8	9	6	S18	14	12
S9	12	9	S19	20	5
S10	14	12	S20	15	11
Mean =	15.5	12.9	Mean =	15.8	8.8

Source of variance	Sum of squares	d.f.	Mean square	F	p
Groups	36.10	1	36.10	2.87	0.1075
Time	230.40	1	230.40	9.38	0.0067
Groups × time	48.40	1	48.40	1.97	0.1774
Subjects (error)	226.40	18	12.58		
Subjects × time (error)	442.20	18	24.57		
Total	983.5	39			

the same. However, the error variances have changed. The total remains the same but a greater part is now due to the 'subjects × time (error)' term, which is used to evaluate the interaction. This error term measures the interaction of individual subjects with time; in other words, it measures the consistency of change.

This result may strengthen doubts you have about the usefulness of statistics. Here the group means suggest that therapy was effective and some treated clients have made substantial gains. If we were treating them clinically (not in an experiment), we would be impressed by their progress. So what has gone wrong? Statistical tests assess the probability that a difference occurs by chance. If clients respond inconsistently, the probability of a chance difference increases. A difference between the groups may occur because the treated group has a few clients who happen to improve and the control group does not. Of course, the clients who make progress may be benefiting from therapy, but, because there are others who do not respond, we will not obtain a significant result. Experiments are not about showing that therapy helps a few clients – they are about showing generally greater improvement in the treated group and being able to generalize this result to other similar clients. Here we can't do this and must conclude that therapy is not effective.

We will return to this problem when we consider the efficacy of therapy at the end of the book. There are two reasons for considering it here, however. First, because it may help you to understand the mysterious workings of analysis of variance. Second, because the outcome is one that is quite likely in the studies of this kind. Although we have to conclude that therapy was ineffective, our dissatisfaction with this result should lead us to examine it in more detail. Suppose the clients who made progress are responding to therapy (and not improving for reasons of their own that we don't know about!). So why did therapy help some clients but not others? One reason may be that the criteria for entry to the experiment are insufficiently strict and that, as a result, the clients differ in their speech-and-language problems. Other possibilities are that the therapy has not been applied uniformly or even that different therapies have been used. In several cases therapy studies have chosen to examine very broadly defined groups of clients and allowed clinicians to select their own therapies. Such studies are an open invitation to clients to respond inconsistently. We will meet them again later.

Other two-factor designs

I have concentrated on the two-factor mixed design because it is so commonly used. However, we should have a quick look at the other two-factor designs. De Nil and Brutten (1991) compared the attitudes to communication of children who stammered and children who were fluent. The children were aged 7, 8, 9, 10 and 11. They hypothesized that children who were dysfluent would have more negative attitudes and would become more negative with age (as one does).

This is a two-factor between-subjects design. The variables are the type of child (with two levels: fluent versus dysfluent) and age (with five levels). As usual I have simplified their experiment (as well as making up the data). The ANOVA table below is for 20 in each group and for the ages 7, 9 and 11 only. The means (high scores represent more negative attitudes) of the groups of children and the ANOVA table are shown in Table 7.5.

Here there are no within-subjects variables; so all the effects are evaluated with the between-subjects (error) term. There is a highly significant difference in attitudes between children who are fluent and dysfluent ($F[1, 54] = 99.63$; $p < 0.0001$) and a significant interaction

Table 7.5 Data and ANOVA table for a two-factor between-subjects design

	7 years	9 years	11 years
Dysfluent children	14.4	17.4	17.5
Fluent children	9.9	8.4	6.0

Source of variance	Sum of squares	d.f.	Mean square	F	p
Type of child	1041.67	1	1041.67	99.63	0.0000
Age	13.63	2	6.82	0.65	0.5251
Type × age	125.83	2	62.92	6.02	0.0044
Subjects (error)	564.60	54	10.45		
Total	1745.73	59			

of type of child and age ($F[2, 54] = 6.02$; $p < 0.01$). Although there is no effect of age overall, the interaction shows that children who are dysfluent become more negative, whereas those who are fluent become more positive. It's likely that we would want to do simple main effects here. We particularly want to know if children who are dysfluent get significantly more negative with age. It will also tell us about change in the fluent group with age and whether the differ- ences between children who are fluent and dysfluent are significant at each age.

Banat et al. (2002) examined whether care staff could estimate the comprehension of adults with learning difficulties accurately. Sentences at three levels of difficulty (with two or three informa- tion-carrying words and higher-language sentences) were taken from the Derbyshire language scheme (Knowles and Masidlover, 1982) and the clients' actual scores were compared with scores predicted by care staff. A two-factor within-subjects ANOVA was used. Nineteen clients participated and were the subjects in the ANOVA. The variables were type of score (actual versus predicted) and type of sentence (with three levels). It was expected that carers' overestimation would increase with the complexity of the sentence.

A significant interaction between type of sentence and type of score ($F[2, 36] = 15.26$; $p < 0.0001$) was found. An analysis of simple main effects showed no difference in scores for two- and three-word sentences. However, predicted scores were significantly ($F(1, 18) = 19.43$; $p < 0.001$) greater than actual scores for higher-language sentences.

Table 7.6 Data and ANOVA table for a two-factor within-subjects design.

		Two-word sentences	Three-word sentences	Higher-language sentences
Clients' % score	Mean	79.47	55.26	32.27
	Std. dev.	16.99	18.29	13.62
Carers' % estimate	Mean	91.58	58.95	68.14
	Std. dev.	7.65	28.65	18.55

Source of variance	Sum of squares	d.f.	Mean square	F	p
Type of score	8538.42	1	8538.42	13.37	0.0018
Type of sentence	26491.39	2	13245.69	47.40	0.0000
Score × sentence	5388.41	2	2694.21	15.26	0.0000
Subjects (error)	8681.53	18	482.31		
Subjects × score (error)	11490.98	18	638.39		
Subjects × sentence (error)	10059.21	36	279.42		
Subjects × score × sentence (error)	6355.88	36	19.30		
Total	77005.82	113			

*Analysis of variance and its big brothers

Analysis of variance is so widely used that you can't get very far reading research, let alone doing it, without knowing something about it. You need to know about it so you can understand results from research, but there is more to it than that. Like other statistical tests, but even more so, knowing about ANOVA helps you design good research. If you know what it does (and especially if you understand interactions), it will help you to decide what data to collect and what design to use.

Analysis of variance is quite hard going. So, when you start to understand it, you are entitled to feel fairly pleased with yourself. Sadly ANOVA is just the baby of the family and its big brothers are less fun to know. Fortunately we only need to meet them briefly. They are analysis of covariance (ANCOVA), multivariate analysis of variance (MANOVA) and multivariate analysis of covariance (MANCOVA)!

We can use ANCOVA in two ways. The first is to control possible confounding variables. I have gone on at length about the problems of quasi-experiments. Because the subjects are not randomly assigned, differences between groups on the DV may be due to confounding variables. Suppose we spot a particular confounding variable that may affect the results. We can check whether this is likely by seeing if the confounding variable and the DV are correlated (see Chapter 10). If they are, we have a problem. Fortunately statisticians have come up with a solution. Analysis of covariance lets us control for the effect of the confounding variable (now called the covariate) statistically. It adjusts the values of the DV to remove its influence. You probably think that this sounds a bit dodgy, and I can't say I blame you. Perhaps an example will help. Campbell et al. (2000) examined the relationship between bone lead levels and language processing in adolescent boys. They divided their sample into four groups with different levels of lead and compared them on language-processing tasks. Significant differences were found between the groups on some tasks. To counter the possibility that both exposure to lead and poor language resulted from social factors, socio-economic status and mother's IQ were used as covariates. The differences between the groups remained. So language-processing levels are not just due to differences in social background. This is still a quasi-experiment, and it's possible that other confounding variables are at work. Nevertheless, ANCOVA has removed an obvious confounding variable and strengthened the evidence that exposure to lead affects language.

Analysis of covariance can also be used to control for differences between subjects and to improve our chances of getting a significant result. It is sometimes used in this way in therapy studies (for examples of its use see Gibbard, 1994; Spector et al., 2003). Clients may vary in the severity of their language disorders, and this may affect how much they benefit from therapy. Milder clients may make greater gains (because they are more able) or more severe clients may do so (because they have more scope for improvement). As we have seen, inconsistent improvement leads to non-significant results. Often the causes of this inconsistency are unknown. Where they are known, however, we can control them by using ANCOVA. In this case we use the initial assessment as a covariate and remove its influence on the outcome. Clients have been randomly assigned, and so we are not using ANCOVA to remove the effect of a confounding variable. Here it reduces a source of variability. As a result, error variance is reduced and a significant result is more likely.

Researchers often use several different DVs to measure the outcome of experiments. Suppose we do an experiment to assess therapy for a group of clients. Having gone to all this trouble, it is reasonable to collect as much data as possible, and conducting several different assessments of their progress only requires a little extra effort. Now why are we doing this and how are we going to analyse the resulting data? We may have chosen our assessments because they measure different aspects of language and will give us a clearer picture of the effects of therapy. On the other hand, we may just be hoping that different measures will increase our chance of getting a significant result. The latter is not recommended. It's quite likely that, if we use a lot of DVs, we will eventually throw up a significant result and it will be a type-one error. The right procedure is to use MANOVA, which lets us enter several DVs in the same analysis and tells us whether there is a significant effect when all of them are considered together (and also whether individual DVs are significant). Gillon (2000) examined the use of phonological-awareness training on phonological awareness, reading and speech production of children with articulation problems. Several measures of phonological awareness and reading development were used, and the data was analysed with MANOVA. Children who received phonological-awareness training made more progress than those who received traditional therapy.

These methods let us do more-complicated experiments, improve our chances of getting significant results and let us investigate data in more detail (MANCOVA combines both in the same analysis). They are complex methods, however. Before using them, you should consult some big books (see, for example, Field, 2000; Tabachnik and Fiddell, 2001). You will quickly find that even statisticians disagree about how and when they should be used. Here we need only mention two practical aspects of their use. The first is that they are hard work. Multivariate analysis of variance requires a larger numbers of subjects than are usually available in small-scale projects, and both MANOVA and ANCOVA require extra testing to assess the DVs and covariates that are used. The second is more important. It is that ANCOVA and MANOVA should only be used after careful thought about the design and purpose of your experiment. With a computer to help you numerous covariates or DVs can easily be added to an analysis. The temptation to do this should be resisted, however. As with more-complex ANOVA designs, variables should only be entered in the analysis when their presence is theoretically justified.

*Chapter 8
Into the storm

Introduction

As leisure pursuits go, Shakespearean tragedies and visiting derelict castles don't score too well these days. So it's a mystery why, when the two occur together, people flock to sit in the cold and see actors stumble about on ramparts. Recently I saw *King Lear* in a castle. As you will know, *King Lear* is a difficult play unrelieved by crossdressing or any of William's little witticisms. Just when you are losing all feeling in your extremities, there is a long period where the actors blunder about in a storm talking nonsense. Fortunately, in the production I saw, a large chunk of this was cut and the audience given hot soup to revive them.

The similarity between all this and books on research methods may already have struck you. The bad news is that it's time to go out into the storm. The good news is that, if this is your first reading, you can skip this chapter. Go and have some hot soup instead. When you read it, you will find that it tries to answer some fundamental questions about statistics. So let's start with a real biggie.

Where did the t-test come from?

When we did the independent t-test in Chapter 5, I tried to convince you that its formula made sense. It contains the things that ought to influence our decision about whether a difference exists in our data (the difference in the means, the standard deviations and number of subjects). Now we take a more sophisticated look at its formula.

We start with the central limit theorem. Suppose a population has a mean μ and variance σ^2 and we draw samples, size n, from it. The frequency distribution of the means of these samples is the sampling distribution of the mean. The central limit theorem tells us that its mean will be μ (the population mean) and its variance will be σ^2/n. This should be familiar. We already know that its standard deviation is σ/√n, the standard error of the mean. The sampling distribution of the mean is normally distributed when the population is normally distributed. When the population is not normally distributed, it tries its best. It becomes closer to a normal distribution as the sample size increases.

Suppose we have lots of samples of 4-year-old normally developing children on the BPVS and plot their means to obtain the sampling distribution of the mean (see Figure 8.1). We now test a sample of 4-year-olds with SLI and compare them with 4-year-olds with normal language. We can do this by comparing the SLI mean with the sampling distribution of the mean (with the means of samples of normally developing 4-year-olds). The sampling distribution of the mean is normally distributed. So we can locate a particular sample on it by obtaining its z-score (just like locating an individual on the normal distribution of other people). We do this by dividing the difference between our sample mean and the mean of the sampling distribution of the mean (which is, of course, the population mean) by the standard error of the mean (the standard deviation of the sampling distribution of the mean). So:

$$z = \frac{\bar{x} - \mu}{\sigma / \sqrt{n}}$$

Where $\bar{x}$ is the sample mean and μ and σ are the population mean and standard deviation and $\sigma / \sqrt{n}$ is the standard error of the mean.

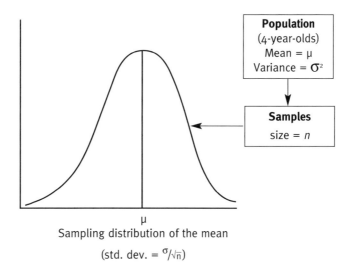

Figure 8.1 The sampling distribution of the mean.

If you have not been distracted by thinking about all those means, you may have noticed that this is the one-sample z-test. Here we are using it to see where our sample mean is on the sampling distribution of the mean. We are doing an experiment whose null hypothesis is that any difference between the two means can be accounted for by chance. Either our sample is from this distribution or it is sufficiently close to its extremes (in the last 5% for a one-tail test or the last 2.5% for a two-tail test) for us to reject the null hypothesis (see Figure 8.2). In fact, we are doing something even smarter than this. The sampling distribution of the mean is made up of samples from the population of 4-year-olds with normal language. If our sample of children with SLI is different, it must come from a different population. Hence we can infer that the two populations differ on the BPVS.

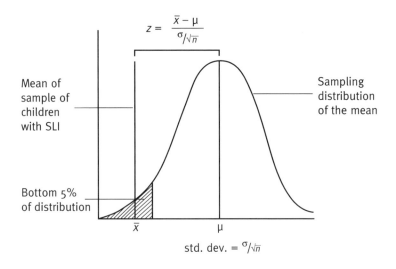

Figure 8.2 Comparing a sample with the sampling distribution of the mean.

Now all this sounds very clever until you notice that we don't know about the sampling distribution of the mean. Without the population mean and its standard error, this is all pie in the sky. When we used the one-sample z-test in Chapter 4, we took advantage of standardized tests that (because they use very large samples) give a good indication of the population mean and standard deviation. Normally we have to compare our sample of children with SLI with another sample of children with normal language and use a t-test to decide whether they come from the same population or not. To do this we need to know by how much samples that really do come from the *same* population differ. Suppose we draw pairs of samples from a population and obtain the frequency distribution of the differences in their means. This is the sampling distribution of the differences between means of samples from the *same* population. It is normally distributed with mean 0 (sample means should be the same), and its standard deviation is the standard error of the difference between means (see Figure 8.3). We can now see where the difference in our two sample means is on this distribution and decide how likely it is that our difference is just one of the ones that might have occurred anyway. First, let's have the equation in words. It is:

$$z = \frac{\text{Difference in sample means - mean of the sampling dist. of differences between means}}{\text{Standard error of the difference between means}}$$

The mean of the sampling distribution is 0; so this formula is actually quite simple. It is:

$$z = \frac{(\bar{x}_1 - \bar{x}_2) - 0}{S.E.}$$

where $\bar{x}_1$ and $\bar{x}_2$ are the sample means and our only problem is knowing the standard error of the differences between means.

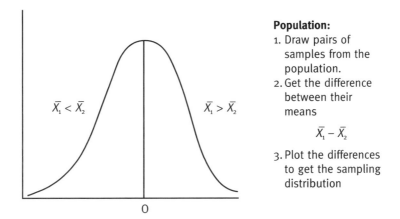

Figure 8.3 The sampling distribution of the difference between two means.

The formula for the standard error of the sampling distribution of the difference between the means takes account of the possibility that the samples differ in size. It is:

$$\text{S.E.} = \sigma \sqrt{\left(\frac{1}{n_1} + \frac{1}{n_2}\right)} = \sqrt{\left(\frac{1}{n_1} + \frac{1}{n_2}\right)\sigma^2}$$

We don't know σ^2 (the population variance), but when did that stop a statistician? They estimate it from the pooled variance of the samples.

$$s_p^2 = \frac{(n_1 - 1)\,s_1^2 + (n_2 - 1)\,s_2^2}{n_1 + n_2 - 2}$$

So the standard error of the difference between two means is:

$$\text{S.E.} = \sqrt{\left(\frac{1}{n_1} + \frac{1}{n_2}\right)s_p^2}$$

We can put this value in the original formula. However, because we estimated σ^2, we must use a t-test not a z-test. So we end up with the formula of the independent t-test:

$$t = \frac{(\bar{x}_1 - \bar{x}_2)}{\sqrt{\left(\frac{1}{n_1} + \frac{1}{n_2}\right)s_p^2}}$$

One- and two-tail tests again

Now that we know about sampling distributions we can make better sense of one- and two-tail tests. When we use the t-test, we compare the difference in the means of our samples with the distribution of random differences in samples from the same population. We call our difference 'significant' if it falls into the 5% of the most extreme outcomes that might occur by chance. If we predict that children with SLI have a lower mean than children with normal language, we put all 5% of extreme outcomes in one 'tail' of the sampling distribution. So, in Figure 8.4a, the area for rejecting the null hypothesis is the 5% at the lower end of the distribution. If we don't make a directional

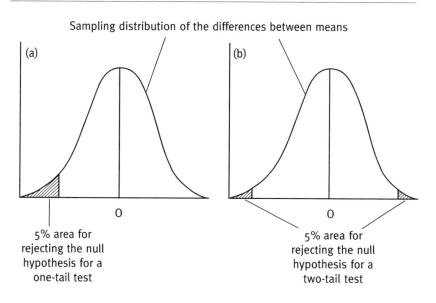

Figure 8.4 One- and two-tail tests revisited.

prediction we must divide the 5% between the two 'tails' making it more difficult to get a significant result (see Figure 8.4b).

Type-one and type-two errors (and the Bonferroni t-test)

All statistical tests carry the risk of a type-one error. The size of the risk is equal to the significance level and can be reduced by using a higher level. We saw in our discussion of planned and unplanned comparisons that statisticians become very agitated about type-one errors. For once they are not just being old fusspots: type-one errors are a serious problem. When researchers fiddle around with their data doing lots of tests, they are likely to make type-one errors. Then they make things much worse by reporting the type-one error as a significant result casually neglecting to tell us about all the tests that produced non-significant results. However, there are occasions when we legitimately need to do lots of tests. So we need a method to ensure that the chance of a type-one error across the whole experiment (called the experimentwise or familywise error rate) is less than 5%.

A common-sense solution is to increase the level of significance so that the chance of a type-one error in the experiment remains 5%. This is what the Bonferroni procedure does. A fuller discussion of it may be found in Rosenthal and Rosnow (1991). A good, if rather extreme, example of it may be found in Kalinowski et al. (1996). They compared people's perceptions of two adult speakers, one fluent, the other dysfluent, using the semantic differential test (Woods and Williams, 1976). This has 25 bipolar adjectives (for example shy/bold) that are rated on a 7-point scale. So Kalinowski et al. needed to do 25 t-tests. To protect against type-one errors they divided the conventional 0.05 level by 25 and used 0.002 as the level of significance. With so high a level of significance a lot of subjects are needed to get significant results. Fortunately they had a lot of subjects and found several significant results.

Exercise 8.1

A therapist reviews the records of children with language delay at his clinic dividing them into those who made good or poor progress. Other information is available about the children, such as the amount of therapy they received, severity of delay, parental attitude and cooperation and age when treated. He compares the groups on each variable to see if they differ significantly on any of them. He hopes to find a variable on which they differ and plans to use it to predict which children will make good progress. What problems arise interpreting the results?

It is not always obvious how many tests were used in an experiment. One reason was given above – researchers do lots of tests but only tell us the results they like. Another reason is that tests may be implicitly carried out. When there are a lot of data, researchers may not know which bits are interesting. When they see the data, the bits that look significant quickly become the bits that are interesting. This is the same problem we had with unplanned comparisons after ANOVA. By selecting the bits we want to analyse we are implicitly carrying out many other tests. Adjustment to the significance level must take account of the number of tests implicitly carried out, not those actually carried out.

The way we approach multiple tests may depend on our hypothesis. Suppose we have a group of children who are late talkers at 2. We follow them up and compare them with their more talkative peers when they are 3. If our hypothesis is that they will be behind in all areas of language, then all the tests we do should be significant. Although type-one errors may occur here, their consequences are less worrying. The overall pattern is convincing. A more likely hypothesis is that we expect them to be behind in some but not other areas of language development. Here we predict which tests will be significant (as in planned comparisons), and we even receive some credit for correctly predicting those that are not. Either of these approaches is acceptable. The more risky alternative is to wait and see what is significant, then find an explanation for it. This is where we may be misled by type-one errors and should avoid this by correcting the significance level for the number of tests conducted. Rescorla et al. (1997), who did an experiment similar to this, found that late talkers were less behind in lexical development than they were in syntax and morphology.

Exercise 8.2

A survey in *Scientific American* recently found that 45% of Americans believe that God created life on Earth sometime within the last 10,000 years. 'Creationists' have been propagating similar beliefs and opposing the teaching of evolution in schools. To support their case they argue that the world has been 'intelligently designed' by a creator to suit our needs. For example, the banana is designed to be easily held and unwrapped, tastes good and even has a sell by date (it goes black). Leaving aside any scientific objections you have to the view that we once cohabited with dinosaurs, can you detect any statistical problems in the example about bananas?

Type-two errors and power

The trouble we take avoiding type-one errors makes it odd that we pay so little attention to type-two errors. These occur when we fail to find a significant result that does exist. Some researchers think that type-two errors cause no great harm. They are unlikely to be published (journals don't like non-significant results); so no one is misled. There is some truth in this; but it's a haphazard way for supposedly smart people to carry on. Moreover, the personal cost of type-two errors is high. We can live with the disappointment of not getting a significant result if that's the way the world is. But, if a significant result is out there, it's a bit dumb to do an experiment with little chance of finding it.

The commonest question asked by people doing research is 'How many subjects do I need?' They know that having too few subjects is the best way to make a type-two error (even if they are not sure what a type-two error is) and know that having more subjects increases their chance of a significant result (by increasing the 'power' of the experiment). Unfortunately the answer to the question may be that

'We don't know' or 'More than you were planning to have' or both. A sensible response to this problem is to look at existing research in the area and to see how many subjects were used in studies that found significant results. Perhaps a similar number will do the trick for us. The statistical version of this is to calculate the effect size from previous research and to calculate how many subjects are needed.

Figure 8.5 shows the relationship between type-one and type-two errors and power. Consider our experiment on therapy for children who are dysfluent again. The left-hand distribution is the sampling distribution of differences between the means of untreated clients (so its mean is 0). We do the experiment and find a difference between treated and untreated clients. We then use the t-test to locate this difference on this sampling distribution. If our difference is in the top 5% (for a one-tail test), we reject the null hypothesis. The rejection area is α, the probability of a type-one error. Now suppose that treatment does work. We will still get varying outcomes in our experiment. The right-hand distribution is the sampling distribution of differences in the means of treated and untreated clients when the null hypothesis is false. The point where we reject the null hypothesis cuts this distribution in two. The left-hand part, β, contains outcomes where we fail to reject the null hypothesis. So β is the probability of a type-two error. The right-hand part contains outcomes where the null hypothesis is rejected. The probability of this is $1 - \beta$, the power of the experiment.

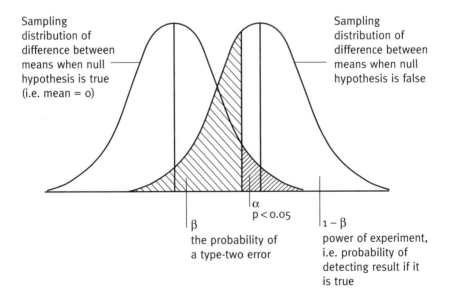

Sampling distribution of difference between means when null hypothesis is true (i.e. mean = 0)

Sampling distribution of difference between means when null hypothesis is false

α
$p < 0.05$

β
the probability of a type-two error

$1 - \beta$
power of experiment, i.e. probability of detecting result if it is true

Figure 8.5 The power of an experiment and type-two errors.

To avoid type-two errors we must increase power. Figure 8.5 shows our options. We could move the right-hand distribution further to the right. Sadly, even statisticians can't pull this one off. The mean of the left-hand distribution is 0, so the distance between the distributions is the mean of the right-hand distribution. This is the mean difference between treated and untreated children when the null hypothesis is false. In other words, it's the effect we are trying to detect – not something we can change. If the distance is large it is easy to find a significant result; if it is small it isn't.

A second option is to increase α (to use a lower level of significance). This is non-starter. The 5% level is widely accepted as a compromise between type-one and type-two errors. Using a lower level (say 10%) will increase power and reduce type-two errors but only at the cost of increasing type-one errors.

A last option remains. We could squeeze the distributions so they overlap less. This means reducing the standard error of the sampling distributions.

$$\sqrt{\left(\frac{1}{n_1} + \frac{1}{n_2}\right) s_p^2}$$

We can do so either by reducing s_p^2, the pooled variance (in other words, by reducing the sample standard deviations) or by increasing n_1 and n_2, the sample sizes.

This is not a very surprising outcome to our little excursion into the world of sampling distributions. We should have done all we could to reduce the sample standard deviations already (by controlling variables and standardizing the procedure). So we seem to have arrived at a conclusion that beginners in research had discovered for themselves – that the way to get significant results is to increase the number of subjects.

Effect size and sample size

Although we seem to have gone by a complicated route to a place we already knew, we have, at least, set the stage for discussing effect sizes and how to calculate the number of subjects required to obtain significant results. Effect size is a simple measure (although statisticians have found many ways of measuring it). We will follow the procedure described by Howell (1997). You can refer to this for further details. In our experiment the effect size is the difference in the mean improvements of the treated and untreated groups divided by the population standard deviation. The numerical difference between the groups will vary with the units we measure it in, so dividing by the population standard deviation reduces it to a common unit. As usual we don't know the population values, and so we estimate them from the values in our experiment (or someone else's experiment if we are trying to find out how many subjects we need). So the effect size, d, is given by:

$$d = \frac{\bar{x}_1 - \bar{x}_2}{s_p}$$

$$\text{where } s_p = \sqrt{\frac{(n_1 - 1) s_1^2 + (n_2 - 1) s_2^2}{n_1 + n_2 - 2}}$$

In Chapter 5 the means for our samples of treated and untreated children were 7.9 and 4.5 and the pooled standard deviation was $s_p = 3.69$; so the effect size was:

$$d = \frac{7.9 - 4.5}{3.69} = 0.92$$

From d we can obtain a measure of power. For the independent t-test, the formula is:

$$\delta = d \sqrt{\frac{n}{2}}$$

Substituting our values in the formula we get:

$$\delta = 0.92 \sqrt{\frac{10}{2}} = 2.05$$

The tables (Appendix 7) tell us that for the $p < 0.05$ level of significance and a one-tail test power equals 0.66.

So our experiment had a 66% chance of rejecting the null hypothesis. This may not surprise you as we have already rejected it! Normally we make these calculations in advance of the experiment, however. We predict the effect size and obtain a measure of power for the number of subjects we intend to use. The calculation then tells us the probability of making a type-two error.

Sixty-six per cent doesn't sound too good. Suppose we want to be certain of avoiding a type-two error and calculate how many subjects we need for 100% power. We find the value of δ from the tables (99% is the best we can do). This is 4.10; so:

$$4.10 = 0.92 \sqrt{\frac{n}{2}} \quad = \quad \frac{n}{2} \quad n\left(\frac{4.10}{0.92}\right)^2 \quad = 40 \text{ (rounded up)}$$

So we need 40 subjects in each group!

An effect size of 0.92 is quite large. Suppose it was only 0.5 and we wanted to be certain of avoiding a type-two error (power = 99% as above). We now have:

$$4.10 = 0.5 \sqrt{\frac{n}{2}} \quad = \quad \frac{n}{2} \quad n\left(\frac{4.10}{0.5}\right)^2 \quad = 134$$

These examples show that the cost, in numbers of subjects, of avoiding type-two errors is large even for large effect sizes. With more moderate ones it becomes silly. Such sample sizes may give you second thoughts about doing an experiment and, in some areas of clinical research, it might be difficult to find the required numbers. Of course, 99% is rather excessive. There is a general agreement that 80% power will do. Even at this more modest level, the number of subjects required to detect small effect sizes is rather scary.

Exercise 8.3

Calculate the number of subjects needed to obtain power of 80% with the effect size of 0.92 in our experiment above.

Power calculations often show that experiments have a relatively small chance of finding significant results. Student research projects are a good example here. However well designed they are, time limitations make it hard to test very many subjects. Often the outcome is that subjects appear to be doing their best to reject the null hypothesis, but the statistical test won't let them (at which point many would-be researchers finally lose patience with statistics). Probably more subjects would have done the trick. The calculations above provide a way of finding out how many more were needed.

Power has been relatively neglected in research until recently. Jones et al. (2002) reviewed research in dysfluency showing that many published studies had low levels of power and that type-two errors were likely. One reason for the increased attention paid to power is the need to obtain research funds. Researchers may be happy to hit and hope in their research design, but people who give out the money are not. They want a result. Non-significant findings are bad news, but findings that might have been significant had more subjects been tested are a waste of money. Applicants for research funds are expected to estimate a likely effect size, calculate the number of subjects required and make their plans accordingly. A good example of this is seen in a study of voice therapy by MacKenzie et al. (2001). They wanted to obtain a high level of power and set the effect size at 0.5. This was rather smaller than effect sizes in the existing literature, and so their strategy was a conservative one. They calculated that 100 subjects per group would give them 94% power. In the event they tested fewer subjects than this, but power was still 81%. At such levels of power it is reasonable to argue that non-significant results correctly indicate that no effect of an IV exists, because the study has a good chance of detecting it if it does.

Power analysis also plays a part in the interpretation of null results. In Chapter 2 we discussed the need to design experiments to show differences and the difficulties we have in showing that, for instance, two different therapies have the same effect. Proving the null hypothesis in experiments is frowned upon because sloppiness by the researcher helps achieve this. The failure to control other variables or to stick to a consistent procedure increases error variance and makes it more difficult to find differences. Power analysis can be used to demonstrate that an experiment had sufficient power to get a significant result if it exists.

This discussion may have convinced you that power analysis is a good idea, but how do we find out about effect sizes? The simplest approach, mentioned above, is to use the effect size from a similar experiment that has already been done. So why, if an experiment has been done before, are we doing it again? In fact, most research areas develop over time. Many researchers contribute by doing broadly similar experiments. These give us a fairly good idea of the effect size in the area. In some areas there are many experiments, and meta-analyses have been conducted. Meta-analysis (see Chapter 14) is a technique for combining results to find the mean effect size for a whole area of research. When available, these do the work for us, both tracking down the previous studies and calculating the effect size.

When no previous research is available, we can select our own effect size. Although, this sounds rather dodgy, we will soon find that we cannot cheat. If we choose a large effect size and need only a few subjects, we may fail to produce a significant result; if we expect it to be small, we commit ourselves to testing many more subjects. Cohen (1988), who has been the main advocate of power analysis, suggests that we use either a small, medium or large effect size giving these *d*-values of 0.2, 0.5 and 0.8. He also gives the percentage of overlap (in the distributions in Figure 8.5) for each of these. Table 8.1 gives the numbers of subjects required per group for a one-tail independent t-test with power of 0.80 (i.e. 20% probability of a type-two error). This just confirms that the cost of power is a large number of subjects, particularly when looking for small effects.

Table 8.1 Number of subjects required for power of 0.80 for a one-tail test

Effect size	*d*	Percentage of overlap	Number of subjects required per group
Small	0.2	85	313
Medium	0.5	67	50
Large	0.8	53	20

Power versus significance

Use of effect sizes changes the way we do experiments. This goes beyond estimating how many subjects we need or discovering that we didn't get a significant result because we had too few. In the good old days results were either significant or not. We worried that significant results might be type-one errors but largely ignored the fact that some, maybe many, non-significant results were type-two errors. Power analyses now mean that many more results can be significant if we can be bothered to run enough subjects.

Looking at it in this way, we can see that significance was a blunt way of deciding which results were important. Now small effects, that experiments of manageable dimensions failed to detect, may become significant results in the hands of ruthlessly determined researchers who are prepared to conduct large experiments. Suppose the treated group in our dysfluency experiment had a mean decrease in dysfluency of only 6.5 (with the untreated group remaining at 4.5 and pooled standard deviation at 3.69). A t-test on these data gives a value of 1.21, which, with 18 d.f., is not significant. The effect size in this experiment is 0.54 and power is only 0.33 (a 67% chance of a type-two error). Suppose we want to increase power to

0.80. A calculation like those above shows that we need 44 subjects per group to do this. Recalculating t (same means and standard deviations) with 44 subjects gives $t = 2.53$ (86 d.f.), which is easily significant ($p < 0.01$).

What are we to make of all this? Clearly large effect sizes are better for all concerned. Researchers can find significant results without too many subjects and clinicians may use treatments with more confidence. In contrast small effect sizes may exhaust the supply of subjects in some clinical groups and the patience of researchers seeking them. Significant results may eventually be obtained, but clinicians may find that the small effects are of little benefit to clients and are outweighed by the expenditure of time required. This sounds like an argument for seeking only large effect sizes. However, there are occasions when patently useful medical interventions are only discovered by testing very large samples. An example is provided by a study of the use of aspirin and thrombolytic treatment with patients after myocardial infaction (ISIS-2) Collaborative group, 1988). Both treatments improved survival rates, and their effects were additive. The differences in survival rates were small but highly significant as over 17,000 patients took part in the study. The benefits of the treatments are clear, and the costs in clinical time and money slight. Small effect sizes are worth pursuing when lives are so easily saved.

Power analysis and SLT

Some of these issues have particular relevance to research in communication disorders. We have seen that power is most easily increased by increasing the number of subjects. It may already have struck you that the large numbers of subjects suggested by power analysis are unrealistic. This is particularly so where subjects must meet a clinical diagnosis for entry to an experiment.

Discussions of power analysis assume that the standard errors of sampling distributions can only be reduced by increasing the number of subjects. This is a reasonable assumption for laboratory-based research, where a careful selection of subjects and control of situational variables should have made the sample standard deviations as small as possible. In clinical research it may be worth trying to reduce subject variance further by the tighter control and stricter criteria for inclusion in the research. Face-to-face therapy makes it difficult to maintain a uniform experimental procedure, and the broad diagnostic categories often used in clinical research make it likely that clients will vary in their response to treatment. These are familiar problems that won't be solved overnight. However, they suggest that it may not be the end of the road if an experiment lacks power and more clients are difficult to find. In clinical research it may be easier to detect therapeutic effects with fewer, more consistent, clients than by trying to increase power by recruiting more clients (although, as we saw in Chapter 2, we must be more cautious about generalizing the findings).

Trying to increase power by including more clients might even reduce power, leading to a nightmare scenario. Chapter 2 discussed the problem of recruiting subjects and the effect that this may have upon the entry criteria of experiments. Power calculations assume that subject variance will remain more or less the same as we increase the number of subjects. However, the need for more clients who are in short supply may lead to the inclusion of some who do not fully meet the entry requirements. It is possible that a vicious circle may occur in which attempts to increase power by increasing the number of subjects are offset by an increased subject variability.

If our research uses a control group of subjects who are in plentiful supply (for example people with normal language skills), we might increase power by increasing the control sample. The calculations of sample size above assumed that samples were of equal size. When unequal samples are used, we replace n in the formula above by the harmonic mean of the sample sizes. This is obtained from the formula:

$$\bar{n}_b = \frac{2n_1 n_2}{n_1 + n_2}$$

where n_1 and n_2 are the sample sizes and $\bar{n}_b$ their harmonic mean. So:

$$\delta = d \sqrt{\frac{\bar{n}_b}{2}}$$

Suppose we compare samples of 10 subjects each using a one-tail test and the 0.05 level of significance. The effect size is 0.5. From the conventional formula we obtain:

$$\delta = 0.5 \sqrt{\frac{10}{2}} = 1.12$$

which gives power = 0.30. Table 8.2 shows the effect of increasing the number of subjects where the new subjects are placed either equally in both groups or in one group, the other remaining fixed.

Table 8.2 Increases in power when extra subjects are added to one or both groups

n_1	n_2	Power	n_1	n_2	Power
10	10	0.30	10	10	0.30
15	15	0.39	10	20	0.37
20	20	0.47	10	30	0.39
25	25	0.55	10	40	0.40

With 10 subjects in each group power is low. Increasing both samples improves power, but increasing one sample (by the same number of subjects) has a much smaller effect. This shows that power is maximized when the groups are equal. The example shows some increase if n_2 rises to 20, but further increases are negligible.

Power analysis has revealed that we often run the risk of making type-two errors in research. This risk is greatest when we try to detect small effects. Journals continue to publish (almost exclusively) statistically significant results; so researchers can ensure that these are obtained by calculating the number of subjects required. This avoids type-two errors but, as the last section suggested, may be misleading for SLT. It reopens the debate about statistical and clinical significance (see Exercise 2.6). In the past researchers have produced statistically significant results and clinicians have sometimes questioned their clinical significance. A more sensible approach might be to decide the minimum change required for a clinically significant result prior to the research and to calculate the number of clients needed to obtain it. A positive result is then both statistically and clinically significant. Failure to find a statistically significant result will indicate that a clinically useful effect was not found. This approach will need an adjustment on the part of

---

Exercise 8.4

A research project compares treated and untreated clients (of any kind you like). The researcher is uncertain how many subjects she needs and has a quick look at the data from time to time. Some treated clients respond well. After a while she decides to analyse the data. The differences are not significant, and so she treats some more clients and re-analyses the data. This might go on for some time and eventually the test is significant. Now it's likely that all researchers have done this at some time and some even know that they shouldn't have. Why shouldn't they?

researchers who may find it difficult to part from the habit of looking for statistically significant results. There is also the problem that clinical significance is a subjective concept. More attention needs to be given to defining what it is for different client groups and to developing ways of measuring it. Almost and Rosenbaum (1998), who assessed treatment for children with phonological disorders, defined a clinically significant change as a 20-point change on the Assessment of Phonological Processes (Hodson, 1986) and calculated the necessary sample size to demonstrate this with 90% power.

Assumptions and transformations

In Chapter 5 we saw that parametric tests may only be used if our data meet certain assumptions. They must come from normally distributed populations that have approximately equal variances (homogeneity of variance), and the data must be on an equal-interval scale. We now look at these assumptions in more detail.

We saw above that the t-test compares the difference between sample means with the sampling distribution of the differences between means. This requires the sampling distribution to be normally distributed. It is normally distributed when the population is normally distributed. Hence the assumption that the populations sampled are normally distributed.

Histograms and comparing measures of central tendency can give an indication of whether data are normally distributed. However, as we saw in Chapter 3, this is difficult when only a few subjects have been tested. Computer programs help us here by displaying the data as a histogram and superimposing on it a normal distribution with the same mean and standard deviation as the sample. The two can then be compared to see if the sample is normally distributed using the exotic (in name, at least) Kolmogorov–Smirnov test. A significant result indicates a departure from normality.

Having established that a normally distributed population is important, most books go on to suggest that it may not matter much after all. The first line of defence is that, with large samples, the sampling distribution is normally distributed even when the population is not. Authors disagree a bit on what a large sample is: some say 30; others, 40. Next they shrug their shoulders and say it doesn't matter much anyway. Howell (1997) noted that 'moderate departures from normality are not usually fatal'. As with people, so with population distributions it seems. This nonchalance is based on the previously mentioned 'robustness' of parametric tests. The evidence for robustness comes from a curious activity known in the trade as Monte Carlo experiments. These involve computers creating a non-normal population and investigating what happens when samples from it are compared. Not very much happens. The chance of type-one errors only increases with fairly extreme departures from normality (but having samples of different sizes with unequal variances as well causes a few problems).

If all else fails, data that are not normally distributed can be transformed. This means that, instead of analysing the actual numbers, we analyse their square roots, logarithms or one of many other possible transforms. The selection of an appropriate transformation can make non-normal data meet the requirement of normality. Logarithmic transformations, for example, are useful with positively skewed data and in situations where the mean and standard deviations of groups are related. Suppose we compare untreated clients with clients who receive either non-intensive or intensive therapy. Improvement increases with the amount of therapy given. However, the greater improvement also reveals that clients vary in their responses to therapy. As the groups' means increase so do their standard deviations and positive skews. A logarithmic transformation will remove the skew and help us meet the homogeneity of variance assumption. Further guidance on transformations can be found in Clark-Carter (1997), Howell (1997) and Tabachnick and Fidell (2001). The rule is that you must select your transformation before seeing how it affects the results rather than doing several and selecting the most satisfactory outcome. I will leave you to work out the reason for this rule.

Clinical data are quite likely to fail the homogeneity-of-variance assumption. Treated groups and clinical groups are likely to be more variable than untreated or non-clinical groups. Books vary in their rules of thumb about unequal variances. Some say the highest variance should be no more than three times the smallest; others say four times. This is not as generous as it sounds. Research reports normally give standard deviations not variances. After you have squared the standard deviations to obtain the variances, the rule seems quite strict.

A test that can tell us whether variances differ significantly would be useful. There are times when we want to show that they do differ. Suppose, for instance, that we compare treated and untreated clients and find no difference in their improvement but a difference in their standard deviations. This suggests that treatment has done something even if it has not improved the group as a whole. The variance ratio or F-test can be used to see whether the variances differ significantly. It calculates the ratio of the largest to the smallest variance. The F-value is looked up with the degrees of freedom of the two variances.

> **Exercise 8.5**
>
> We compare a group of 10 treated children who stutter with 10 untreated children. The mean changes in the number of dysfluencies of the two groups are 4.7 and 4.5. Clearly treatment has had no effect. However, their standard deviations are 1.42 and 3.41. Should we be curious about this difference?

Normally we want to show that variances don't differ. Here we use the F-test to decide whether the variances are homogeneous. Researchers have done this for many years. Recently, however, statisticians have become concerned that the F-test is unreliable in situations where the data are not normally distributed. As a result they prefer to use Levene's test. This requires more arithmetic than the F-test; so we won't go into it here. However, many computer programs automatically use Levene's test to discover whether data meet the homogeneity requirement and, when they don't, give an alternative (lower) significance level based upon a reduction of the degrees of freedom for the test.

The last of our three assumptions was that the data are measured on a fixed-interval scale. Rating data may look numerical, but they are not fixed-interval data and should not be analysed with parametric tests. This is bad news for SLT. We often resolve our problems about measuring behaviour by asking people to indicate their level of agreement with statements offered to them (see Chapter 11). This lets us measure things like quality of life, depression and the stress of caring for people with communication problems but produces non-parametric data. So, if we are strict about the fixed-interval rule, we must use non-parametric tests.

There was a time when statistics texts were, if nothing else, united on this issue and, as it was often difficult to decide if samples came from normally distributed populations and had homogeneous variances, the presence or absence of interval data was often decisive in the choice of test. Times have changed. Some texts still insist on interval data (see, for example, Bowling, 1997; Hinton, 1995; Field, 2000). Others recognize the problems that this presents and concede that rating data are often treated as if they are interval data (see, for example, Polit, 1996). Others seem to have no problem with it at all (for example Howell, 1997; Howitt and Cramer, 1999). If you are the sort of person who likes a compromise, you might take Clark-Carter's (1997) advice. Many measures ask people to rate a series of statements. If each is rated on a 5-point scale, the total score will be quite large. Clark-Carter suggested that we can use parametric tests when it is greater than 20.

The above deals with the assumptions for parametric tests from Chapter 5. However, there is a further assumption we have not covered because it applies only to within-subjects ANOVAs. This is the assumption of sphericity. Suppose we monitor the progress of a group of clients we are treating. We assess them before treatment and at monthly intervals for 3 months. So time of assessment is a variable with four levels. If we subtract each client's initial score from that client's score after the first month, we will get a changed score. These will vary across clients, and we could calculate their variance. Suppose we do this for all possible pairs of levels (there will be six sets of scores). The sphericity assumption is that these variances are homogeneous.

If sphericity is not present, the results of the ANOVA may be incorrect. This applies to one-factor within-subjects ANOVAs and to any within-subjects variables in more complex ANOVAs. This is looking pretty serious, and it won't be much fun working out all the variances either. Fortunately most computer programs have ways of dealing with this. Normally they use Mauchly's test. If this is non-significant, we are in the clear; if it's significant, the sphericity assumption is false and something must be done about it. This usually means reducing the degrees of freedom so that a significant result is less likely. There are two common procedures for this, known as the Greenhouse-Geiser and Huyn-Feldt corrections. In each we multiply the degrees of freedom by a value (normally less than 1 and referred to as 'epsilon'). Again, computer programs do this for us; so we don't have to worry about it. However, you might wonder why there are two methods that produce different adjustments to the degrees of freedom. There has been much statistical scratching of heads about this. Opinion seems to be that the Greenhouse-Geiser correction is rather too conservative and the Huyn-Feldt correction rather too lax. So what do you do when one gives a significant result and the other doesn't? Field (2000) suggested taking the mean of the two significance levels. Statistics is not an exact science!

Fixed and random effects

Suppose we conduct a study of treatment of dysarthric speech. We treat several speakers who have dysarthria (others acting as untreated controls), and, to assess their progress, we have listeners hear and try to identify words in samples of the clients' speech before and after treatment. The number of items correctly identified gives us a measure of their intelligibility. This design is not easy to use. We need many listeners and different speech samples (so listeners don't keep hearing the same words), and listeners should not know whether they are hearing pre- or post-therapy or treated or untreated samples. Working out who hears what and in what order can be quite complicated. Despite this, the design is appealing. We want to show that treatment has made the clients' everyday communication more intelligible. Surely any reasonable person would think we have achieved this if a random sample of listeners (naive about dysarthric speech) find the post-therapy speech of the treated clients easier to understand? Surely we can now say that treatment will make other speakers with dysarthria more intelligible to other listeners? Reasonable people might think so, but statisticians won't like it.

The problem here is that we have two sets of potential subjects in our experiment. We could let the clients be the subjects. Their pre- and post-treatment scores will be the means of the listeners' scores. Alternatively we might let the listeners be the subjects, each with a pre- and post-score, which is the mean of the speakers. If we are cunning, we will let whichever group is larger be the subjects to get a better chance of a significant result. This is likely to be the listeners, and, if they are not significant, there are lots more listeners out there to be called upon! Your experience of research methods so far will probably tell you that you are not going to get away with this. The problem first emerged in a discussion of reaction-time experiments with different types of word stimuli by Clark (1973), who referred to it as the 'language as fixed effect fallacy'. The data in these experiments were the mean reaction time of each subject to groups of words. This removed the variability in reaction time to different words. Words became a fixed factor, and statistical generalization from the sample of words to other words became invalid. This was precisely what researchers had in mind; so the situation was not a very satisfactory one.

Suppose we let speakers be the subjects in our experiment and analyse the mean scores of the listeners. Here speakers are a random factor and listeners a fixed factor. The result may support the experimental hypothesis but the means conceal the variability in listeners, making it inappropriate to generalize the finding to other listeners (in an extreme case the difference in the means might be due to one sensitive listener, not to listeners generally). We can only generalize this result to the same listeners hearing other speakers with dysarthria. The reverse applies if the listeners are the subjects. Now speakers are a fixed factor and we can only generalize to other listeners hearing the same speakers. If we do both analyses and both are significant, we can generalize to other listeners for the same speakers and to other speakers for the same listeners but not to both other speakers and listeners.

A statistical solution to this was offered by Clark (1973). Briefly we need to do both analyses and then combine the F-values to obtain min F'. The formulae for doing this and for determining the degrees of freedom of min F' and a further discussion of the issue may be found in Pring and Hunter (1994). Min F' can only be significant if both the analyses are significant (and sometimes not even then). It's quite common for this research design to be used with only a few speakers (because relevant clients are in short supply). Therefore it may be difficult to obtain significant values for both results. In such cases we must hope that the findings can be replicated by other researchers with other similar clients and other listeners.

Chapter 9
Analysing categorical data

Introduction

I was recently wondering whether there might be a gender difference in preferences for quantitative and qualitative research. To test this hunch I looked at my books on research methods and classified them as either quantitative or qualitative (not hard as it turned out – few cover both areas) and then looked at the gender of their authors. The results are shown in Table 9.1.

Table 9.1 Some data on gender and preferences in research methods

	Qualitative methods	Quantitative methods
Female authors	13	5
Male authors	17	34

Tables like this are called contingency tables and the data are called nominal or categorical data. Instead of giving us a score on a measure of behaviour, the subjects are members of a category. It looks like there is a relationship between the two: female authors write fewer books on research methods generally but are better represented in the qualitative section. Of course, we need a statistical test to decide if the authors are in these categories by chance or whether the probability of their being there by chance is low enough that we can reject the null hypothesis and claim a significant result. The test we use is called chi square (χ^2).

Chi square is a useful and widely used test. You can see one reason why in my example. The data are easily obtained. The subjects don't actually have to do anything, and researchers get off lightly too (although you might have to do a bit more than walk to your bookcase). As a result we can quickly test an idea by looking at data or clinical records that are to hand. For example, we might wonder whether children with language impairment respond better to therapy if treated early. We should be able to find data on this in clinical records. We can classify children as being treated early or late (by age when treatment began) and see how they responded to therapy. Table 9.2 gives three possible outcomes. In the first there appears to be a relationship between good responses and early treatment, in the second there is no relationship and in the third good responses are more likely with late treatment.

Table 9.2 Three possible arrangements of subjects sorted by the early/late therapy and good/poor response to therapy variables

	Good response	Poor response		Good response	Poor response		Good response	Poor response
Early	23	15	Early	15	23	Early	10	28
Late	8	34	Late	16	26	Late	25	17

Working out chi square

An SLT working with people who have had laryngectomies is interested in factors that help them adjust to their illness. Clients completed questionnaires to measure their psychosocial adjustment and the extent of their social contacts and the support this gives them. They are assigned to the categories 'good/poor adjustment' and 'good/poor social support'. In Table 9.3 the row and column totals and the total number of subjects are also included. We need these to calculate chi square.

Table 9.3 Data on adjustment to laryngectomy by level of social support

	Good social support	Poor social support	Row totals
Good adjustment	36	12	48
Poor adjustment	9	13	22
Column Totals	45	25	70

The scores in Table 9.3 are called the observed scores; we now need to calculate the expected scores. These are the numbers of subjects we expect in the cells of the table by chance (when no relationship exists between the variables). The expected score for each cell is:

$$\text{Expected score} = \frac{\text{row total} \times \text{column total}}{\text{grand total}}$$

So for the first cell of the table:

$$\text{Expected score} = \frac{48 \times 45}{70} = 30.86$$

Table 9.4 Expected scores for adjustment and social support

	Good social support	Poor social support
Good adjustment	30.86	17.14
Poor adjustment	14.14	7.86

The expected scores are shown in Table 9.4. There are two things to notice about them. First, they are a purely mathematical distribution of the subjects. We don't actually expect there to be fractions of people in the cells. Second, they add up to the whole numbers of people in each row and column. This means we could short-cut the calculation; once we have one score, we could get the others by subtraction from the row and column totals (but it's better to calculate the others and use the totals to check your calculations).

Chi square can now be calculated from the formula:

$$\chi^2 = \sum \frac{(O - E)^2}{E}$$

Where E = the expected scores and O = the observed scores. It's a good idea to do the calculations in a table until you are confident of what you are doing (see Table 9.5).

This value is looked up in the chi-square tables (Appendix 8). The degrees of freedom for chi square are the number of rows $-1 \times$ the number of columns -1 or $(r - 1) \times (c - 1)$. Most of the time we have two rows and two columns (a 2×2 chi square); so the d.f. = 1 and the table values are:

$$p = 0.05 \quad 3.84, \quad p = 0.01 \quad 6.64, \quad p = 0.001 \quad 10.83$$

The value obtained for the example above (see Table 9.5) exceeds the table value for the $p < 0.01$ level of significance.

Table 9.5 Working out chi square

O	E	$(O-E)$	$(O-E)^2$	$\dfrac{(O-E)^2}{E}$
36	30.86	5.14	26.42	0.86
12	17.14	-5.14	26.42	1.54
9	14.14	-5.14	26.42	1.87
13	7.86	5.14	26.42	3.36
				$\sum \dfrac{(O-E)^2}{E} = 7.63$

Exercise 9.1

Work out chi square for the figures given above about the gender of writers of research-methods books. Is there a significant relationship between these two variables? What conclusion might you draw from this?

Some heavy warnings about using chi square

There are several problems to be aware of when using chi square despite its obvious usefulness. One problem is that we must define the variables. In the case of my research-methods books this is straightforward – both variables fall into two distinct categories. In other cases we have to choose cut-off points that 'create' the data. Suppose we choose an age to divide children into early- and late-treatment groups and a level of progress to define good and poor responses. We do a chi square and just fail to produce a significant result. It is tempting to see if we can improve on this result by moving the cut-off points a little so that the odd subject slips into a different category. Hopefully I don't have to tell you what a deceitful and depraved practice this is. The temptation to cheat can be avoided by having an arbitrarily fixed cut-off point, such as performance on a standardized test, which is decided in advance and can't be fiddled.

A further problem is that chi square is nearly always used in situations where the IV has not been manipulated. An alarm bell should already be ringing in your head. As a result confounding variables will be present and caution is needed drawing conclusions from the results. In our comparison of early- and late-treated children we would, at the very least, want to know why children were treated early or late. Perhaps the late-treated children had more severe problems that had not responded to earlier treatment or the early-treated cases may have been given preference and received more treatment as a result. Likewise, the data on laryngectomy (which are loosely based on research by Blood et al., 1994) only allow us to conclude that social support and good adjustment are related and not that the former causes the latter. Clients may well benefit from good social support; on the other hand, clients who are well adjusted are probably more likely to maintain social contacts.

Chi square is often used to ferret around in data to discover more about what went on. Suppose we do an experiment comparing treated and untreated children. The result was not significant, but some treated children improved and others did not. In such cases it's impossible not to look at the data and discover (or invent) a reason why some children did well and others didn't. Our intention here is a good one. Finding a reason may be important. Unfortunately there are always some children who improve for reasons of their own. If we look long and hard at them, we might see something they have in common and use a chi-square test to show that treatment works for left-handed children! You might find something more plausible that they have in common, but, no doubt, you get the point. This is another good way of making a type-one error.

Despite these dire warnings, we would be crazy not to learn from the data of experiments that have not worked or from the many hours spent keeping good clinical records. So go ahead – see what you can learn. Then test your hypothesis by setting up a new experiment. It's surprising how the prospect of carrying out an experiment undermines enthusiasm for wild ideas about left-handed children!

Using chi square with data from a single subject

All our examples of research so far have been of groups of subjects. Some areas of research in SLT use single cases, and chi square is often used to analyse the data. As far as I can find, the 'big books' have not expressed an opinion upon this unusual use of chi square. It's possible that statisticians are right now shaking their heads about it. Nevertheless, chi square has been widely used on single-subject data; so a precedent has been set. Nowhere is this more the case than in cognitive neuropsychological studies, and these provide many good examples. Here we often want to show that a client can process one class of stimuli better than another. Suppose we ask a client to read regular and exception words (PALPA test 35 – Kay et al., 1992) and obtain the results given in Table 9.6.

Table 9.6 Data from a client reading regular and exception words

	Regular words	Exception words	
Correct	24	16	40
Incorrect	6	14	20
	30	30	60

It looks like the client reads regular words better than exception words. Regular words can be read either visually or phonologically, while exception words require a visual approach. So a client who is better at regular words is reading phonologically and is a surface dyslexic.

Exercise 9.2

Carry out a chi square on the data in Table 9.6. You will find it easy to calculate the expected frequencies as the columns have the same number of cases. At issue here is whether the scores could have arisen by chance or whether there is a relationship between right and wrong responses and the type of words indicating surface dyslexia

---

It's interesting to reflect for a minute on the PALPA tests. Essentially each test is an experiment and tests a hypothesis (for example that any difference in the reading of regular and exception words is unlikely to be due to chance). You might then wonder whether the results of these experiments might not be explained by confounding variables. For instance, regular words might be used more frequently than exception words. People with aphasia are better with frequent words, which might explain the result. Fortunately the designers of PALPA knew all about confounding variables. In each test huge efforts were made to control other variables. The regular and exception words, for example, are matched for frequency, imageability, grammatical class and number of letters, syllables and morphemes.

Chi square with large contingency tables

So far we have only used chi square with 2×2 contingency tables. We can use it with larger tables. Suppose we ask a client with aphasia to name pictures and expect naming to decline with frequency. We select three groups of 20 words of high, medium and low frequency each with 20 pictures and obtain the result shown in Table 9.7.

Table 9.7 Some data on naming words of different frequencies

	High	Medium	Low
Named	17	14	9
Not named	3	6	11

We can analyse these data with chi square. The calculations take a little longer (there are six cells), and the degrees of freedom increase to $(c - 1) \times (r - 1) = 2 \times 1 = 2$.

In theory chi square can analyse any size of contingency table, but we need to use our common sense here. There is no point having extra rows or columns if they do not tell us anything. The more we have, the more difficult it is to know where a significant result is significant! In the above little is gained by having three levels of frequency; it might have been better to have had more pictures at the high and low levels. This is supported by the fact that the high-versus-medium data and the medium-versus-low data are not significant if analysed alone. Even when a large contingency table is justified on theoretical grounds (there are three or more levels of a category that differ in a theoretically meaningful way), we still face the problem of finding out where a significant effect is coming from. This means doing further tests, which means more work and possible type-one errors.

One-sample chi square

Suppose we test a person with aphasia who seems not to understand written words. We might want to know if he can distinguish real written words and non-words (lexical decision) (see PALPA tests 24–27). We give him 30 real words and 30 non-words printed on cards and in a random order and ask him to sort them into words and non-words. Forty-one cards are correctly sorted and 19 incorrectly. Here chance is a factor. A client who responds randomly will score about 30. So does 41 correct indicate some ability at the task or is it a chance result? Here the expected scores are 30 correct and 30 incorrect, and the observed scores are 41 correct and 19 incorrect. We can use chi square to decide whether the observed scores differ from the expected (chance) scores.

This is significant at the $p < 0.01$ level (see Table 9.8); so we may conclude that our subject retains some ability to distinguish real words from non-words. This is a one-sample chi-square test. Essentially there is only one category on which responses differ, and we are testing whether their arrangement within the category can be explained by chance.

Table 9.8 Calculations for a one sample chi-square

O	E	$(O-E)$	$(O-E)^2$	$\dfrac{(O-E)^2}{E}$
41	30	11	121	4.03
19	30	11	121	4.03
				$\sum \dfrac{(O-E)^2}{E} = 8.06$

One of the most useful PALPA tests assesses whether clients understand spoken or written words. The client must match each word to one of five pictures. These are:

- the correct target;
- a close semantic distracter;
- a distant semantic distracter;
- a visually similar distracter;
- an unrelated picture.

A possible result is shown in Table 9.9 and the calculation is shown in Table 9.10. Note that the expected score is 8 as there are 40 trials and 5 responses. We can use a one-sample chi square to see if these scores differ from chance.

Table 9.9 Data from a client matching spoken words and pictures

	Target	Close semantic distracter	Distant semantic distracter	Visually similar distracter	Unrelated picture
Observed score	17	9	6	3	5
Expected score	8	8	8	8	8

Table 9.10 Working out a one-sample chi square with five cells

O	E	$(O-E)$	$(O-E)^2$	$\dfrac{(O-E)^2}{E}$
17	8	9	81	10.1
9	8	1	1	0.1
6	8	-2	4	0.5
3	8	-5	25	3.1
5	8	-3	9	1.1
				$\sum \dfrac{(O-E)^2}{E} = 14.9$

This one-sample chi square has c − 1 degrees of freedom. So we look up the tables with d.f. = 4. The table values are 9.49 and 13.28 for the $p < 0.05$ and $p < 0.01$ levels of significance, so this result is significant at $p < 0.01$.

This tells us that the scores differ from chance. However, we don't know which categories cause the significant effect. This is like the situation with ANOVA. There an overall test might be significant, but we needed comparisons to discover what was significant. This led to concern about type-one errors. The same applies here. Whenever we go tripping through data with gay abandon carrying out tests as we go, it's possible that we will keep going until we find a type-one error.

There is a solution to this problem. Assessments like PALPA are highly focused and should be used to address specific problems. It's likely that we wanted to know whether the client had any understanding of the words and whether his errors were semantically related to the target. Here we have planned the tests in advance so we need not worry about type-one errors. The first compares correct responses with all errors (17 correct versus 23 wrong); the second compares semantic and non-semantic errors (15 versus 8). You will do this in Exercise 9.3. Be careful with the expected frequencies.

Exercise 9.3

1. Carry out the two tests described. The first looks at whether the client performs above chance at getting the right target and the second looks at whether there are more semantic errors than expected by chance.
2. To further illustrate the usefulness of chi square in trawling medical records here is an example that has nothing to do with SLT. Evans et al. (2000) examined deaths from coronary heart disease by day of the week in Scotland. Analyse my made-up figures and see if deaths vary with the day of the week. What might you conclude from this?

Sunday	Monday	Tuesday	Wednesday	Thursday	Friday	Saturday
10	18	9	8	9	7	9

Some further points about chi square

An alternative formula for chi-square

There is an alternative formula for the calculation of chi square. It is:

$$\chi^2 = \frac{N(ad + bc)^2}{(a + b)(c + d)(a + c)(b + d)}$$

where N is the total number of subjects and a, b, c and d are the scores in the cells of the contingency table as shown below.

Table 9.11 Values used in the alternative formula for chi square

	Good social support	Poor social support	Row totals
Good adjustment	a	b	$a + b$
Poor adjustment	c	d	$c + d$
Column totals	$a + c$	$b + d$	N

Using the values from Table 9.3, we find that:

$$\chi^2 = \frac{N(ad - bc)^2}{(a + b)(c + d)(a + c)(b + d)} = \frac{70(36 \times 13 - 12 \times 9)^2}{48 \times 22 \times 45 \times 25} =$$

$$\frac{70 \times 129600}{1188000} = 7.63$$

Some people prefer this formula because you don't have to calculate expected frequencies. However, for reasons explained below, we may need to know the expected frequencies.

Chi square is for independent data

Chi square is for independent data. Subjects may only contribute once to the data and the grand total must equal the number of subjects (or items). This is a nuisance. Table 9.12 shows a client's performance naming a set of pictures on two occasions. It looks like he improved, and the data look suitable for a chi square. As the data are not independent, the test can't be used, however. Fortunately there is another test we can use.

Table 9.12 Data from naming pictures on two occasions

	First test	Second test
Pictures named correctly	8	15
Pictures not named	17	10

The McNemar test

The McNemar test is a version of chi square for within-subject designs. To use the test we must reorganize the data into the form shown in Table 9.13.

Table 9.13 Data for use with the McNemar test

		Second assessment		
		Correct	Wrong	Totals
First	Correct	6	2 (b)	8
assessment	Wrong	9 (a)	8	17
	Totals	15	10	

In Table 9.13 the row and column totals are the values in Table 9.12. However, the test uses the values inside the table, which show how items changed. We need the number of items that have gone from wrong on the first test to right on the second and vice versa. These are labelled *a* and *b*. Note that while these values can be converted, by adding up the rows and columns, to those in Table 9.12, the reverse is not true (more than one set of scores can add to the appropriate row and column totals). So to use the McNemar test you must keep a record of how the client performed on individual items.

The formula for the test is: $\chi^2 = \dfrac{(|a-b|-1)^2}{a+b}$

Where $|a-b|$ indicates the difference between *a* and *b* (it's always positive).

So for the data above: $\chi^2 = \dfrac{(|a-b|-1)^2}{a+b} = \dfrac{(|9-2|-1)^2}{11} = 3.27$

If we test someone on two occasions, some items will change by chance. These are as likely to go from right to wrong as from wrong to right, however. The McNemar test assesses whether the change is due to chance (in both directions) or if there is a trend (mainly in one direction). The value of chi square is looked up in the normal way. The value (3.27) is lower than the table value (3.84) at the $p < 0.05$ level; so the second test score is not a significant improvement.

Chi square and percentage data

Consider the data on adjustment and social support after laryngectomy. The table for these data was unclear because the numbers of subjects in the good/poor adjustment and good/poor social support categories are different. Table 9.14, which gives the percentage of subjects in each cell, is a clearer way of presenting the data.

Table 9.14 Data from Table 9.3 in percentages

	Good social support	Poor social support
Good adjustment	51%	17%
Poor adjustment	12%	18%

Having presented the data like this, it's easy to carry on and do the chi square on the percentage figures. Don't. Chi square doesn't know they are percentages. It assumes that we had more subjects than was the case, and we may obtain a significant result where we should not have done.

Yates' correction

Many statistics books, particularly older ones, give slightly different formulae for chi square than those given here. These formulae include a continuity correction called Yates' correction. They are:

$$\chi^2 = \sum \frac{(O-E-1/2)^2}{E} \quad \text{and} \quad \chi^2 = \frac{N(|ad-bc|-N/2)^2}{(a+b)(c+d)(a+c)(b+d)}$$

Statistical opinion has now moved against the use of Yates' correction. Non-statisticians can welcome this on three grounds. First, the reasons for using it were largely incomprehensible. Second, it was often the source of errors during calculation of the test. Finally, not using it is more likely to give a significant result!

The problem of small expected frequencies

Chi square is said to be inaccurate when the expected frequencies are small. Many books suggest that a 2×2 chi square should not be used if any of the expected frequencies are less than or equal to 5. We need the expected frequencies to decide if we can use chi square; so we should make a habit of using the expected frequencies formula.

The surest way to avoid this problem is to have plenty of subjects. Nevertheless, sooner or later we will find ourselves in a dilemma about whether we can use chi square or not. An irritating instance is where we devise our own test material. For instance, many people with aphasia have trouble with function words. To assess this problem, we devise a test of reading function words and homophonic content words (such as 'or' and 'oar'). The shortage of homophonic words means that we have only 10 items in each group. Our client's performance is shown in Table 9.15.

Table 9.15 Data on reading function and content words

	Function words	Content words	Row totals
Correct	3	9	12
Incorrect	7	1	8
Column totals	10	10	20

Two of the expected frequencies are below 5; so can we use chi square? Conventional wisdom suggests not, but this is another issue on which statisticians are getting less rigid. Rosenthal and Rosnow (1991) stated that chi square may be used with expected frequencies as low as 1 as long as the total number of subjects/items is 20 or more. Howell (1997) noted that expected frequencies should be above 5 but admitted this is a conservative rule and one he 'occasionally violates'. He says that using chi square is unlikely to cause type-one errors but may lead to type-two errors due to lack of power. When the big books disagree, it's hard to know what to do. We start by considering the alternatives. (Note that the example uses matched pairs of words, and so we might consider using a McNemar test.)

Fisher's exact test

Fisher's exact test is used in place of chi square when expected frequencies are small. Its calculation is less than straightforward, however. The formula is:

$$p = \frac{(a + b)!(c + d)!(a + c)!(b + d)!}{a!b!c!d!N!}$$

where a, b, c and d are the totals in each cell and N is the total number of subjects. The explanation mark indicates that the totals are factorial where, for example, $10! = 10 \times 9 \times 8 \times 7 \times 6 \times 5 \times 4 \times 3 \times 2 \times 1$. So for our data above:

$$p = \frac{12!8!10!10!}{3!9!7!1!20!}$$

This takes some calculating. The number 20! is large enough to give your calculator a headache, and who wouldn't make a mistake carrying out such a calculation? Nor is this the end. Fisher's test is not called 'exact' for nothing. It calculates the exact probability of a particular outcome, not whether the outcome is statistically significant. To decide this we must calculate the probabilities of more extreme outcomes and add these together, hoping the total will be less than 0.05.

It's easy to conclude that Fisher was having a bad day at the office when he invented this test. It's my impression that the test was very rarely used before computer programs became available to do it for us. Now that they are available it's often used even when chi square is appropriate. Nor have I had much success persuading clinicians to have a computer ready on the off chance that they might want to do a Fisher's exact test! In everyday use it looks like we will have to risk using chi square even when expected frequencies are a bit on the small side.

Chi square and its tails

The chi-square tables are for a two-tail test. In the examples above a directional hypothesis was often tested; so a one-tail test might have been used. This is clearly the case when clients read regular and exception words. We don't give this test out of idle curiosity; we expect an advantage for regular words. Despite this, the test is usually used in its two-tailed form. This is because it is often used to explore data without a clear hypothesis. Our use of the test, particularly with single-case data, is sufficiently unorthodox and potentially open to type-one errors that it's probably better (and simpler) if we continue to use chi square as a two-tail test.

Chapter 10
Correlation and
regression

Introduction

So far, research design has been all about controlling variables. We do this in experiments by random assignment and by keeping a strict grip on procedure. In quasi-experiments we can't randomly assign, but we still try to keep variables under control. In correlational research the reverse applies. We want them to vary so that we can look at the relationships between them. Two methods are used: correlation and regression. Correlation is used to measure the relationship between variables and to discover if it is statistically significant. Regression lets us predict one variable from another. Simple correlation and regression look at relationships between pairs of variables. Multiple regression predicts one variable from lots of others.

Let's go back to our experiment with children who stammer. That some children were assigned to the untreated group was a concern. A less worrying approach might be to treat all the children and see if a relationship exists between how much therapy they receive and their improvement. In other words, we see if amount of therapy and improvement are correlated.

Suppose we have data on 20 children. A first step in correlation is to draw a scatterplot. We put the number of therapy sessions on the x axis and the amount of improvement on the y axis. This gives us an idea as to whether the variables are related. Figure 10.1 shows three possible scatterplots. In (i) there is no relationship. In (ii) improvement increases with therapy. The variables are positively correlated (their values increase or decrease together). This is the outcome we were hoping for because it seems to show that therapy worked. In (iii) improvement decreases as therapy increases. Here the variables are negatively (or inversely) correlated (one increases as the other decreases).

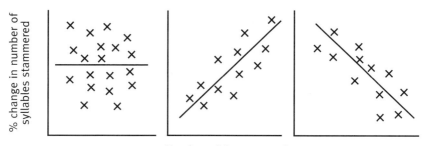

Number of therapy sessions

Figure 10.1 Different possible scatterplots of the relationship between sessions of therapy and improvement.

You have probably realized that there is a problem with correlation. We do not manipulate the IV (therapy); so confounding variables may affect the DV (improvement). We don't know why children got different amounts of therapy. Therapists might give more to children who they see improve (casually abandoning those who don't). Here therapy and improvement are positively correlated, but we can't conclude that therapy causes the improvement. Alternatively some children might make rapid progress and be quickly discharged; others who don't progress stay on to receive more treatment. This gives a negative correlation, which suggests that therapy isn't working. This shows that we have to be very careful when interpreting the results of correlational research. It also means that the correlational approach is rarely used to examine the effects of therapy.

In the scatterplots, I have drawn a line to indicate the trend of the data. In (i) it is horizontal because there is no trend. In (ii) it slopes upwards to the right, indicating that fluency increases with therapy. In (iii) it slopes downwards to the right, indicating that the change in fluency decreases with therapy. This line is handy because, if we know its mathematical formula, we can predict the change in fluency for a given amount of therapy. I have just drawn in the lines, but it's possible to get the formulae and make predictions. This is what regression does.

The scatterplots do not show a perfect relationship between the variables (all the points would be on a line where such a relationship exists). This is obviously reasonable. Changes in the children's fluency are affected by other variables as well. To assess the relationship we obtain the correlation coefficient. It's always between −1 and +1: −1 and +1 are perfect negative and perfect positive correlations respectively. Zero means there is no correlation. So we hope to find a figure as close to −1 or +1 as possible, depending on whether we want a negative or a positive correlation. We then test whether this correlation may have occurred by chance. We assess the probability of this and, if p < 0.05, we reject the null hypothesis. Correlation, like other statistical tests, comes in one- and two-tail versions. If we predict the direction of a correlation, we use a one-tail test; if we don't, we must use a two-tail test. As usual we decide this in advance. When no good theoretical reason exists for a directional hypothesis, we must use a two-tail test.

Exercise 10.1

Here are some examples of correlation. Would you expect a positive or negative correlation? Make sure you understand why there is a correlation in each case.

1. Yaruss et al. (2002) surveyed the opinions of people who stammer. One question asked them to rate the success of their therapy and the competence of the SLT conducting it. The paper reports the correlation between these ratings.
2. Moeller (2000) assessed the vocabulary of children with hearing loss on the Peabody Picture Vocabulary test (PPVT) when they were 5 years old. She correlated their PPVT scores with (a) their age when they began an intervention programme and (b) a rating of family involvement in the programme (high scores = good involvement).
3. Mimura et al. (1998) gave language assessments to people with aphasia following left hemisphere damage. They assessed them at 3 months and 9 months post-onset and looked at the correlation between their improvement and changes in cerebral blood flow (CBF) in the (a) left and (b) right hemispheres.

When can we use correlation?

Scatterplots are useful because they warn us about situations where correlation would be inappropriate or misleading. Correlation may only be used when variables are linearly related; so we use a scatterplot to check that this is the case. In Figure 10.2 the variables are related but the relationships are not linear and can't be assessed using correlation.

In correlational studies we want variables to vary. It's easy to see why. If the clinic in our dysfluency study had operated a totally egalitarian approach to therapy, it would have been impossible to

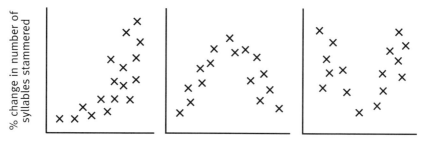

Number of therapy sessions

Figure 10.2 Some non-linear relationships between variables.

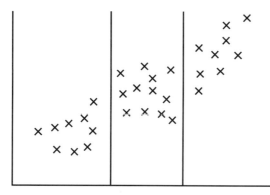

Figure 10.3 Why we need a wide range of values to calculate a correlation coefficient.

investigate whether the amount of therapy was related to progress. A less extreme version of this problem is shown in Figure 10.3. The data appear to show a fairly strong correlation, but, if we only have the data from the middle section, we are unlikely to find this out (the reverse, where we only have data from the two ends, is also misleading, but this tends to exaggerate the correlation).

Sometimes variables are only correlated in part of their range. Figure 10.4 shows data about children's ages and the size of their vocabulary. There is a correlation in the middle range of ages but not at the ends. Here we won't get a significant correlation if we use all the data but would if we use only the middle values.

I have repeatedly warned you about sifting through your data before deciding which bits to analyse and so you may feel that it's cheating to look at scatterplots. However, they are an exception. In Figure 10.4 the correlation coefficient would probably be non-significant and tell us little. The scatterplot gives us a picture of the relationship

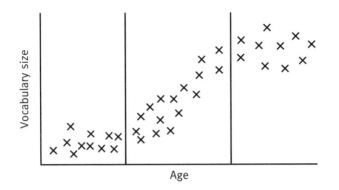

Figure 10.4 Data on vocabulary size in children of different ages.

between the variables. This is probably more important than the correlation anyway.

Outlying values (see Figure 10.5) are a problem. They may dramatically affect a correlation especially when we only have data on a few subjects. In (i) there is no correlation for the main group of subjects, but the outlier will increase the coefficient. In (ii) a strong relationship is spoilt by one subject. This problem may occur in clinical research where individuals sometimes produce eccentric scores. You will want to know who the extreme case is. This is acceptable if it helps you to understand what went on. However, it does not allow you to decide that the subject was odd and should be excluded (it's easy to find 'oddness' in any subject who is ruining data). Turfing troublesome subjects out of your study is against the rules. The best solution is to avoid using correlation with small numbers of subjects where outliers might strongly influence the outcome.

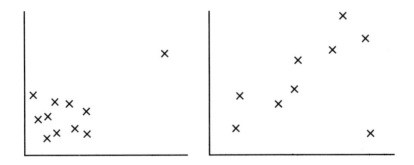

Figure 10.5 The effects of outliers on the correlation coefficient.

The Pearson product-moment correlation coefficient

The Pearson product-moment correlation is used with parametric data. The correlation coefficient, r, is found from the formula:

$$r = \frac{n\sum xy - (\sum x)(\sum y)}{\sqrt{(n\sum x^2 - (\sum x)^2)(n\sum y^2 - (\sum y)^2)}}$$

where x and y are the values of the variables and n the number of subjects.

Ma and Yiu (2001) designed an assessment of the problems faced by people with voice disorders. Voice impairments may be assessed by acoustic analyses. These do not tell us how much they affect clients' everyday life, however. The new assessment (the VAPP or Voice Activity and Participation Profile) quantifies the 'limitation of activities' and 'restriction in participation' (World Health Organization, 1999) due to voice disorders. Ma and Yiu used the Pearson product-moment correlation to examine the relationships between their assessment and acoustic measures. The assessment gives an overall rating by clients of the severity of their voice problem and an activity limitation score (ALS) and a participation restriction score (PRS). The ALS and PRS were significantly correlated with severity but unrelated to acoustic measures. This suggests that there is a dissociation between impairment (measured acoustically) and the disability and handicap that result. It also suggests that the VAPP may give clinicians a better indication of the treatment a client needs.

Table 10.1 gives made-up scores for 10 clients. Answers were given by indicating a point on a 10 cm visual analogue scale (see Chapter 11). To simplify the calculation I have given mean scores to the nearest centimetre. High scores indicate more severe problems. Table 10.1 lets us calculate the values needed for the formula. I have used them to calculate the correlation coefficient between rated severity and ALS.

Table 10.1 Made-up scores for 10 subjects doing the VAPP

	Rated severity (x)	ALS (y)	PRS	xy	x^2	y^2
Client 1	4	8	3	32	16	64
Client 2	2	5	3	10	4	25
Client 3	8	6	8	48	64	36
Client 4	3	2	7	6	9	4
Client 5	4	6	7	24	16	36
Client 6	9	7	8	63	81	49
Client 7	8	9	6	72	64	81
Client 8	3	6	4	18	9	36
Client 9	9	10	8	90	81	100
Client 10	5	8	7	40	25	64
	55	67	61	403	369	495

$$r = \frac{n\sum xy - (\sum x)(\sum y)}{\sqrt{(n\sum x^2 - (\sum x)^2)(n\sum y^2 - (\sum x)^2)}} = \frac{10 \times 403 - 55 \times 67}{(10 \times 369 - 55^2)(10 \times 495 - 67^2)}$$

$$r = \frac{4030 - 3685}{\sqrt{(3690 - 3025)(4950 - 4489)}} = \frac{345}{\sqrt{665 \times 461}} = 0.623$$

The tables for the Pearson product-moment correlation (Appendix 9) give the required values of r for different levels of significance and for one- or two-tail tests. The degrees of freedom for the Pearson test are $n - 2$. Looking in the tables for 8 d.f., we find the values 0.549 for a one-tail test and 0.632 for a two-tail test at the $p < 0.05$ level of significance. Since activity limitation would be expected to increase with severity, a one-tail test is appropriate here, and the result is just significant. It is not significant for a two-tail test.

Exercise 10.2

Find out whether rated severity and the PRS scores in Table 10.1 are significantly correlated.

*Where did the correlation formula come from?

On the basis that when you have to take some nasty medicine it's better to know what it is, we should know where the Pearson correlation formula comes from. Correlation is based on covariance where the covariance of x and y is:

$$\frac{\sum (x - \bar{x})(y - \bar{y})}{n - 1}$$

Notice that this is similar to the formula for the variance itself. The variance of x is:

$$\frac{\sum (x - \bar{x})^2}{n - 1}$$

The difference is that we multiply pairs of differences of x and y from their means rather than squaring the differences of x from its mean.

This gives us a measure of whether x and y co-vary. If they are positively related subjects who are above the mean on x, they should be above the mean on y. The same applies for values below the mean. The covariance formula will give a positive value because, most of the time, we are multiplying either two positive or two negative numbers. When x and y are inversely related, subjects will be above the mean on one and below the mean on the other. Here positive and negative values are multiplied and the formula will give a negative value. If values of x and y are unrelated, they will be randomly arranged around their respective means. The formula will be made up of random positive and negative values and will sum to somewhere near zero.

So far so good. However, covariance will vary with the units used to measure x and y. To overcome this we standardize the differences between x and y and their means by dividing by the standard deviations of x and y. The result is r, the correlation coefficient.

$$r = \frac{\text{The covariance of } x \text{ and } y}{\text{std. dev. of } x \times \text{std. dev. of } y}$$

$$\text{so } r = \cfrac{\cfrac{\sum(x - \bar{x})(y - \bar{y})}{n - 1}}{\sqrt{\cfrac{\sum(x - \bar{x})^2}{n - 1} \times \cfrac{\sum(y - \bar{y})^2}{n - 1}}} \qquad \text{or } r = \cfrac{\sum(x - \bar{x})(y - \bar{y})}{\sqrt{\sum(x - \bar{x})^2(y - \bar{y})^2}}$$

As we changed the formula for variance from the defining to the computational version (which was easier to work out), so we can change (by a bit of mathematical wand waving) the formula for the correlation coefficient to:

$$r = \frac{n\sum xy - \left(\sum x\right)\left(\sum y\right)}{\sqrt{\left(n\sum x^2 - \left(\sum x\right)^2\right)\left(n\sum y^2 - \left(\sum y\right)^2\right)}}$$

Exercise 10.3

Suppose we want to compare estimates of children's language ability by parents and teachers. We ask them to do a language assessment in which they predict the performance of the children. We can now compare the scores of parents and teachers using a t-test. We could also look at the correlation between their scores. What might you conclude if both, one or neither is significant?

Interpreting a correlation coefficient

We have already seen that a fatal error in interpreting correlation is to assume that one variable causes changes in the other. This issue is so important that it's worth having another example of the problem. There is a lot of evidence that children with language disorders also have social and emotional problems (see Botting and Conti Ramsden, 2000). Suppose we find a sample of children at risk for language disorder and give them a language assessment and a test of socio-emotional problems and find that the scores are correlated. Does this mean that one causes the other? A plausible case may be made in either direction. Language problems may lead to peer rejection and academic failure resulting in socio-emotional problems. Alternatively the presence of social and emotional difficulties may restrict opportunities for language development. A third possibility is that both result from a common neurological problem. Each explanation is possible but none are proven by correlation.

If we cannot make statements about causation from correlation, what can we conclude? In Exercise 10.2 there was a significant correlation of 0.686 between rated severity and PRS scores. This is a strong correlation, but it is some way short of perfect (which would be $r = 1$). The size of r needed for a significant result decreases as the number of subjects increases. With 30 subjects, the value of r for a one-tail test is only 0.306. So what can we conclude from a significant correlation of only 0.306?

In the scatterplot of a perfect correlation all the subjects are on a straight line. As the points on the diagram spread out around the line, so the correlation coefficient decreases. This dispersion of the points is due to the influence of other variables. In our example on therapy and dysfluency, a correlation of 0.306 with 30 clients means that improvement was related to therapy but that other variables had a strong influence as well.

We can find out how much variation in improvement is due to therapy by squaring the correlation coefficient (r^2 – some books call this the coefficient of determination). This is the proportion of the variance in improvement accounted for by the amount of therapy given. For a correlation of 0.306 it is 0.093. So only 9.3% of the variance is accounted for by therapy; the other 90.7% is due to other variables. If nothing else this should stop us getting too carried away by significant correlations. That the result is significant is important, but we must remember that other variables still account for most of the variance. Notice that I said that 9.3% of the variance was 'accounted for' by therapy. It's very easy to become confused here. Books use different phrases ('accounted for', 'explained by' and, when we use regression, 'predicted by'). The one thing we should not say is 'caused by'.

The Spearman rank-order correlation coefficient

Just as there were parametric and non-parametric tests for comparing groups of scores, so there are parametric and non-parametric correlation coefficients. The Spearman rank-order correlation coefficient is used with data that do not meet the demands of parametric tests. Like other non-parametric tests, it ranks the data. In some circumstances this can be quite useful. For example, the Spearman coefficient is less affected by outliers than is the Pearson test. To do the test we must rank each set of scores separately starting with the lowest score (we first rank the rated severity scores, then the ALS scores). Ties, as usual, are given the mean of the ranks that they would have received. Next we calculate D, the differences in each pair of ranks and square and add them to obtain $\sum D^2$. In Table 10.2 these calculations are carried out on the rated severity and ALS scores from above.

Table 10.2 Scores and calculations for the Spearman correlation coefficient

	Rated severity (x)	ALS (y)	rank of x	rank of y	D	D²
Client 1	4	8	4.5	7.5	-3	9
Client 2	2	5	1	2	-1	1
Client 3	8	6	7.5	4	3.5	12.25
Client 4	3	2	2.5	1	1.5	2.25
Client 5	4	6	4.5	4	0.5	0.25
Client 6	9	7	9.5	6	3.5	12.25
Client 7	8	9	7.5	9	-1.5	2.25
Client 8	3	6	2.5	4	-1.5	2.25
Client 9	9	10	9.5	10	-0.5	0.25
Client 10	5	8	6	7.5	-1.5	2.25
						$\sum D^2 = 44$

We now use the formula $r = 1 - \dfrac{6\sum D^2}{N(N^2 - 1)}$

to calculate the correlation coefficient.

$$r = 1 - \frac{6\sum D^2}{N(N^2 - 1)} = 1 - \frac{6 \times 44}{100(100 - 1)} = 1 - \frac{264}{900} = 0.733$$

Then we look up the table value (Appendix 10) of r for N, the number of subjects and for a one- or two-tail test.

Regression

Suppose there is a significant correlation between therapy and increased fluency. We can use this relationship to make predictions; here, we ask how much improvement we expect to see if we gave a child a particular amount of therapy.

This is what regression does. It calculates a formula (the regression equation) to predict one variable from the other. It does this by drawing a line through the points on the scatterplot. In Figure 10.1 I drew these lines in a rough-and-ready way; regression does it mathematically. It uses the formula for a straight line, which takes the form $y = a + bx$. The formula predicts y (the amount of improvement) from x (the number of sessions). Regression uses the data to obtain the values of a and b that give the best estimate of y. In other words it calculates the formula of the line that best 'fits' the points on our scatterplot. In case you have forgotten, a is the value of the intercept (the point where the line cuts the y axis, where $x = 0$) and b is the slope of the line (also called the regression coefficient).

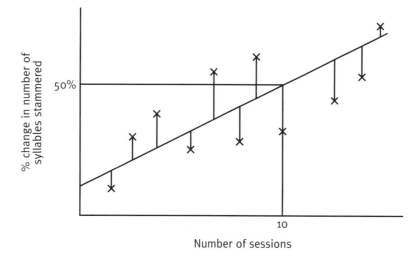

Figure 10.6 The method of least squares regression.

Figure 10.6 shows some points on a scatter plot and a regression line. To show how the regression line predicts improvement I have marked in the prediction for 10 therapy sessions, which is a 50% improvement. As you can see one child did have 10 sessions but didn't manage a 50% improvement. This will happen as long as the relationship between the two variables is less than perfect. In fact, none of the points on the scatterplot is actually on the regression line. Each subject has both a true score (y) and a score (y') predicted by the regression formula. The regression line is calculated by minimizing the differences between actual and predicted scores ($y - y'$) (these differences are called residuals). Some differences are positive and some negative, which gives statisticians an excuse to square them. So we obtain the regression line by minimizing the squares of these differences, and the method is called the 'method of least squares'.

You may think this has not taken us very far. As non-mathematicians we could spend a long time staring into space and be no nearer to knowing how to minimize the squares of these differences! It turns out to be easy, however, and, if we have worked out the correlation coefficient, we already have the information we need. The best-fitting line occurs when:

$$b = \frac{n\sum xy - (\sum x)(\sum y)}{n\sum x^2 - (\sum x)^2}$$

This gives us b; now we need a. Fortunately the regression line is quite accommodating here. It always passes through the point on the graph that represents the means of x and y. So we can put into the formula our value of b and the means of x and y and solve it to find a.

Exercise 10.4

Work out the regression equation that predicts ALS from rated severity in the data in Table 10.1.

In the example above we used the regression equation to predict improvement from a given number of therapy sessions. For any two correlated variables there are two regression equations each predicting one variable from the other. This sounds rather complicated but we need not worry about it. In practice we normally know one variable (x) and want to predict the other (y); so it is obvious which equation we need. All this talk of predicting one variable from another makes it very easy to believe that the known variable is causing the change in the other variable. The answer is still the same on this one. It might be, but we have not proved this.

Before we continue, it's worth sorting out our terminology. When we use regression we are trying to predict one variable from another or, in the case of multiple regression, from several others. Traditionally books have called these 'predicted' and 'predictor' variables. More recently they have started to call them 'dependent' (DV) and 'independent variables' (IV). I am going to use the latter terminology, which is similar to that used in experiments. We have to remember, however, that here the independent variables are not manipulated.

Our example of regression above is a rather unlikely one. There probably is a relationship between the amount of therapy and changes in dysfluency, but the variability in children's responses to therapy means that it is unlikely to be a strong one. The day when clinicians consult a regression equation to decide how much treatment to give may be some way off (but, before you heave a sigh of relief, have a look at Jacoby et al., 2002). So let's look at an example from the literature on specific language impairment (SLI). It's an unusual example but one that illustrates nicely how the regression equation works. It uses regression to try to unravel a theoretical issue about SLI.

Experiments have compared the reaction times (RTs) of children with SLI and typically developing children. Suppose we ask them to do different reaction-time tasks. As the tasks get more difficult the RTs of both groups will increase. Figure 10.7 shows three possible relationships between the mean RTs of the groups on different tasks. The means of typically developing children are on the x axis and those of children with SLI on the y axis.

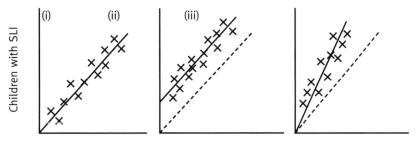

Figure 10.7 Three possible regression lines for the relationship between the RTs of typically developing children and children with SLI.

Each scatterplot shows a strong correlation between the reaction times (the points are tightly clustered around the regression line). As a result the value of r^2 will be large and the RTs of either group should be highly predictable from those of the other. In the regression equation $y = a + bx$, y is the RT of children with SLI and x the RT of typically developing children. In scatterplot (i) the two groups have similar RTs, which increase equally with task difficulty. As a result the regression equation reduces to $y = x$. The intercept (a) is 0 and the slope of the regression line (*b*) is 1 (here both variables are measured in the same units so an equal change gives *b* the value 1). The other scatterplots show situations where children with SLI are slower than typically developing children. In (ii) they are slower by a fixed amount. The regression line is parallel to the original one (shown on the scatterplot). It has a slope of 1 and cuts the y axis above 0. The regression equation here is $y = a + x$. In (iii) they are slower by an amount that increases with task difficulty. The regression line is steeper than the original (again shown) and $b > 1$. The intercept is 0; so the regression equation is $y = bx$.

We can now use RT data to find the actual regression equation. In this example the intercept value, a, is a purely mathematical quantity (because an RT of 0 is not possible). Nevertheless, the value of a (and whether it is greater than 0) and of b (and whether it is greater than 1) will let us decide which of the relationships in Figure 10.7 is correct.

Research findings have favoured the third outcome in Figure 10.7. This is consistent with the 'generalized slowing' hypothesis (Kail, 1994). It proposes that RT tasks are made up of different processing subtasks, all of which are affected in SLI. As task demands increase more subtasks are required. Reaction times increase for all children, and an increasing disadvantage is seen for the group with SLI. Several studies (Kail, 1994; Windsor and Hwang, 1999; Miller et al., 2001) have confirmed the hypothesis. Very high correlations exist between the RTs of the two groups, and over 90% of the variance in RTs in SLI can be predicted from the RTs of typically developing children ($r^2 > 0.9$). In their regression equation, Miller et al. found that a did not differ significantly from 0 and that b was significantly greater than 1 as expected from the hypothesis and shown in Figure 10.7 (iii). This was true for both verbal and non-verbal RT tasks, despite the fact that the children had similar non-verbal IQs. Children with general learning deficits were also tested. The slowing effect was stronger for these children as shown by a higher value of b in their regression equation.

Partial correlation

Two things about correlation and regression may be irritating you. The first, as I keep reminding you, is that we can't conclude that because two variables are correlated one causes a change in the other. The second is related to this. Correlation is used to show that two variables picked out of a complex situation are related. We are bound to wonder about the other variables, however. Suppose we find a significant negative correlation between age and language recovery after a stroke. The older clients are, the poorer their recovery. Other variables obviously influence recovery. The severity of the stroke is likely to be one, and it may be correlated with age as well. Other variables – therapy, the client's motivation, the support they receive from carers – affect recovery and may all be correlated with one another. Sometimes researchers measure many variables and report the correlations between all of them. This may not be very helpful. Typically it only manages to show that most of them are significantly correlated with one another.

So we are back where we often find ourselves in the behavioural sciences: struggling to understand a complicated situation. As you might have guessed, it's going to take some statistical wizardry to make much progress. First, let's look at partial correlation. Suppose we want to know whether age and recovery are related but realize that severity will confuse the relationship. Partial correlation allows us to calculate the correlation between age and recovery removing the effect of severity (sometimes called partialling out or statistically controlling the effect of severity). It is a useful technique in its own right and is important for the role it plays in multiple regression, which is covered in the next section.

Venn diagrams provide a useful way of describing relationships between variables (even if they do evoke unhappy memories of mathematics teachers). In Figure 10.8 (i) the circles represent the variance in recovery and age. The overlap in the two circles is the amount of variance in recovery accounted for by age. The remainder of the recovery circle is variance accounted for by other variables. In Figure 10.8 (ii) severity is added to the diagram. It also accounts for some variance in recovery. In this diagram age and severity account for independent parts of the variance in recovery, and the total amount of variance explained is their sum. If the world worked like this, life would be much easier (and multiple regression would be a cinch). In fact, age and severity are likely to be correlated with one another as shown in Figure 10.8 (iii). Now part of the variance in recovery is shared between them, and the total variance accounted for is less than the sum of their parts.

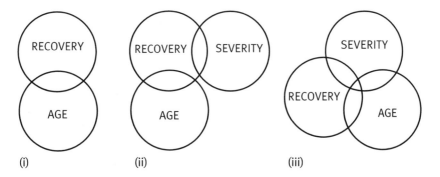

Figure 10.8 Venn diagrams of the relationship between age, recovery and severity.

Partial correlation lets us examine the relationship between age and recovery with the effect of severity removed. The partial correlation of Y with X_1 with X_2 controlled is indicated by $r_{y1.2}$ and is obtained from the formula:

$$r_{y1.2} = \frac{r_{y1} - (r_{12} \times r_{y2})}{\sqrt{(1 - r_{12}^2) \times (1 - r_{y2}^2)}}$$

where r_{y1} and r_{y2} are the correlations between Y and X_1 and X_2 and r_{12} is the correlation between X_1 and X_2. In the example above let the correlations of age and severity with recovery be 0.50 and 0.40 and the correlation of age and severity be 0.60. The working-out of the partial correlation of age and recovery is shown below. Its significance can be looked up in the Pearson tables (Appendix 9). Here we use $n - 3$ d.f.

$$r_{y1.2} = \frac{r_{y1} - (r_{12} \times r_{y2})}{\sqrt{(1 - r_{12}^2) \times (1 - r_{y2}^2)}} = \frac{0.50 - (0.60 \times 0.40)}{\sqrt{(1 - 0.60^2) \times (1 - 0.40^2)}} = \frac{0.26}{\sqrt{0.74 \times 0.84}} = 0.33$$

This formula lets us calculate the partial correlation between two variables removing the effect of a third. When the effect of one variable is removed, the correlation is called a first-order partial correlation. The effects of more than one variable may be removed. When two are removed, the correlation is a second-order partial correlation, and so on. In this terminology the correlation between two variables is called the zero-order correlation or bivariate correlation.

As you would expect, the partial correlation is smaller than the original correlation of age and recovery. This can be seen in Figure 10.9, which reproduces Figure 10.8 (iii) in a general form. Here X_1 and X_2 are the IVs (age and severity) and Y is the DV (recovery). The zero-order correlation is represented by the overlap between the circles Y and X_1. The variance accounted for is $(a + b)$ and the proportion of variance accounted for is $(a + b)/(a + b + c + d)$. When we calculate the partial correlation of Y and X_1, we remove the variance accounted for by X_2. X_1 now accounts only for a. As a proportion of the variance in Y that remains after the effect of X_2 is removed, this is $a/(a + d)$. Although we won't bother calculating it, we can also work out $a/(a + b + c + d)$. This is the proportion of the total variance in Y that is accounted for by X_1. This is needed in multiple regression and is called the semi-partial (or part) correlation of Y and X_1.

Partial correlation is often used in studies of child development to remove effects of age or IQ. Suppose that we want to see if phonological awareness helps children learn to read. We measure phonological

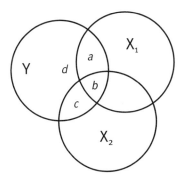

Figure 10.9 Venn diagram of the relationship between X_1 and X_2 and Y.

awareness and a year later assess reading and find that they are correlated. An obvious confounding variable is the children's general
cognitive ability. Smart kids are likely to be good at phonological
awareness and reading. Here partial correlation can be used to
remove the effect of general ability and to see if a significant correlation remains. This does not establish a causal relationship (other variables remain), but it rules out one alternative explanation. Of course,
we can approach this particular problem experimentally by looking
at the effects of training in phonological awareness. Children are
randomly assigned to groups who do or do not get training. Here the
IV (training) is manipulated. Studies of this kind have shown that
training leads to better progress in reading (Bradley and Bryant,
1983; Hatcher et al., 1994).

Kay-Raining Bird et al. (2000) used this approach to study phonological awareness and reading in children with Down syndrome.
There is disagreement whether reading difficulty in Down syndrome
is a direct result of poor phonological awareness or whether the children are forced to learn by some other non-phonological means
(Cossu et al., 1993). Kay-Raining Bird et al. assessed phonological
awareness and reading over 4 years and 6 months. Reading
progressed more than phonological skills, suggesting that the children were using other strategies. Nevertheless, phonological ability
and reading were related after the effects of age and mental age (the
children varied widely on both) were removed. This suggests that
phonological-awareness training may still help their reading.

*Multiple regression

Multiple regression is a complicated statistical technique. If you want
a full account of its mysteries, you will need to consult one of the
'big books'. No one does multiple regression without a computer; so

books base their accounts around examples of printouts from statistical packages. Here I will describe what multiple regression does with the help of a few examples.

In the last section I suggested that there was a correlation of 0.50 between age and recovery after a stroke. Although a high correlation, the proportion of variance accounted for (r^2) is only 25%. We also saw above that a correlation can be significant without accounting for much variance. This is often the case (our example on RTs in children with SLI was unusual here) and explains why simple regression is not used much. Age and recovery may be correlated, but we won't get far predicting recovery from age alone. We can obtain a better prediction by including other variables. This is what multiple regression does, and it is very popular as a result. We can use it to predict a DV from several IVs and to find out how much variance each IV accounts for. In addition multiple regression is very accommodating and allows us to include categorical variables (for example gender or social class) among the IVs. On the negative side, it does require that the data meet a number of assumptions. I will just mention the most immediately relevant of these (the others are in the 'big books'). Multiple regression requires a lot of data. Typically books recommend that we should have between 10 and 15 subjects per IV.

Multiple regression calculates a regression equation for us. The equation takes the form:

$$y = a + b_1x_1 + b_2x_2 + b_3x_3 + \text{.......} + b_nx_n$$

Here there are several IVs (the formula allows for any number up to n), and we can predict the value of y if we know the values of b (the regression coefficients) and a. The regression coefficients can be positive or negative and can vary substantially in size. The last point is confusing because it seems reasonable that the importance of an IV should be reflected in the size of its regression coefficient. This is not the case. Independent variables are measured in different units, and changes in some will be numerically much larger than in others. To clarify this an alternative version of the regression equation is often used. In this the IVs are standardized (transformed so their means = 0 and their standard deviations = 1). The formula is called the standardized regression formula. It is:

$$y = \beta_1x_1 + \beta_2x_2 + \beta_3x_3 + \text{.......} + \beta_nx_n$$

When variables are standardized, the regression equation has no intercept with the y axis so a drops out of the equation. The regression coefficients are replaced by standardized regression coefficients indicated by β (sometimes called β weights). Computer programs give us both versions of the regression formula. The latter has the advantage that it gives a more immediate impression of the importance of the IVs.

Multiple regression gives us R, the multiple correlation coefficient. This is the correlation between y and all the IVs. It finds R by correlating the actual values of the DV with those predicted by the equation. If the prediction is good there will be little difference between these and the multiple correlation coefficient will be large. R only takes values between 0 and 1 (but individual IVs may be positively or negatively correlated with y).

R^2 is the proportion of variance accounted for. Unfortunately R^2 is a biased estimate and must be adjusted downwards. Computer programs give an adjusted value (called adjusted R^2 or shrunken R^2). They also give the significance of R^2. You may be surprised to find that they do this by calculating an F-ratio of the explained variance divided by the unexplained or error variance (this is because, somewhere beyond our comprehension, ANOVA and multiple regression are all tangled up in a vast mathematical conspiracy). The formula for this is:

$$F = \frac{\dfrac{R^2}{k}}{\dfrac{(1 - R^2)}{(n - k - 1)}}$$

where n = number of subjects and k = number of predictor variables.

Suppose we want to study the language of children with cochlear implants. This is not an experimental situation. We can't fool around randomly assigning children to 'implants' or 'no implants'; in fact, we can't even control when they have their implant or what happens to them afterwards. We can assess their language ability (say at 5 years of age) and collect data on variables such as age at implant, how long they have had it, the training they receive and measures of their cognitive abilities, social background and parental involvement. Then we can use multiple regression to see how well these IVs predict language at 5 years (the DV).

We need a regression equation that includes variables that are good predictors. We could put all the IVs into the analysis at once, but it's more likely that we will 'develop' the equation by putting in and, sometimes, taking out IVs in turn. Suppose we put in the variables we expect to be good predictors. The analysis gives us R^2 and tells us whether it is significant. If R^2 is not very large, we can include further IVs. This will result in a new regression equation and a potential increase in R^2. Look at Figure 10.9 again. X_1 predicts part of the variance in Y ($a + b$). X_2 also predicts part of the variance ($b + c$). Together they predict ($a + b + c$) (the zero correlation of X_1 and Y squared plus the semi-partial correlation of X_2 and Y squared). It's worth including X_2 in the regression equation if the extra variance explained (c) is significant. Multiple regression tells us whether it is. This lets us identify the variables that give the best prediction. Frequently one or two IVs make a big contribution, and adding further ones makes little difference.

The amount of variance accounted for by our IVs may be disappointingly small. Variance that is not accounted for is due to unexplained individual differences (error variance). If our prediction is not good enough, it's up to us to discover further variables that will improve it. Practical considerations will play a part in this. Information on some variables is much more easily obtained than on others. We are likely to go for the best prediction we can get using readily obtained information.

It's not worth including an IV if it is highly correlated with another IV. This has a statistical name – multicollinearity. We can see why in Figure 10.9. If X_1 and X_2 are highly correlated, their circles will overlap substantially and they will account for more or less the same variance in Y. Multicollinearity should be avoided – first, because it's not going to improve our prediction and, second, because it gives computers a headache. To do so we look at the correlations between the IVs before doing a multiple regression analysis and only include one of any pair that are highly correlated (0.85 or above).

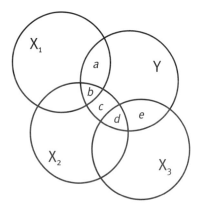

Figure 10.10 Venn diagram of the relationship of three IVs with Y.

Researchers are often more interested in which variables are good predictors than in the overall prediction (R^2). Our cochlear implant example illustrates this. Here we don't want to predict outcomes passively. We want to discover which IVs are associated with good outcomes so that we can improve practice with future clients. This isn't going to be easy, however. Look at Figure 10.10. Our Venn diagram now has three IVs. Each accounts for some variance in Y. Deciding on their relative importance is tricky, however. Do we judge them by their total contribution to R^2 or by their unique contribution (the part which is independent of other IVs). In Figure 10.10, the total contributions of the IVs are quite similar but their unique contributions differ. Their contributions will also depend on the order in which they are entered in the regression equation. Whichever goes in first will appear to account for more variance as it will 'claim' its shared variance with other IVs. The one that goes in last will only have its unique variance.

There are different approaches to this problem. In simultaneous or standard multiple regression all the variables are entered and each is assigned its unique variance. So X_1 is assigned a, X_2 is assigned c and X_3 is assigned e; b and d contribute to R^2 but are not attributed to an individual IV. This treats all IVs equally and evaluates their contributions independently of the other variables in the equation.

Hilari et al. (2003) used simultaneous multiple regression in a study of factors that contribute to quality of life in people with chronic aphasia. They adapted a quality-of-life measure to make it more appropriate for clients with communication problems. This was given to a large sample of people with dysphasia and their scores were used as the DV in the multiple regression. They then examined which other variables made significant unique contributions to the prediction of quality of life. Measures of communication disability, emotional distress, activity and the presence of other comorbid conditions all did so; measures of cognition, age and social support did not. The total predicted variance (R^2) was 52%.

Schmidt and Lawson (2002) used simultaneous multiple regression to analyse data on early communication between parents and very low birth weight children. They analysed videos of parents and children and looked at how much variance in verbal IQ at 3 years of age could be accounted for by different types of interaction. Not surprisingly, the children's ability at 2 years of age accounted for the largest part of the variance (42%). The level of parents' attention-focusing behaviours and of the child's shared attention each contributed smaller but unique and significant proportions of the variance (9% each), however.

Stepwise multiple regression enters IVs individually using the total amount of variance attributed to each to decide the order of entry. The IV with the largest total contribution is entered first. Other IVs are then entered according to their share of the remaining variance. In Figure 10.10, X_1 accounts for most variance and is entered first. It gets its unique variance and its shared variance with X_2 ($a + b$). X_3 now accounts for more of the remaining variance and is entered next. It gets ($d + e$). Finally X_2 is entered and gets c. Each IV is entered in turn, and the process stops when further IVs do not significantly increase R^2. The stepwise approach is used when the priority is prediction. It tells us which variables predict the DV, disregarding whether their contributions are unique or shared variance. Cannito et al. (1997) investigated spasmodic dysphonia. The presence of dysfluency in spasmodic dysphonia is controversial. Some authors believe it is a symptom of the dysphonia; others deny this. Cannito et al. found that clients were frequently but not invariably dysfluent and that dysfluency was not clearly related to the severity of the dysphonia. Listeners rated the severity of the dysfluency and stepwise multiple regression was used to investigate which variables predicted their ratings. The variables included several measures of fluency. By far the largest proportion of the variance (62%) was accounted for by the number of dysfluencies per 100 words. This figure includes variance shared with other measures of dysfluency, none of which entered the regression equation. Other significant IVs were speech rate and number of reading errors and these with the number of dysfluencies per hundred words accounted for 77% of the variance. The study concluded that dysfluency is not a defining feature of the disorder but features strongly in clinical judgements of it.

In hierarchical multiple regression the researcher decides the order in which variables are entered. As in stepwise regression, IVs entered first will be assigned more variance. In Figure 10.10 we might enter variables in the order X_1, X_2, X_3. Then X_1 will get ($a + b$), X_2 will get ($c + d$) and X_3 will get e. Hierarchical regression is used where the researcher has a particular reason – practical or theoretical – to enter variables in a predetermined order. It may be used in studies of child development where some variables take precedence over others because they occur earlier in development. Geers (2002), who conducted research similar to the example on cochlear implants above, divided her IVs into three groups, which were entered in turn reflecting their presumed order of influence on the children. The first group contained variables related to the individual children and their families and accounted for 20% of the variance in language scores. Variables related to the implants and to the children's education were then entered in turn adding 24% and 12% of the remaining variance.

It can also be used to 'control' or partial out the effects of variables. Knight et al. (1997) developed a measure called the Care Burden Scale to assess the effect caregiving has on personal, social and family life. Carers of people with multiple sclerosis completed the scale and other measures, and hierarchical multiple regression was used to see which affected the carer's quality of life. Client age, gender and years since diagnosis and the carers' work status were entered first because they were assumed to be independent of subsequent IVs. R^2 was not significant. Then measures of the distress caused by the illness, ability of the carer to cope and social support were entered. R^2 remained non-significant and only became so when the Carer Burden Score was entered. This suggests that the burden of caring has a stronger influence on carers' quality of life than either the distress of the illness itself or the support available to them. This approach might be used to assess the effects of therapy. Here we might enter other IVs that affect progress first and then see what remaining variance is accounted for by the therapy that clients received.

Bishop (2002) used a similar approach (proposed by DeFries and Fulker, 1985) to distinguish genetic and environmental influences on SLI in a twin study. Measures of phonological short-term memory (non-word repetition) and auditory processing were obtained, and regression was used to predict one twin's score from the other. Whether the twins were MZ (identical) or DZ (fraternal) was then entered in the analysis (a categorical variable coded as 1 or 0 in the data). An improvement in prediction is evidence of a genetic influence. Bishop found a genetic influence on short-term memory but not on auditory processing. This suggests that the two are separable deficits that may individually or in combination contribute to SLI.

Exercise 10.5

1. Blood et al. (2002) asked SLTs working in schools to complete a job satisfaction survey and used hierarchical multiple regression to find out which variables predicted job satisfaction. Thirty-six per cent of the total variance was accounted for, and the SLTs' job satisfaction was significantly associated with spending longer in their current job, having a small caseload and being older. Comment on the outcome of this study.
2. It has been suggested that people who are bilingual find it easier to learn a further language than people who are monolingual. Describe a way of investigating this using multiple regression.

Finally we look at logistic regression. Although this sounds like another member of the regression family tree, it is based upon a different mathematical approach. For our purposes the similarities between logistic and multiple regression are more important than the differences. In logistic regression we use several IVs to predict a DV, as in multiple regression. Here, however, the DV is a categorical variable, and we try to predict it with a series of IVs, which may be either continuous or categorical. Logistic regression is increasingly popular in SLT (and other health research) because we often want to predict dichotomous outcomes. Examples might be whether clients will respond well or poorly to therapy, whether children will become chronically dysfluent or not or whether language impairment can be predicted from earlier measures of a child's abilities. As in multiple regression, we may want to know whether a group of IVs accurately predict a DV or whether individual IVs are good predictors.

Earlier I suggested that clinical decisions were unlikely to be influenced by regression analysis. Here are two examples where logistic regression is banging on the clinic door. Jones et al. (2000) and Kingston et al. (2003) used it to predict how many sessions children require to become fluent with the Lidcombe program (see Chapter 15). Children who had successfully completed the programme were put into groups that required more or fewer than 10 sessions. Logistic regression was used to predict group membership. The children's initial severity was a significant and strong predictor of the number of sessions. Time since onset was a marginally significant predictor (surprisingly, longer times were associated with fewer sessions). Gender and the children's ages were unrelated to the number of sessions.

A study with even clearer relevance to clinical practice is that by Catts et al. (2001). They used logistic regression to predict reading problems in children from their performance on language assessments in kindergarten. Here the primary aim was prediction rather than the contributions of individual IVs. Consequently stepwise logistic regression was used. Tests of letter identification, phonological awareness, rapid naming and sentence imitation and the years of education received by the children's mothers were significant predictors. Catts et al. (2001) provide a regression equation to give the probability that a child will be more than one standard deviation below the mean in reading from these variables, and discuss its clinical application.

Chapter 11
Measurement

Introduction

You might have noticed that art galleries and museums are going in for increasingly smarter cafés these days. Clearly the public is finding culture hard work and needs to be rewarded with afternoon tea. As it's such an important attraction, it would be silly not to find out if the customers are satisfied. Last time I went, I was given a form with boxes marked 'excellent', 'good', 'fair' and 'poor' to rate the quality of the food and drink, value for money, service and cleanliness.

In this book I have written about how difficult it is to measure things like satisfaction with therapy, the stress of caring for people with communication problems or the quality of life of people with aphasia. So are they really any harder to measure than the quality of the bread pudding? The common element is that we want to measure people's attitudes, opinions and feelings. The usual way of doing this is to present people with a series of questions or statements about the thing we want to measure and have them indicate their level of agreement with them. Many tests like this exist, and a glance at the SLT literature shows that research is highly dependent on them. Suppose, for instance, that we want to assess the levels of stress that people experience. There are physiological measures of stress, but these are not very convenient if we want to monitor it over time and in everyday-life situations. Rating scales allow people to give us their own view of the stress they are experiencing. Blood et al. (1997) wanted to examine the relationship between stress and dysfluency. They used two measures of stress: the Social Readjustment Rating Scale (Holmes and Rahe, 1967), which measures overall life stress, and the Daily Stress Inventory (Brantley et al., 1987), which measures its daily fluctuations. They found no difference in life stress between people who were fluent and non-fluent, but there was a relationship between day-by-day levels of stress and dysfluency.

Obviously I have been misleading you about the difficulties of measurement. It's not difficult to devise measures of complicated things like stress; the problem is whether they are accurate or not. In this chapter we look at the design and use of tests and assessments. The study of tests is called psychometrics. I must confess that psychometrics is not the most fascinating part of the behavioural sciences. But it is important. If measures are not accurate, there is no point using them. Psychometrics consists of techniques for selecting test items, presenting them, standardizing tests and assessing reliability (do we get the same score when a test is re-administered?) and validity (does a test measure what it claims to measure?). I will concentrate on tests like those described above; however, much of the content of this chapter also applies to language assessments (especially the section on reliability and validity) and questionnaires (especially the sections on selecting and presenting items).

Selecting test items

The first step in devising a new test is to generate potential items. It's usually easy to think of the first few, but after this the going gets tougher. Suppose we are designing a measure of quality of life. We will want a test that is comprehensive and includes as many areas in which quality of life may be affected as possible. A test made up of items suggested by one or a few people is likely to be biased towards their view of what needs to be measured; so it's a good idea to consult as many people with knowledge of the area as possible. Clinicians working with a target group of clients, other experts and the clients themselves are all likely to be consulted. There is no set way of doing this. We might consult them individually or by using focus groups. We might ask them to generate items themselves or to approve of and find omissions in those already selected. Often, researchers do both, asking them to generate items and, later, to judge a first draft of the proposed measure.

Other tests can be a further source of items. This may seem an odd suggestion – if a test already exists, why do we need a new one? It's often the case, however, that tests need updating and improving. In these cases, individual items from older tests may still be useful. We may also want to develop an existing test for use with a special group of clients; here we may include items from the original test combining them with new specialized items.

A general feeling is that measures should be brief to make them easier to administer. This is particularly the case where clients with communication disorders find the test difficult to understand or where clients suffer from a loss of attention or fatigue. Two factors argue for longer tests, however. One is that brief measures may fail to cover all aspects of what is being measured. Here, brevity may be achieved but at the expense of reducing validity. In their discussion of questionnaire design Rust and Golombok (2000) suggested identifying all the relevant areas to be addressed and giving them weightings to reflect their importance within the test. We can then decide the total number of items the test will include and divide them accordingly. The other consideration is that longer tests are more reliable. All measurement involves some degree of error. By including more items in a test we help to average out the sources of error (much as we do by having more subjects in an experiment), and this makes the test more accurate.

A further concern in test construction is that a measure should look valid. It should look like it is testing the thing that it claims to test. Measures that achieve this are said to have content validity and face validity. Both are largely subjective. The use of experts in selecting items and in judging their suitability and the comprehensiveness of the test in general contribute to its content validity. Face validity concerns the general impression made by the test. It's likely that people will take tests more seriously if they make sense and ask questions that clearly acknowledge their needs and problems. It also helps if they have the impression that the researcher knows what he or she is doing. There are cases where we might want to conceal the purpose of a test and so sacrifice face validity. Tests of undesirable traits might need to disguise their purpose to prevent people from making more socially desirable responses. With any luck there will be few occasions where we need to do this in SLT research.

Care must be taken to make test items clear to those who are being tested. Items should be screened to make sure that they are not ambiguous, that the language used is clear and avoids jargon or technical vocabulary that will be unfamiliar to those doing the test. Streiner and Norman (1995) suggested that tests should not demand a reading level greater than 12. In the case of tests to assess clients with communication disorders further steps may be needed to ensure that they can comprehend and respond accurately to the items.

A search for test items is likely to produce more than are necessary for the intended length of the measure. We then need a means of choosing between items. The best procedure here is to give all the items to a large sample of the intended respondents and examine their responses. Some simple rules can help us eliminate items. At this early stage it's likely that we will have some items that are very similar. If clients confirm this impression by responding to them in the same way, some can be eliminated. All the items must discriminate between individuals. If everybody scores the same on an item, it cannot do this and should be eliminated. A rough guide is to only include items where between 20% and 80% of clients respond in the same way. Obvious instances of items that fail this rule are ones where people with high and low scores on the test overall respond in the same way.

A few items may be eliminated immediately by common-sense use of these rules, but to do the job properly we will need some statistics. First, however, we must distinguish two sorts of measures. Consider measures of quality of life again. Some give an overall score; others are divided into subsections and give separate scores for different areas of quality of life. In the former all the items are measuring essentially the same thing, and we expect scores for one item to be correlated with those for other items and with the overall scores on the test. Items that fail to do this are not measuring the same thing as the rest of the test.

One method of examining the reliability of a measure is to correlate the score from one half of its items with the other half. This is split-half reliability. (We look at this later). A high correlation shows that people are responding consistently to the two halves. A low one shows that either the items are dissimilar or that clients are responding erratically to them. In either case the test is unreliable. Many years ago statisticians came up with a more complicated way of doing this. Not content with one correlation, they decided to get the mean correlation of all the ways that a test could be split into two halves. This calculation does not sound like much fun. Two formulae are used. The Kuder–Richardson formula 20 (KR-20) (Kuder and Richardson, 1937) is used with dichotomous responses (yes/no, true/false). Cronbach's alpha (Cronbach, 1951) is used for items with more than two responses. Most measures have multiple responses, and so Cronbach's alpha is more widely used. Now take this process a step further. With the help of a computer, we can take each item out of a test in turn and calculate alpha for the remaining items. If alpha increases when an item is removed, it is out of line with the others and we can improve the test by removing it. If a test has subsections, we have to carry out the process for each subsection.

Test subsections may be created deliberately. Here the test designer deliberately identifies necessary subsections and selects items for each subsection. On other occasions, however, a test designer will generate a lot of items and then divide them into subsections statistically by analysing the responses to them. They do this with factor analysis, which sorts items into groups by looking at people's responses to them. Items with similar responses go into the same group. In effect we are detecting items that measure common factors and that form different subsections within the test. Here the statistics end and it is up to the test designer to identify what the factors are and to give sensible-sounding names to the subsections that result. This may not be as easy as it sounds.

This process serves two purposes. First, it improves the test by identifying different factors and giving users the opportunity to evaluate them separately. Second, it allows us to reduce the number of items. Candidates for deletion are items that don't belong in any subsection (but we may wonder if they are important and consider adding items to create a further subsection) and items in a subsection with more than its share that can stand losing a few.

The process of developing tests by throwing questions at people and factor analysing their responses dates from the early days of personality testing. Researchers had mixed motives here. They wanted to sort items into groups to develop the test. They also hoped that the personality traits revealed by the test would sort the people into groups too. Unfortunately (or not, depending on your point of view) factor analysis did not cooperate. Different researchers came up with different numbers of traits. Despite this setback, factor analysis and related techniques are useful in test development. For example, Deary et al. (1995) devised an assessment for globus pharyngis, a condition where clients complain that something is stuck in their throat but show no organic pathology. Analysis showed that the test revealed three factors. The condition may be psychosomatic and the role of SLTs is controversial; nevertheless, the test allows them to assess its severity and response to therapy. The same approach has been used with quality-of-life measures. Cella et al. (1996) devised a measure of quality of life in multiple sclerosis. Analysis identified six subtests. This sort of analysis also tells us the proportion of the variance accounted for by each factor. Hence it tells us which factors (subtests) contribute most to the overall measure.

As you may have concluded by now, the problems of creating new tests are sufficiently daunting that we will want to be sure that it is necessary before we start. Obviously this includes checking thoroughly to see whether anyone else has already created a similar test. Finding a test not only saves work but also means that data on other clients or on non-clinical controls may already be available for comparison with our own findings.

A related issue concerns the use of generic and specialist tests. Some tests are sufficiently general that they are used in many different health settings and with different client groups. These include measures of health status such as the SF-36 (Ware et al., 1993) and measures of psychological well-being, such as the Hospital Anxiety and Depression Scale (Zigmond and Snaith, 1983). The psychometric properties of such tests have been thoroughly investigated, and they are easily available. As a result they are widely used in many areas of research, including research by SLTs.

The comparison of generic and specialist tests is particularly relevant to the assessment of quality of life. Generic tests let us compare a client group with other groups. Wilson et al. (2002) used the SF-36 with clients with dysphonia. This allowed them to compare their clients with controls. They concluded that dysphonia had an adverse effect on quality of life and that clinicians should be aware of this when assessing and treating these clients. Generic measures are less satisfactory when specific disabilities affect particular aspects of quality of life. The failure of some tests to address the impact of communication problems on quality of life is a good example here. It is likely to diminish their accuracy and their face validity when used with clients with communication disorders. This has led to an increase in the availability of client-specific measures. In some areas researchers can now choose between competing measures, each claiming advantages over others.

Exercise 11.1

Consider how you might select items for:

1. a test of occupational stress among SLTs.
2. a test of the distress caused by having tinnitus.
3. a quality-of-life measure for people with multiple sclerosis.
4. a test of functional communication in aphasia.

Presentation

Having selected our test items, we must decide how to present them. The choice of methods is governed by personal taste, mythology and a little research evidence. The favourite is to use a Likert scale. Here we ask people to answer questions or indicate their agreement with statements, offering them several possible responses. There are a number of ways of getting their responses. Some are shown in Figure 11.1.

Perhaps the most common is a 5-point scale (i). Subjects are offered statements and indicate their level of agreement by ticking

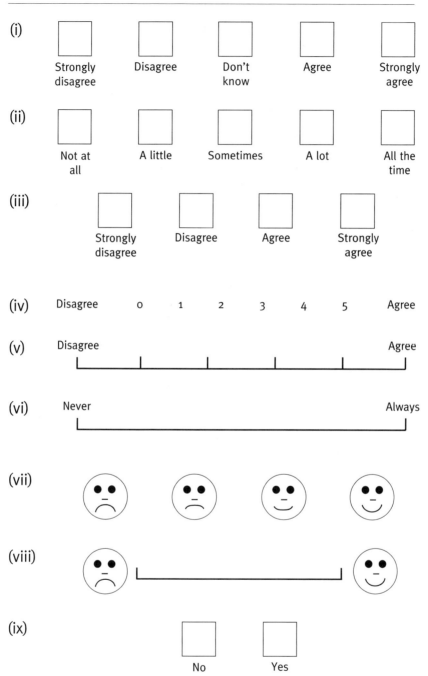

Figure 11.1 How to ask questions.

the appropriate box. Responses are then converted to numbers using a 1-5 (or 0-4) scale, and a total score for the test or for a subtest is obtained by adding across items. The verbal labels can be chosen to suit the form of question. Version (ii) might be used where clients are asked to indicate the extent to which they experience symptoms (see Wilson et al., 1991) or the extent of their handicap or loss due to illness or communication problems (see Cella et al., 1996).

It's easy to imagine that the form of the scale will effect people's responses. For instance, it's possible that people avoid using the 'strongly agree' and 'strongly disagree' categories opting for the milder 'agree'/'disagree' or that they avoid making a choice by opting for the middle 'don't know'. Streiner and Norman (1995) referred to the former as 'end aversion'. They suggested that it may be avoided either by not using such extreme terms for the end points or by increasing the number of categories on the scale but expecting the ends to be rarely used and disregarding them when they are (for example a 7-point scale becomes a 5-point one). The problem with either is that there will always be occasions when clients do want to use the extremes. Over use of the 'don't know' option can be avoided by using a 4-point scale with no midpoint as in (iii) (see Pound et al., 1993).

Five-point scales are popular, but more categories can be added. As they increase so may the problem of naming them and the suspicion that clients are losing track of what they mean anyway. In fact, there is evidence that the reliability of measures increases with the number of categories offered up to about seven. There is also evidence that the number of categories between which people can distinguish is pretty close to seven. All of this suggests that five categories is about right and that more than seven is probably not a good idea.

An easy let-off for the test designer is to use options like those in (iv) and (v). Here the end points are named but the respondent is left to sort out the categories in between (see Deary et al., 1995). Since the categories no longer need names, there may be a temptation to have a lot of them. Equally respondents may be tempted to make life easier for themselves by biasing responses towards the named end points.

The visual analogue scale (vi) has only named endpoints. Respondents indicate where they are on a line of fixed length (say 10 cm). This approach seems to be growing in popularity (see Stern et al., 1997; Ma and Yiu, 2001). Researchers may like it because it feels more precise. This may be a false impression, and its popularity may decline when the time comes to measure the responses. The use of visual analogue scales is sometimes adapted to measure change. Here clients are shown their responses before treatment and asked to indicate how much they think they have changed.

Smiling and frowning faces (vii and viii) may be used to facilitate responding by clients who have difficulty using standard Likert scales. They may be useful with children and clients with communication problems.

Typically measures of this kind are designed for completion by the client. This allows them to set their own pace and saves time. It may not be possible with some SLT clients, however.

In general it seems desirable that a measure should use the same form of presentation for all its items. This makes life easier for respondents, and any calculation of the overall test score is also easier and clearer. Likewise, it is best if subtests use the same method and have a similar number of questions. Neither is necessary, however, and should not be pursued to the detriment of the test generally. Some items obviously demand a particular form of response, most notably those that can only be answered yes/no or true/false (ix). Methods can be found for combining scores from different sorts of items and for comparing subtest scores. The SF-36 is an example of a test with a rather complicated presentation. It includes items with four- and six-category responses and yes/no responses. It has several subtests with different forms of presentation and numbers of items and requires a scoring algorithm to obtain an overall score. None of this appears to have affected its popularity!

Reliability and validity: an introduction

For those of us who sometimes confuse reliability and validity, a recent radio interview may be helpful. The interviewee, Denis, represented a company that was selling plots of land on the moon and could provide customers with a passport for travel to inspect this real estate. Denis, who was himself the ambassador to the Moon, a position with the title Head Cheese, was busy marketing a new product that revealed to buyers their alien genealogy. To cut a long story short, it was a test tube of powder that, when spat on, changed colour to reveal which part of the universe you came from. Denis claimed to be from the Pleiades. Just as the credibility of this story began to wane, Denis revealed a surprising knowledge of the psychometric properties desirable in such a test. It was reliable, he assured us, as he had carried it out several times with the same result, but he conceded that it was going to be hard work checking its validity. The tests we use in SLT have more practical, if more mundane, objectives. We still need them to be reliable and valid, however.

You may have noticed that correlation made an appearance in our discussion of item selection. Correlation is also used to measure test reliability and validity (but when used for reliability, it is called a reliability coefficient). We need to correlate performance on the test on different occasions or when used by different people to assess its reliability and with performance on other measures to test its validity. Two preliminary points should be made. The first concerns the test of correlation to be used. In Chapter 10 we used the Pearson and Spearman correlation coefficients for parametric and non-parametric data respectively. Most measures use rating scales, and so a Spearman correlation seems appropriate. In fact, Streiner and Norman (1995) suggested that the Pearson coefficient may be used and that it produces accurate results even when the data are not normally distributed. The second point concerns significance. As we saw in Chapter 10, quite low correlations are significant when, as is likely here, large numbers of subjects are employed. We need much higher correlations when assessing reliability and validity. Typically we want figures in excess of 0.8.

Reliability and validity are important in all forms of measurement. This includes measures of physical quantities. We overlook this because typical household equipment, such as clocks, scales and thermometers, are sufficiently accurate for their purpose. They are not adequate for scientific purposes, however. Here more precise instruments, are required and their reliability is essential. In the behavioural sciences we are accustomed to less accurate forms of measurement and issues about reliability and validity loom large. This applies to all the measures we use from formal language assessments down to counts of events (dysfluencies, eye contacts) in research data. In the former, reliability and validity have been assessed and are usually high. In the latter, we often have to assess reliability ourselves.

Measures of reliability

The most obvious way to assess reliability is to test people twice and compare their scores. This is test-retest reliability. There is an obvious problem with this method. It is unclear what interval should elapse between the two administrations of the test. If too short an interval is used, reliability may be overestimated because clients remember items and answer them in the same way. If too long an interval is used, clients may change and reliability will be underestimated. The interval can be judged, to some extent, by how rapidly clients are expected to change. Nevertheless, a lot of guesswork is involved. Despite these problems, test-retest data are important if they are available since they are the only direct measure of the stability of a test over time. Similar considerations may govern the use of a test. Some tests specify an interval between uses. This is to avoid clients remembering their previous responses and to allow time for change to occur (because test users want to detect change rather than measure reliability).

An alternative to test-retest reliability is parallel- or alternative-forms reliability. This capitalizes on the fact that some tests have alternative versions. If clients can stand doing both, we can correlate the scores and obtain a reliability coefficient. This may sound too good to be true. Given the effort to construct a test, it may seem unlikely that anyone will produce two versions. However, some tests do have alternative forms, usually because they recognize that users will want to assess change over short periods of time.

An adaptation of the parallel-form approach is split-half reliability. Here we correlate the score from one half of the test items with that from the other (typically we compare odd with even numbered items). This gives the reliability of half of the test rather than the reliability of the test as a whole. It underestimates the latter, as reliability increases with the number of items in the test. We can calculate the overall reliability (r) from the split-half reliability (x) with the formula

$$r = 2x/(1 + x)$$

As we have seen, use of the Kuder–Richardson formula 20 or Cronbach's alpha is an extension of split-half reliability. They help in the selection of items and estimate reliability by measuring the internal consistency of the test. They have become increasingly popular now that computers can perform the calculations.

It's also important that tests produce the same results when a clinician tests a client on separate occasions or when different clinicians test the same client. These are intra- and inter-tester/rater reliability. The former is assessed in test-retest reliability. The latter is difficult to test because it may involve the client repeating the test. Inter-rater reliability is particularly important in research studies that involve counts of behaviours or ratings by observers. Here we need to show that the data are reliable and do so by showing that different raters agree. We look at means of doing this in Chapter 13.

A reliability coefficient of 0.8 or more tells us that a test is reliable but does not tell us much about the accuracy of an individual score. As with all statistics, a client's score is our best estimate of their true score. But how accurate is it? We can gain an indication of this from the standard error of measurement (SEM). This is the standard deviation of the distribution of scores we would get if we kept repeating the assessment on the client. Of course, we are not going to do this. Not only would the client become bored but his or her scores would rapidly change anyway as he or she learned how to do the test! Fortunately we can calculate it from the reliability coefficient:

$$SEM = \sigma \times \sqrt{1 - r}$$

where σ is the standard deviation of scores on the test and r is the reliability coefficient. We can now calculate a confidence interval for a person's score on a test. Suppose the test has a reliability of 0.9 and converts raw scores to a scaled score with a standard deviation of 15 (as in the BPVS and the CELF-R). Then:

$$SEM = 15 \times \sqrt{1 - 0.9} = 4.74$$

This demonstrates that quite a large margin of error exists even in tests that are highly reliable. If someone scores 100 on the test, that person's 95% confidence interval is:

$$100 +/- 4.74 \times 1.96 = 90.7 \text{ to } 109.3$$

This may shock people who treat tests scores too seriously. I confess that it took me a long time to realize that they were as potentially inaccurate as this suggests. I suspect that many other test users are unaware of this even though some tests report their SEM and even give confidence intervals in their manuals. It means we should be cautious about thinking a client is as good or as bad as a test score suggests. It also means that we should think twice before claiming that clients have improved when we retest them and they produce a moderately higher score than before.

The SEM also has implications for research. It's common for scores on standardized tests to be used as criteria for including clients in research projects. Children with SLI, for example, are often required to score below a standard score on a language assessment and above it on a non-verbal assessment. This is done to show that the children differ on the two tests and, therefore, have a specific deficit. Confidence intervals, like the one above, question whether many of these children really differ on the tests. Use of a larger disparity in the criterion scores might make this claim more credible. Unfortunately it would also make finding children who meet the criteria more difficult.

In Chapter 4 I pointed out that we can only accurately use standardized tests if we follow the procedure used during standardization (and described in the test manuals). The same is true of reliability.

Reliability is tested on a particular sample of people, and the test is conducted in the standard manner by clinicians experienced in its use. The reliability of the test is only maintained if we use it in the same way. We should avoid testing clients for whom it was not designed and should (as always) follow the standard procedure. Tests are not designed for use by naive clinicians and, in some cases, may require training before they are used. In general reliability is assessed under optimal conditions. Even small departures from this may affect the reliability of tests in clinical use.

Measures of validity

We have seen that the first step in establishing the validity of a test is to examine its content. Content and face validity are not assessed statistically. They are established by a consensus among experts and users of the test that the designers have got it right. They are important but alone are insufficient to establish the validity of a test.

The main method of assessing the validity of a measure is to compare it with other measures of the same thing. This is criterion validity. You may guess that other measures are often, but not always, other tests. This raises again the issue of how a new test can be better than an older one if the older one plays an important part in its validation. Of course, it can be better in different ways. It might be more comprehensive or more modern in the things it tests and the language it uses. Leaving this issue aside, we would expect two tests of the same thing to be correlated. This correlation gives us a quantitative measure of the test's validity. Comparison of the test scores with currently available data is called concurrent validity. Here we give clients the test along with other tests and correlate the results. Predictive validity is used if a test predicts a future outcome that can be used to validate it. This form of validity is commonly used with tests of ability or aptitude or selection/screening tests. Accurate prediction of a later outcome is a convincing demonstration of validity but has the disadvantage that we may have to wait some time to get it.

Validation of a measure is often a cumulative process. Showing that scores on a new test correlate with those on an older one helps but hardly convinces. Typically test designers will assemble stronger evidence than this by showing that it correlates with several other measures. When a test has different subtests, each may be compared with different existing tests. Discriminant validity may also be used. Here we demonstrate that test scores correlate with some but not other measures. This helps to define precisely what the test is measuring. Good tests also gain validity through use. Practitioners find that they can trust them and that further data become available on their predictive validity.

When no obvious criterion is available for validation, we may resort to construct validity. Personality tests are, perhaps, the best examples of construct validity. A researcher may believe that a certain personality trait exists and design a test to measure it. Here the test is assessing a theory of personality; the theory may be controversial, and no other measure of the proposed trait may exist. Here validation is sought by using the test to identify people with and without the trait. Then we can create experimental tests to see if their behaviour is consistent with the predictions of the theory.

Exercise 11.2

Consider how you might assess the validity of tests to:

1. measure communication problems in dementia.
2. predict children's language from parental reports of their early (< 2) symbolic skills.
3. measure parents' attitudes to pre-school speech and language services.

Reliability and validity: some examples

Not all these forms of reliability and validity are likely to be used with any given test. The major standardized tests of language are as thoroughly assessed as any. The CELF-3 is a good example. Data on its reliability and validity were collected during the standardization process. In Chapter 4 we saw that it has 10 subtests, which are combined to give composite scores for receptive and expressive language and an overall language score. Cronbach's alpha was used to measure the internal consistency of each subscale and of the composite scores for each age of child tested. The reliabilities for the three composite scales are mainly in excess of 0.9.

Test-retest reliability was also assessed. Children at four ages were retested by the same clinician up to a month after their first assessment. Reliability coefficients are given for each subtest and composite score. Those for the total language score range from 0.86 to 0.94. The standardization procedure required two clinicians to mark each test. Most of the tests are objective and unlikely to result in disagreements between markers. Inter-rater reliability was examined, however, for those tests where marking was more subjective.

The CELF-3 was designed to include language skills that are 'well documented in the literature addressing language disorders'. This, and the extent of the consultation during its development from the CELF-R (see Chapter 4) contribute to its content validity.

Concurrent validity was tested by comparing scores on the CELF-3 and CELF-R at different ages for normally developing and language disordered children. Correlations for the composite scores ranged from 0.68 to 0.83. Scores on the CELF-3 and the WISC-III were also compared. As expected the tests are correlated and a stronger relationship exists with verbal IQ (0.75) than with non-verbal IQ (0.60). Predictive validity was also assessed. The test correctly identified 85% of a sample of children with a language disorder but only 57% of children without one. Finally construct validity was assessed by factor-analysing test scores. Although the test has separate subtest scores, its claim to measure general language ability was supported by showing that one dominant factor in the analysis accounted for 53% of the variance in scores.

Tests like the CELF are developed with commercial considerations in mind and with the expectation that they will be widely used. They need to conduct thorough reliability and validity studies. Other specialist measures may be investigated less thoroughly and with smaller samples of clients. An example of a well-investigated specialist measure is the VAPP (Ma and Yiu, 2001), which we met in Chapter 10. It was designed to assess the limitation of activities and restriction in participation (WHO, 1999) due to voice disorders. Cronbach's alpha was used to examine item consistency and the effects of removing items from the test. Internal consistency was 0.98 and all items were retained because none reduced this figure substantially. Test-retest reliability was 0.86. Validity was examined by correlating scores with another measure of voice handicap. We also saw that the scores for activity and participation were correlated with one another and with clients' rated severity of their voice disorder. None of these was significantly correlated with acoustic or perceptual measures, which assess the severity of their impairment. This confirmed the clinical view, endorsed by the WHO model, that personal and environmental factors influence activity and participation and divorce them from any direct relationship with impairment. These findings also add to the construct validity of the VAPP.

Traditionally clinicians have viewed parental reports of their children's language with suspicion. They are assumed to be inaccurate because parents are untrained in assessing language and less than objective in their judgements. Such reports would be valuable to clinicians, and so finding that they are valid would be useful. The

MacArthur Communicative Development Inventory is a means of obtaining clear data from parental reports. Parents are given lists of vocabulary and sentences and indicate whether their children use them. The validity of these reports can be assessed by correlating the data with measures taken in clinic. Studies of normally developing children (Dale, 1991), children with Down syndrome (Miller et al., 1995) and children with language impairment (Thal et al., 1999) have found evidence that the reports are valid.

Finally we should consider whether all tests must be reliable and valid. On the surface this seems a silly suggestion; after all, textbooks on psychometrics are adamant that they should be. The PALPA is an example of a test whose reliability and validity are unknown. So how does it get away with it? The issue has been discussed by Wertz (1996) and Kay et al. (1996). Let's look at its validity. Kay et al. ask us to consider the non-word reading test. Clearly it tests non-word reading. If we claim nothing more for it, then we need not test its validity. The picture-naming test is a more debatable example. There is no dispute that it measures picture naming. Does it also measure the difficulties that clients have finding words in conversation? It may do, but we would need to test the validity of this. In other words, validity is only necessary when a test claims to measure something more general than the skills required to complete the test itself. Most tests do claim to do this; PALPA, for the most part, does not.

Chapter 12
Asking questions

Introduction

In the next two chapters we look at ways of asking people about their behaviour and of observing them behaving. Longer accounts of these methods can be found in textbooks that deal with qualitative research (see, for example, Bowling 1997; Denscombe, 1998; Bryman, 2001; Robson, 2002). As I explained in Chapter 1, I am not fond of the habit of dividing research methodologies into quantitative and qualitative camps. There are two reasons for this. The first is that too many people become over-excited about the virtues (and vices) of each form of research. I suggested before that each is particularly good at investigating certain types of research questions. People who stick with one or the other may miss opportunities. It is important to put prejudices aside (something social scientists are supposed to be good at) and ask which is more appropriate for the research you want to do.

A second reason is that, in practice, it may be difficult to draw a line between the two approaches anyway. This difficulty is reflected in the next two chapters, which are not entirely about qualitative methods. Each follows the same approach, moving from more-to-less structured methods of doing research. In each, structure can be imposed by limiting the range of people's responses. We can ask them questions where they must choose from predetermined responses or use open-ended questions where they decide what is important. In observational studies we can define specific behaviours in advance and record how frequently or under what circumstances they occur. Alternatively we can just observe their behaviour – even join in with it – and try to make sense of it as we go along.

When to use a questionnaire and when to interview

The commonest ways of asking people about their behaviour are by questionnaire and by interview. Researchers' intuitions will usually tell them which method is better in a given situation. Several factors may influence the choice. One practical consideration concerns the number of people we want to talk to. Questionnaires can be sent to respondents, who can then usually complete them themselves. They are well suited to survey research where large numbers of people are contacted. Arndt and Healy (2001), for example, contacted 500 therapists in their survey on the extent and nature of language problems in children who are dysfluent. Postage costs should be borne in mind here and (as you will know if you have received unsolicited questionnaires yourself) there is the possibility that a lack of interest might combine with the form slipping down the back of the sofa to reduce the response rate. Poor response rates are common in survey research. We will come back to them later.

Interviews are used when we want to allow respondents to express their feelings in greater detail. Here we may want to vary the questions for different individuals, responding to their previous answers and encouraging them to give further information. It's possible to interview people by telephone, but this runs counter to the spirit of getting close to them and discovering more about them. Consequently researchers prefer to interview face to face. This might involve travel, and the interviews themselves are often time-consuming. All of which suggests that a relatively small number of people will be involved. In the study by Roulestone (2001), which examined how therapists select children for therapy, 11 SLTs provided most of the data, and Yorkston et al.'s (2001) study of the experiences of people with multiple sclerosis was based on inter-views with just seven clients.

The numbers of people to be contacted, therefore, is a consider-ation in the choice of method. This is not, in case you are wonder-ing, a matter of laziness on the part of the researcher – if anything, a small number of interviews and the analysis of the data they produce are harder work than a survey – it's about the objectives of the research. Surveys are versatile. They can collect facts about the respondents, measure their opinions and attitudes or ask them to do tests and assessments such as those described in Chapter 11. Surveys have been used in SLT research to consult therapists about their clinical practices and clients about their experiences of ther-apy. They might be conducted or sponsored by the government to assess the implementation of policy (see, for example, Lindsay et al., 2002b, on SLT provision in educational settings). More often they look at particular types of clients or therapies. Culton and Gershwin (1998) asked therapists about practices in laryngectomy; Parkinson and Rae (1996) asked about their use of counselling, and Winter (1999) asked about provision for bilingual children. Clients are also surveyed. Hayhow et al. (2002) asked adults who stammer about its effects on their lives and their experiences of therapy, while Iversen-Thoburn and Hayden (2000) asked people with laryngectomies about their use of esophageal speech, and Kersten et al. (2002) surveyed young people with stroke about their needs. In such cases the populations may be quite small (see Boyd and Hewlett's 2001 study of male speech therapists for an extreme example!), and the sample may be representative of them. In contrast, interviews with small numbers of people are unlikely to be representative of the population. Interviewers rarely intend that they should be, however. Their objectives are normally to understand the experiences of those interviewed rather than to collect data that is strictly representative of the populations to which they belong.

A further issue concerns the use of open or closed questions. The former encourage respondents to think about and discuss their answers; the latter restrict them to giving short responses or ticking boxes. Questionnaires tend to use closed questions to collect specific information. Closed questions are easier for the respondent to understand and are likely to produce clear answers (particularly if a multiple-choice format is used). Respondents normally fill in questionnaires themselves, and so the latter is an important consideration. Having said this, it's hard to resist the temptation to ask respondents to 'explain your answer' or to 'add further comments'. A problem here is that responses may vary. Respondents may say little or nothing or ramble on for pages. They may misunderstand the question or decide that the questionnaire is hard work and that they don't have time to do it after all. The exercise may be self-defeating because the responses are so variable and because deciphering them is so difficult and time-consuming. This is often a source of disappointment to new researchers using questionnaires. If open-ended questions are important, an interview is a better option. There a skilled interviewer can obtain more information by further questioning while keeping the respondent within the area of interest. In other words, there is a trade-off between the depth of the enquiry and the size and representativeness of the sample of respondents.

Questionnaire design

Many books provide useful guides on designing questionnaires. Much of what they have to say sounds like good old common sense and may encourage the belief that questionnaire design is not difficult. Nevertheless, it is surprisingly easy to get wrong. Two general rules apply. Plan ahead and pilot test as much as possible. Planning ahead includes thinking clearly about the purposes of the questionnaire and the research questions you want to answer. It will help you to get the right questions and to avoid asking silly or unnecessary questions that increase the length of the questionnaire and irritate the respondents. Pilot testing is important because questionnaires are normally one-off events. Once you have put them in the post, it's too late to add or change a question or clarify the instructions. Pilot testing can establish that people can follow the instructions, understand the questions and are not offended or exhausted by answering them. The aim here is to get feedback. So check how they have dealt with the questionnaire and how they have answered the questions. Be prepared to change or remove questions that don't work well. Ask them about the general appearance of the questionnaire and the impression it creates and find out about any problems they had understanding the instructions.

There are similarities between designing a questionnaire and the procedures described in the last chapter for creating tests. Much that was said there about getting experts to help select questions applies here. So does the general advice about length and the wording of questions. Questionnaires are rarely subjected to the sort of statistical analysis that tests are, however. We are unlikely to standardize a questionnaire or to examine the internal consistency of its items. They are usually designed for a particular piece of research and may not be used again by other researchers. Researchers don't worry very much about the reliability and validity of questionnaires. This may be reasonable in cases where the questions are mainly factual and where there is no apparent reason for people to answer misleadingly. It is less reasonable where researchers want to know about people's opinions and attitudes. Here it is better to use an established measure if one is available.

There are two further problems with large postal surveys. First, how do we get a random sample of respondents? Second, how many of them will reply? Sampling clinicians is not too difficult as national professional bodies have lists of those qualified. Fimian et al. (1991) randomly selected 2,000 clinicians from ASHA records. Arndt and Healy (2001) randomly sampled 50 clinicians in each of 10 states.

Random client samples are more difficult to obtain. In some cases organizations exist to support and represent clients. Not all clients join such bodies, however; so membership may not be random. Hayhow et al. (2002) sent their questionnaire to all dysfluent members of the British Stammering Association. Another alternative is to contact clinicians about clients on their caseloads.

Clearly it is not easy to get a random sample in these circumstances. This is not the crime it was in experimental research, however. Some researchers are quite straightforward about it and use 'convenience' samples. Yaruss et al. (2002) wanted to question people who stammer about their use of support groups. The groups are largely informal, and it would be difficult to reach their members. Instead they surveyed members who attended a conference. This was not a random sample, but it avoided a lot of inconvenience.

A further reason for not worrying about the randomness of the sample is that many people don't respond anyway. Surveys of the general population may have particularly poor rates of response (< 25%). Surveys of special populations may do somewhat better because they ask about things that are of direct interest to them. Despite this, most of the surveys quoted in this chapter had response rates below 50%. The respondents in Yaruss et al. (2002) appear to have been a keen bunch, and yet only 41% replied. Hayhow et al. (2002) only had a 26% response rate.

Low response rates are frustrating for researchers. A greater concern, however, is that those who respond are not representative of the population. Confounding variables will be present if those who do respond differ in some systematic way from those who don't. Fimian et al. (1991), who asked clinicians about occupational stress had a 31% response rate. It's possible that the questionnaire encouraged clinicians who experience a lot of stress to respond, thus producing data that were not representative of all clinicians.

It's a good idea to give people a fixed time in which to respond. This avoids waiting around wondering whether further questionnaires will be returned. The researcher can then either analyse the responses received or take action to increase the response rate. Arndt and Healey (2001) asked for replies within 2 weeks and then sent a second questionnaire to non-responders. This approach reduces bias by encouraging non-responders to respond. The alternative – to contact a new group of people – might just perpetuate a response bias because similar people either respond or don't respond again. This approach makes it difficult to maintain confidentiality. Fimian et al. (1991), who wanted responses to be confidential, used a different approach. They calculated descriptive statistics on their sample and showed that these were not substantially different from known data for all SLTs.

Analysing data from questionnaires

Data from questionnaires rarely require complicated forms of analysis. The tests we have already covered may be sufficient. Often, the most important data can be reported using descriptive statistics. Thus Iversen-Thoburn and Hayden (2000) reported the mean times taken to become proficient using different methods of alaryngeal speech. Kersten et al. (2002) gave the percentage of respondents who reported various unmet needs (and SLT was prominent among them), and Winter (1999) reported that 59% of therapists worked with bilingual clients.

We may want to compare the answers given by different groups of respondents. Typically we divide respondents into groups by their answers to one (usually factual) question. For instance, we might divide therapists into those with more than or less than 5 years' experience and compare their answers to other questions to see how they differ. If the answers are yes/no responses, we can use chi-square tests. If they are measures of attitudes or opinions (a Likert scale), we can use Mann-Whitney tests. There are problems here, however. Questionnaires produce masses of data, and it may be tempting to go on doing tests until you think you have found something interesting. Once we have divided our therapists into two groups, we can compare their responses on any or all of the other questions. If this doesn't lay the golden egg, we may be tempted to go back and divide them in some different way and try again. The first problem here is that by doing lots of tests we increase the chance of making type-one errors. Even if we just eyeball the data and do the tests that look interesting, we are implicitly doing the tests that don't look interesting! The second problem is that we are likely to produce a confusing mixture of significant and non-significant results that it will be difficult to make sense of anyway. All of this goes back to the need to plan ahead. Questionnaires must have a clear purpose. Proof that they have one is that we can state in advance what we want to find out. This helps us decide what questions to ask in the first place and what analyses to do when we get the answers.

Interviews

Eastwood (1988) suggested that SLTs were ignoring alternative approaches to research. Her view that the profession might benefit from using qualitative research methods was a timely reminder of this neglect. At the time quantitative approaches to research held sway and there was frustration that, as a result, many areas of interest to clinicians were inaccessible. Subsequently there has been a considerable expansion in the use of qualitative methodologies, nowhere more so than in the use of interviews. This approach has proved both useful and congenial to clinical researchers. Interviews have been used to examine the perspectives of clients living with communication disorders and with chronic illnesses and to discover their reactions to therapy. Parents and carers have been interviewed to learn more about the problems of helping children with language or learning disorders and of caring for the elderly. Even clinicians have not escaped. Interviews have been used to examine their clinical practices and decision-making.

Interviews may seem similar to (and as much fun as) conversations. They require planning and experience to be successful, however. Interviews are often described as being 'semi-structured' and 'in- depth'. These terms summarize the attractions of the interview as a research methodology. The terms 'structured', 'semi-structured' and 'unstructured' are used, somewhat inconsistently, to indicate points on a continuum. Structured interviews give respondents little opportunity to expand on their answers and may have few advantages over questionnaires. Unstructured interviews are at the other extreme. Usually the interviewer does little more than introduce the topic and give occasional cues to the respondents, who are allowed to take the discussion in whichever direction they wish to. The semi-structured approach is a popular compromise. The interviewer sets the rules and has decided the agenda (but experienced interviewers do so discreetly). They will have a list of topics to cover and will want each participant to respond to all or most of them.

The in-depth nature of the interview reflects the fact that participants are encouraged to expand their answers and are allowed to part from the script when the interviewer decides this is appropriate and that something of interest may result. A skilled interviewer can balance the competing demands of covering the topics on time and letting respondents tell the story as they see it. Analysis of interview data (see below) consists of picking out themes and illustrating these by quoting from the material. Where there is no structure in the material, this can be a formidable task. By planning a list of topics and ensuring that each participant responds to them, the semi-structured interview makes this task a little easier.

Studies using interviews in SLT have often had very small samples and appear to be unconcerned about whether they are random or not. After all the fuss about needing large random samples in experimental research, this may strike you as odd. Small samples are often justified by the difficulty of finding appropriate respondents and the time required to interview them and analyse their data. There is a danger that data from small samples may represent the views of a minority of the possible respondents, however. It is often argued that sample sizes in qualitative research should be determined by the data themselves. When interviewing more people fails to reveal any new themes within the data, there is no need to go on interviewing. Such a rule has the weakness that a few interviews with a homogeneous group of respondents may terminate the research before more diverse views can be sampled.

There are several reasons for the use of non-random samples. The first is practical. Random samples are easily obtained when the relevant population can be identified and is available for sampling. Qualitative researchers often want to contact groups of people with unusual experiences or knowledge. They may be few in number and hard to find. In extreme cases researchers may ask people they interview to identify others whom they know to have similar experiences – a practice known as 'snowballing'. In other cases participants may be contacted by means that are unlikely to result in random samples. Crichton-Smith (2002) contacted many of her adults who stammer through a newspaper advertisement. Knox et al. (2000) interviewed the families of children with a learning disability. They recruited their sample by invitation, stating the aims of the research. This may have attracted respondents with strong feelings, and so the researchers were cautious about generalizing the findings to other families.

A further reason for abandoning random sampling is that it is inefficient. Qualitative researchers point out that random samples merely collect many typical participants. They argue that less-typical people provide more-interesting data. This deliberate targeting of special groups is called 'purposive sampling'. Michallet et al. (2001) interviewed spouses of people with severe aphasias. Their sample was not representative of all spouses of people with aphasia but did include those with experience of living with partners with very limited communication. This may result in more striking and informative, if less representative, data. Parr et al. (1997) also used purposive sampling. Their large sample of people with dysphasia was deliberately structured to ensure that certain groups were represented.

Samples may also be chosen for theoretical purposes. This reflects the fact, mentioned in Chapter 1, that qualitative research often plays an important part in developing theories. Theoretical samples consist of groups of people selected because they provide a test of an emerging theory. Grounded theory (Glaser and Strauss, 1967) provides a formal description of the process by which qualitative data are interpreted and hypotheses generated and tested by further theoretical sampling. It is discussed further below.

These reasons provide a convincing case for non-random sampling. It's easy to get the feeling, however, that qualitative researchers might choose a non-random sample even when a random one was staring them in the face. Bowling (1997) is among those authors who suggest that there are times when random samples can be used and offer the advantage that the findings can be generalized to the population sampled. A policy of explicitly stating when samples are random or intentionally non-random might be appropriate here. The difference in quantitative and qualitative approaches to sampling may be overstated. We saw in Chapter 2 that experimental researchers are rarely explicit about the population to whom their results may be generalized. In practice both types of research often duck the issue and leave the reader to decide whom to generalize the results to. This usually results in generalization to a larger population than that sampled. A large black hole exists between truly random and deliberately non-random samples. Within it there is greater overlap between quantitative and qualitative practices than either likes to admit.

Skills and procedures

Although interviewing represents an appealing approach to research, it would be foolish to think that it will be problem free. Effective interviewing is a skilled performance, and experience is necessary to obtain the best results. Semi-structured interviewing may be the most demanding form. Here the interviewer must affect a smooth compromise between covering a range of topics while allowing the respondent to present their personal view. This must be achieved while monitoring the time and disposition of the respondent so that, where possible, the experience is enjoyable.

It is likely that some people are intuitively better interviewers than others. Nevertheless, there is scope for improvement in all of us. Large-scale research projects often train their interviewers. Performance may be practised and monitored, advice given by experts and opportunities offered to watch other interviewers at work. This not only improves skills but also ensures a greater consistency of approach within the project. Smaller projects may use a single interviewer and have few of these advantages. It's important to pilot the interview before starting. Researchers may be reluctant to do this because they are impatient to get on and because it may use up some (hard-to-find) respondents needed for the research. Here, practice with proxy respondents may be useful. Performance should be videotaped and studied and respondents, proxy or real, invited to comment on the interview.

As in all research, planning is important. This extends to seemingly trivial details, such as ensuring that the room is appropriate and comfortable and greeting respondents and putting them at ease on their arrival. Video or audio equipment must work on demand, without breaking down or running out of tape, and must preserve a clear record of the interview without being intrusive or disconcerting to respondents. Bowling (1997) suggested that the intrusiveness of the recording techniques may be tested by switching off the equipment and continuing chatting to see if anything new emerges. Bryman (2001) felt that some interviewees fail to adjust to being taped and suggested making notes on things they say when the tape is switched off. Respondents must be informed of the content of the interview and must consent to it. They should be assured that their views, expressed in the interview, will be respected and that the information they give and their identity will remain confidential. Where personal or difficult issues may be raised, they should be informed in advance. This may affect their willingness to participate but is preferable to any loss of rapport or the giving offence during the interview. The length of the interview should be estimated and respondents informed. Interviews may be long, in some cases exceeding 2 hours (see Michallet et al., 2001; Crichton-Smith, 2002). A break may be needed but will lead to a loss of continuity; light refreshments may be appropriate!

Interviewers must be attentive listeners. The clearest sign of a failed interview is one where the interviewer talks too much. Questions should be short and clear. A balance must be struck between being specific and being vague. Neither is desirable. The former may result in brief, factual and uninformative responses; the latter, in confused responses. Questions should not imply that a particular answer is right or more socially acceptable. Interviews in which respondents tell interviewers what they think they want to hear are of no value. This point reflects a general need for interviewers to be non-judgemental and to have respect for their respondents and their views. Interruptions should be infrequent and used mainly to encourage more-detailed answers or to ask for clarifications. Robson (2002) distinguished between probes and prompts. Probes seek further explanation or expansion. They may range from encouraging non-verbal cues such as short silences or quizzical expressions to requests to repeat or expand upon points. Prompts are more explicit. They may suggest possible answers and are used when a respondent has difficulty finding a response. They should be offered as possibilities that can be accepted or denied so as to avoid putting words into the respondent's mouth. Close monitoring of replies is necessary. Ambiguous or contradictory responses must be clarified during the interview.

Interviews are invariably audiotaped or videotaped for detailed analysis. Nevertheless, interviewers may wish to make additional notes as they proceed. This is, inevitably, a tricky business. Care is needed not to interrupt the flow of the interview or distract the respondent. In some instances (see Yorkston et al., 2001) two interviewers may be used – one to conduct the interview and the other to make notes.

Not the least of interviewers' problems is that they may omit important questions. Semi-structured interviews normally ask a range of questions, and the expectation is that respondents will answer all or most of these. Robson (2002) suggested that an interview schedule should be used and gave an example of one. This lists the main questions and suggestions for supplementary questions to obtain more detail. It can be consulted and questions ticked off during the interview. Parr et al. (1997) and Glogowska and Campbell (2000) gave the interview guides that they used to ensure that important areas were covered systematically. Most books recommend that the initial questions should be straightforward and non-controversial. They serve the dual purpose of obtaining general information about the respondents and making them feel at ease before the serious part of the interview. Similarly, the final questions are usually low key to promote a cordial end to the proceedings. The intervening questions form the main part of the interview. Questions may be asked in a fixed order or the order may remain flexible, changing to improve the flow of individual interviews.

It's a general rule that interviewees should be treated as, and perceive themselves to be, the expert on the issues on which they are interviewed. This helps to smooth the way. It's obviously the case, and it doesn't hurt for interviewers to remind themselves of this periodically. They are there to find out what the 'experts' know, not to assume that they know more. Nevertheless, it's obviously important that interviewers come across as sincere and well informed. In SLT, interviews may be with other clinicians where shared knowledge of therapy issues is assumed, or with clients where sensitivity and an appreciation of their feelings and difficulties are essential. An easy way to fail is to ask dumb questions. To ensure this is not the case it's worth thinking hard about the content of the interview. This means getting advice on the questions and how best to ask them. Consultations with other clinicians, experts and clients are important, and focus groups may be used to establish the main themes of the interview (Knox et al., 2000; Roulestone, 2001).

Analysing interview data

Analysis of interview data is hard work. The material is studied to detect common themes, and the research is reported by outlining the themes and illustrating them with extracts from individual interviews. These extracts are important. They give a flavour of the data and help to convince the reader that the correct themes have been identified. The first step is transcription. This is a lengthy business. Bowling (1997) suggested that 2 to 4 hours of transcription time are required for each hour of interview. Bryman (2001) put it at 5 hours plus. The time will depend upon the material, the quality of the tape and other factors. Allow plenty of time and expect it to take longer. Transcription usually involves repeated listening to the tapes, and the transcriber may develop ideas about the data while doing this. In this way transcription and analysis merge and the labour involved is reduced. Despite the work involved, most researchers are fairly obsessive about their data and feel that transcriptions should be a complete record of what is said in the interview. In fact, transcripts often go beyond what is said and use symbols to indicate other audible but non-verbal events. Silverman (1993) gave a list of symbols used to indicate pauses, intake and outlets of breath and changes in tone, volume or stress.

The transcription is used to identify themes in the data. This interpretative stage is the most controversial part of the methodology, described by Bowling (1997) as 'a strength and a weakness' of the approach. Skilful interpretation can provide valuable information. It's easy to imagine that misinterpretation might occur, however. The process is a creative one, and individual researchers often find it difficult to describe how they reached their decisions. We will return to this below, but first let's look at an example of the analysis of interview data.

Yorkston et al. (2001) interviewed people with multiple sclerosis. They used the WHO 1999 model, which divides disabilities resulting from illness into impairments, limitations in activities and restrictions in participation. While the first two can be assessed with standard tests, the impact on communicative participation is better addressed by interviews. This allowed clients to describe their communication in their own words and through descriptions of their personal experiences. Three main themes relating to changes in communication, participation in communication and the unpredictability of communication were identified, each with subthemes. Extracts are used to illustrate and support the themes identified. The study is impressive because it succeeds in giving insight about the clients and presents findings that have important implications for therapy. Clients were more concerned about participation than their impairments or limitations upon their activities. In some cases quite mild impairments had major effects on their lives. In contrast, therapy is often offered at the levels of impairment and activity. This mismatch suggests that clinicians should assure clients that they aim to improve participation and should monitor the effects of therapy upon it.

The process of analysing the data and extracting themes is a laborious one. Traditionally it has been done by constructing charts or by using index cards so that similar extracts from different respondents can be brought together and cross-referenced. The option of using computer programs to categorize extracts and to retrieve relevant sections rapidly is now popular. Researchers are undecided on the merits of the two approaches. Some argue (as they do with quantitative data) that a hands-on approach gives greater insight into and familiarity with the data. The advantages of the computerized approach increase with the volume of the data to be processed and with the complexity of the coding system used. It is particularly good at rapidly retrieving the context in which coded extracts occur and can play an important part in helping to develop theories from the data. A description of the use of a computer program and a discussion of its advantages and disadvantages may be found in Morison and Moir (1998).

Yorkston et al. (2001) analysed their data in two stages. The first categorized extracts using the client's own descriptive terms. Thus items might be coded as being 'in the past'. Later, after repeated reading and study of the material, coded items were grouped into the more abstract themes listed above. The first process is time-consuming. The second demands a thorough knowledge of the material and an ability to conceptualize its content. There may be conflicts between the need to organize the data and the desire to maintain the individuality of the respondent's accounts. Individuality may be preserved by letting many different themes emerge from the data. In practice this approach may be overwhelming, however. Developing more abstract themes gives the conclusions greater generality and is important if the aim is to develop theoretical accounts from the data.

The way in which the analysis is conducted will depend upon the objectives of the research. The role of qualitative research in developing theories has already been mentioned. Where this is the objective, researchers may have few preconceptions about their data and expect to search through in-depth to discover what themes occur. In other instances they may start from a particular hypothesis about the situation they are investigating and seek to prove it or expand upon it. The latter imposes greater structure on the investigation. It will affect the type of questions asked, and the themes extracted from the data are likely to be influenced by the initial hypotheses. Pope et al. (2000) called these approaches inductive or deductive. In the inductive approach, themes are extracted gradually from the data. In the deductive approach, the themes are derived from hypotheses proposed before or in the early stages of the analysis. The distinction is far from absolute, however. It is unlikely that any researchers use a totally inductive approach (have no preconceptions about their data). Nor should those using a deductive approach close their eyes to any new or unexpected themes that may arise. Researchers themselves are rarely explicit about the approach they have used. The former is the more traditional; the latter has been increasingly used in areas of applied research, particularly in health settings.

Grounded theory provides the most popular account of the inductive approach. The term is used because hypotheses are 'grounded' in the data themselves rather than being defined prior to the analysis. Grounded theory is a general account of qualitative data analysis (not just of interview data). Infighting among proponents of the approach has led to different accounts of the theory since its original proposal by Glaser and Strauss (1967). Bryman and Burgess (1994) suggested that few researchers use it in its entirety. Its influence has been on the general approach to data analysis rather than as a precise method. An account of the theory can be found in Bryman (2001). At the heart of the technique is a continual interchange between the data and the conclusions drawn from it. Data are analysed and provisional hypotheses drawn. These are then tested against continuing analysis of the same data or of new data from further interviews. Glogowska and Campbell (2000) interviewed 16 parents about the treatment of their children who had language disorders. Sets of four interviews were conducted and analysed in turn, allowing later interviews to check the interpretation of the earlier data and to develop new lines of questioning. This approach may be extended to identifying and interviewing particular types of respondents who offer a strong test of the emerging interpretation. The general aim is to focus the ongoing research more precisely and to test potential conclusions as the research develops. The concept of theoretical saturation is important. By asking new questions and interviewing new respondents, the research aims to find out all there is to know. At the end of this procedure no new themes should be emerging from the data.

One form of deductive analysis is the framework approach described by Ritchie and Spencer (1994). It was developed for applied research in areas of social and health policy and has been used in SLT research (see Parr et al., 1997; Glogowska and Campbell, 2000; Crichton-Smith, 2002). Applied research is often funded by the government and used to investigate current policy and to improve provision. As a result it may begin with specific hypotheses, and the interviews will have a 'topic guide' to indicate areas of questioning. The method was described with several examples in Ritchie and Spencer (1994). The researchers first familiarize themselves with the data. Where there are a lot of data or where, as is common in commissioned research, a deadline must be met, this process may only consider some of the data. During familiarization, the researcher will begin to identify a thematic framework representing the main themes within the data. Given the more structured nature of the interview, it is likely that some themes will relate directly to items on the topic guide. New themes will arise, however, and researchers must look for more general and more abstract themes that link areas of the data. Themes and subthemes are numbered and used to index the remaining data. An adequate thematic index should allow most of the remaining data to be indexed. Sections of the transcript may require several different indices, and their concurrence can help to identify more general themes. Once indexing is completed, charts can be made to link the extracts that belong to different themes, allowing further refinement and interpretation to take place.

Problems and solutions

Issues about the reliability and validity of findings apply in qualitative as well as quantitative research methods. However, researchers seldom offer much reassurance that their findings are either reliable or valid. It is often said that qualitative research methods are valid because they examine and try to explain real-life events. This is misleading. The events may be real, but the theories proposed to explain them are subjective interpretations of the data, and confirmation that the researcher's interpretation is right would be welcome.

In general reliability is assessed by showing that other researchers would reach similar conclusions if they conducted the same research. One obvious source of disagreement is the coding of interview data. It should be possible to show that independent scorers agree on coding. Crichton-Smith (2002) reported 94% agreement between the author and a second independent scorer. Many other papers offer little evidence that coding is reliable, however. Moreover, it is likely that agreement will decline as coding moves from the transcript of the interviews to the more abstract themes upon which theories are based. Of course, reliability is rather more than this. It applies to the interviews as well. Participants in interviews react to one another. If two interviewers ask the same questions of the same client, there is no guarantee that they will get the same information. Clients may be more or less reticent or interpret questions differently when asked by different interviewers. Studies have given little attention to this problem. Size may be the obvious solution. Studies with several interviewers and a number of respondents in effect treat the interaction as a random variable. Individual interviews may vary but the overall standard should be acceptable. Conversely studies with few respondents and a single interviewer might be less reliable.

These largely unacknowledged problems of reliability make it important that the validity of the findings is demonstrated. If a study is unreliable, it may lack validity. Quite simply, if researchers differ in conducting the interview or coding the data, their conclusions will differ; both cannot be right.

One method of validating data from interviews uses the respondents themselves. Who better to ask if the findings are true? Robson (2002), who prefered the term credibility to validity, pointed out that if the respondents believe the findings are credible they must be true! This is respondent validation or member checking and is widely used. Yorkston et al. (2001) and Chrichton-Smith (2002) asked their respondents to validate their findings. Michallet et al. (2001) recruited 10 further spouses of people with aphasia to validate the findings from their original interview data. Respondent validation may be used at the end of the interview process, as in the examples above, or may be part of an ongoing analysis using grounded theory.

In some cases respondents may not only be asked to validate research findings but to suggest things that are missing from the explanation (see Michallet et al., 2001). This approach caters for the possibility that a theoretical account is true but not the whole truth. A similar objective is served by the attention given to negative evidence. This is evidence that does not fit an emerging story. It may consist of clients who give different answers to questions or clients with an entirely different tale to tell. It is obviously important, but how important? Quantitative research has an advantage here. Statistical tests assess not only the size but also the consistency of differences between subjects. No such 'objective' criteria are available to the qualitative researcher, who must assess whether a small amount of evidence must change an otherwise consistent theory or not. The absence of negative evidence helps to validate research findings. This absence becomes more impressive as the number and variety of respondents interviewed increases. Its importance is again seen in grounded theory, where the testing of theories through further data collection is, in effect, a search for possible negative evidence.

Interviews (and other qualitative methods) are popular because the researcher comes close to the action. Researchers must be aware, however, that this very closeness to the data offers them the opportunity to influence both the responses given and the coding of the interview material. The need for awareness of bias is called reflexivity. The researcher must acknowledge their prejudices and bear them in mind when conducting and interpreting interviews. Judging when prejudice ends and overcompensation begins will not be easy, however. Glogowska and Campbell (2000) acknowledged that their interviews with parents of children with language disorders might be affected because the interviewer was an SLT. They asked non-SLTs to check the interpretation of the data to counter this potential bias.

A further problem is that the analysis of interview data must to a great extent be taken on trust as the procedures involved are not easily described to readers of the research. This contrasts with quantitative methods, where the methodology and statistics are normally described in detail and are open to criticism from other researchers. Ritchie and Spencer (1994) pointed out that one of the advantages of the framework approach is that it defines a common methodology. This tries to make the methods of analysis more disciplined and explicit and reflects the need for greater openness in applied research where findings may lead to important changes in policy. The progressive refining and testing of hypotheses against new data in grounded theory also provide an opportunity for a clearer account of the research process. However, Bryman (2001) noted that researchers often claim to have used grounded theory but do not make this apparent in accounts of their research.

Researchers often use a multi-method approach to research. Thus interviews may be used alongside questionnaires or observation, and qualitative and quantitative methods may be combined within the same research project. This approach is attractive because it can provide more comprehensive data. Similar findings from different approaches can also be used to validate the conclusions of the research. This approach to validation is called triangulation. Although it has been widely discussed (see, for example, Erzberger and Prein, 1997), Mays and Pope (2000) noted that its role as a test of validity is controversial. They were wary of the view that one approach may compensate for weaknesses in another and that differences in information from different approaches can be resolved. Nevertheless, they commended it as a means of increasing the comprehensiveness of the research. An example of the multi-method approach may be found in Glogowska et al. (2002) who compare data from a randomized control trial of SLT for pre-school children with data from a questionnaire and interviews with their parents. In line with the view of Mays and Pope, the aim in this study appears to be for comprehensive data rather than validation via triangulation.

Focus groups

Focus groups share many of the advantages of interviews but speed up the process by studying several respondents at a time. Their current popularity as research tools should not disguise a disreputable past. They have been used for many years in market research and, more recently, by political parties that, having rejected the idea that policy should be based on political principles, have used them to find out what voters want. Famously the Labour Party used them to sound out Conservative voters. They obviously made their point. This has given focus groups a bad name; so let's concentrate on their role in research.

Speeding up the process is not the main attraction for serious researchers. For them, groups are valuable because they stimulate discussion and allow issues to be investigated in greater depth. Focus groups are not group interviews in which each person is asked and answers questions. They are relatively unstructured conversations between participants who react to one another's views. Disagreements occur commonly but can be used to make participants delve deeper into their feelings about issues of interest. For these reasons, focus groups are particularly good at detecting negative evidence.

Focus groups have problems as well. Books often refer to focus-group leaders as mediators or facilitators (not interviewers). This reflects their diminished role. They will usually have a topic list, as in interviews, and a range of prompts to stimulate and guide the discussion. However, groups are less easy to manage, and decisions about when to intervene or change direction may be difficult. As a result focus groups may be preferred by researchers who want less- rather than more-structured discussion. Groups involve a loss of confidentiality and some participants may be inhibited and minority views may not be heard. However, Kitzinger (1995) suggested that groups might disinhibit some participants in a way that interviews cannot. The procedures for data analysis are similar to those for interviews but may be more difficult. Transcription is particularly troublesome as participants interrupt and talk over one another, and identification of speakers may also be a problem.

There is some disagreement about the best number of participants to have in focus groups. Increasing the numbers may increase the possibility that some participants will opt out of the discussion. As a result some suggest that six is a reasonable number; others seem less concerned and suggest 10 or even 12 as a maximum size. One reason for planning to use larger numbers is purely practical. Gathering that many people together at one time is not easy; plan for 10 and you may end up with nearer six anyway. We normally expect focus groups to produce healthy and helpful disagreement between participants. It's possible, however, that participants may compromise and move towards a consensus that does not truly represent individual views. This suggests that research projects should use several groups so that different opinions are properly represented.

A good recent example of using focus groups in research is a study by Paradice and Adewusi (2002). They used seven focus groups to obtain the views of 51 parents about the educational provision for their children with speech and language problems in mainstream schools. As its title suggests, the study found disquiet among parents regarding their children's education. They regarded good provision as more a matter of luck than educational policy and were critical of the lack of resources, including the availability of SLTs. As well as providing an analysis of the main themes supported by quotations, the paper provides a lengthy appendix detailing the issues raised in each of the focus groups.

Chapter 13
Observational research

Introduction

All research involves observing people's behaviour. The approaches described in this chapter take this to the extreme, however. Observational research, as its name suggests, attempts to directly observe and interpret behaviour. When successful, it has advantages over interviewing, which may be affected by selective recall or deliberate attempts to mislead the researcher. Observing behaviour sounds like fun and, as with interviewing, appears to draw on skills we are accustomed to using in everyday life. Of course, we are not going to get away with just importing our casual (probably inaccurate) everyday methods into research. Observational studies must be more systematic and must find ways of demonstrating that the conclusions drawn from the observations are correct.

Like interviewing, observation comes in different forms, and these impose different degrees of structure on the research. The major distinction is between systematic (or structured) observation and participant observation. The former is widely used in social and in developmental psychology and in studies of animal behaviour. It often results in quantitative data, which can be analysed statistically. Although it is normally used to study naturally occurring behaviour, it can be used experimentally by placing participants in a controlled environment and observing their behaviour (the DV) as aspects of the environment (the IV) are changed. In all observational studies there are concerns about the effects that the observer may have on the behaviour of those observed. Systematic observation has the advantage that observers may conceal their presence by watching from a distance or by using video recordings. Where this is not possible, they should try to become a normal and unthreatening part of the environment by accustoming the subjects to their presence over time. In either case the observer avoids interactions with the subjects that might influence their behaviour. A structured approach is also used in the data collection. Predetermined target behaviours are identified, and the observer records these as they occur.

Kaderavek and Sulzby (1998) used a systematic approach to observation to monitor joint book-reading sessions between parents and young children. Their paper presents the observational protocol that was developed as a result of this research. Observers were asked to watch for examples of specific behaviours that indicated positive and negative aspects of parental help to the child, the child's responsiveness and of the social and emotional climate of the interaction.

Systematic observation is often used to analyse the behaviour of individual clients. Forman et al. (2002) used it to study self-injurious behaviour in a man with profound intellectual disabilities. Different theories exist of the roles of staff behaviour and of the client's own use of self-restraining behaviours in promoting or regulating instances of self-injurious behaviour. Observation of the client was conducted in his natural environment. Instances of two forms of self-injury, three types of staff intervention and two methods of self-restraint were recorded. A sequential analysis was used in which events prior to and after an instance of self-injury were examined to discover its causes.

Systematic observation can also be used to assess the effects of interventions. Best et al. (1993) studied children with poor communication in nurseries. Treated children joined small groups in which communication was encouraged through play. They improved more than untreated children both on formal language assessments and on data obtained by observing their communication in the nursery. Chadwick et al. (2002) examined carers' knowledge of dysphagia management strategies with clients with learning disabilities. Carers underwent training, and their knowledge was assessed by interview and by observation of them caring for clients. Surprisingly their performance outstripped their knowledge. Chadwick et al. suggested that much of their knowledge consisted of procedural memories that are adequately performed but are difficult to verbalize. The finding has important implications for the assessment of training in such areas.

Assessments of functional communication have increasingly used an observational approach. The ASHA FACS (Functional Assessment of Communication Skills for Adults) (Frattali et al., 1995) consists of 43 different behaviours in four different domains and is scored through observation of the client. Davidson et al. (2003) conducted an observational study of elderly people with and without aphasia. Many similar communication activities were seen in each group, but the people with aphasia had more limited social situations and fewer conversational partners. The data were also used to validate the ASHA FACS. Thirty-four of the items were observed in the people with aphasia and 39 in the controls. An observational approach may also be used to assess adults with learning difficulties. Dormandy and Van der Gaag (1989) pointed out that neither aphasia nor developmental language assessments are appropriate for this client group and explore the use of observational (subtests of the Communication Assessment Profile (CASP), Van der Gaag, 1988) and formal assessments (elicited conversation and formal picture description tasks). The observation task specifies a range of communication skills, which are observed and rated by the assessor. Clients obtained higher scores on it reflecting their greater ability in natural situations. Formal methods were also recommended, however, to elicit a wider range of language structures.

At the other extreme are studies where the researcher is a participant. Here the aim is to observe more varied behaviours of people in social groups or organizations. The observer must enter the participants' environment (though they hope to do so as unobtrusively as possible). This is not easy and may lead to uncertainty about whether the participants' behaviour has been influenced or whether some behaviours have been 'censored' during the period of observation. The origins of participant observation are in sociology and in social anthropology, and it has commonly been used to study how social or political groups or organizations work. Organizations have strong and persistent influences on people's behaviour that may only be recognized by observers from outside. The researcher's aim is to produce an account of this that reflects and explains the participants' behaviour and experiences.

The comparison of the two forms of observation is similar to that between questionnaires and interviews. Questionnaires and systematic observation are normally used where we already have some understanding of a situation. We may have a theory of what is going on and know what sorts of information we want. As a result they ask specific questions, which may be answered by asking about or observing specified behaviours. Participant observation is similar to interviewing in that observers may observe any or all behaviours and will select and combine their observations in an effort to develop a theory of why an individual behaves or a social group operates in the way it does.

Studies that use participant observation may be very time-consuming and difficult to pull off. As with interviewing, large amounts of data result and analysis is a formidable task. When they are successful, they can be spectacularly so, however. Social anthropological studies where an observer spends long periods living in and observing other societies provide classic instances of its use. Here the time taken serves to make observers trusted figures who do not inhibit normal behaviour. It allows them to observe complex behaviours whose purpose may only become apparent when set in their context. Closer to home, these studies have often been most effective when researchers penetrate organizations or groups whose members practice idiosyncratic behaviours that they may wholly or partly conceal from society at large. Early studies such as those of Festinger et al. (1956) on a religious cult, and of Goffman (1961) and Rosenhan (1973) on mental hospitals, illustrated the potential of the methodology. In the former the authors joined a cult whose beliefs, unwisely but not atypically, included a prediction that the world would end on a certain day. Contrary to logic, the failure of this prediction confirmed rather than undermined members' beliefs. Festinger et al. proposed that people have difficulty dealing with dissonant cognitions and resort to faith rather than logic in reconciling them. The study is still widely quoted (often as an example of unethical practice, which modern squeamishness would forbid – this sort of thing is now left to journalists). The Goffman and Rosenhan studies exposed (and may have improved) the practices of mental institutions. Goffman's study was instrumental in showing how greatly behaviour is influenced by 'total' institutions. In Rosenhan's, observers faked psychiatric symptoms to gain entry and showed that getting out was rather more difficult. One alarming aspect of the latter was that other clients were rather quicker at detecting normality than were the professionals.

Participant observation appears to be more popular than systematic observation in many areas of clinical research. The tradition of investigating 'exotic' institutions continues. Brooks and Brown (2002) used participant observation to penetrate the mysteries of the NHS. They suggested that eliminating 'ceremonies' that unnecessarily preserve demarcations between those working in it can bring about organizational change. Examples are provided to illustrate ceremonies that preserve boundaries. Sanger et al. (2000) examined communication between female juvenile delinquents. Assessments of prison populations have shown that many have poor communication skills. Sanger et al. sought further evidence of this by observing communication between teenage girls in a correctional facility. Observation was first conducted from a distance. Participant observation and discreet recording of conversations was introduced when it was judged that the girls would accept this. Twenty-two per cent of those observed were thought to need therapy.

Participant observation is especially useful for researching situations that are inaccessible using other methods. Westby (1997) investigated the view that children with learning disabilities or from culturally diverse backgrounds fail in school because they don't know the rules. Specifically their background may have failed to prepare them for the independent and self-regulating approach to learning that schools try to foster. An observational study was conducted of a school and described the changing demands made on the children at different ages. It has also been used to investigate home care (Briggs et al., 2003) and different forms of residential care (McAllister and Silverman, 1999) for clients with dementia. Booth and Booth (2002) used observation to investigate the role played by men in the lives of mothers with intellectual disabilities. Their findings countered the stereotype that they were a nuisance and showed that a majority played constructive and supportive roles.

Systematic observation

The problems of observing behaviour become apparent when we try to do it. Different behaviours happen at the same time, and they don't stop happening while the observer draws breath. Systematic observation tackles this problem by specifying those behaviours that the observer must watch for. Normally observers have a list of behaviours (called a behavioural schedule) on which to record target behaviours as they occur. The target behaviours must be clearly defined (their definitions are called behavioural codes). Bakeman and Gottman (1997) suggest that two features are essential to systematic observation. The behavioural codes must be clearly specified in advance, and the observer or observers must have demonstrated their reliability in using them.

The choice of the behavioural codes is fundamental. Systematic observation normally tests a hypothesis, and behavioural codes are selected that are relevant to that hypothesis. As with all research think before you start and keep things as simple as possible. A clear hypothesis helps by defining behaviours that are relevant and should restrain the over-excited researcher from including a few others just because they might be interesting. Asking observers to record many behaviours is counterproductive. Most observers (even with the aid of video recordings) can only watch for a few behaviours at a time. The problem is not merely that they are watching for too many things. The more there are, the less likely it is that different behaviours can be discriminated easily. The general rule should be to have a few behaviours clearly distinguished by their behavioural codes. In their study of children in nurseries Best et al. initially intended to ask observers to identify types of utterance (for example questions, comments and so forth), but pilot testing indicated that this was unlikely to be feasible. Rather than have observers produce more-detailed but less-reliable data, they opted for simpler measures (numbers of interactions, initiations and turns in an interaction), which were more easily observed.

Pilot testing is useful in a number of other ways. It can be used to check whether the behaviours are sufficiently obvious to the observer. Behaviours that require too much interpretation by the observer are no good. Even if they reach the right decision, they might miss other behaviours while making up their minds. Pilot testing may reveal obvious omissions from the original schedule or that two behaviours frequently occur together making it unnecessary to include them as separate behavioural codes. Other behaviours may occur very rarely. We should think twice before including these, as their infrequent appearance in the data may be difficult to interpret.

Decisions must be made about when and how to organize observational sessions. These are likely to be quite long. They should be of similar length and occur in similar circumstances for each participant. Observation may be continuous, or time sampling may be used. In the latter, the observer is alerted (usually by a taped signal) at fixed intervals and records the behaviour that is occurring at that time. There is no magic formula here; decisions about the style and timing of the observations should be made to suit the behaviours to be observed and the circumstances under which observers perform best. Continuous observation is useful when we want information on the duration of behaviours or the sequence in which they occur. Normally the period of observation is predetermined, and the data may be the number of times the behaviour is observed or, where duration is measured, the percentage of time devoted to the behaviour. Time sampling may be easier for the observer. It is useful for unambiguous behaviours whose presence or absence can easily be determined at the point of sampling. The data are clear and can be analysed easily, and the reliability of observers (see below) can be readily assessed. Compromises between the two approaches can be struck. Time sampling with a very short interval is similar to continuous observation. Alternatively the observer may be asked to record those behaviours that occur in the interval between signals rather than at the point when they occur. In either case the signal acts mainly as a convenience to observers, helping them to organize the recording of their observations.

The use of an observation schedule and the training of observers in its use go a long way towards ensuring that the data from systematic observation are reliable. Nevertheless, checks on reliability are necessary. Where more than one observer is used, we need to check that they agree by comparing their data on the same subject. In small-scale projects a single observer may be used. Here a second observer should observe part of the data so agreement can be compared. It's not sufficient to just show that observers come up with similar numbers from their observation. We need to show that they agree on the classification of individual behaviours. Time sampling helps because observers' decisions are made at the same time and are directly comparable. Measurement of agreement is not straightforward, however. Suppose we ask two listeners to decide whether a child with an articulation disorder is accurately producing a sample of 100 words. Table 13.1 gives two versions of the level of agreement between the two observers (or the same observer on different occasions).

Table 13.1 Agreement between two therapists on a child's articulation errors

(i)   (ii)

	Second observer	
First observer	Right	Wrong
Right	0	1
Wrong	1	98

	Second observer	
First observer	Right	Wrong
Right	49	1
Wrong	1	49

The most obvious measure is percentage agreement. In each case it is 98%. This is misleading, however. In (i) the observers agree when the child makes an error with great consistency. In (ii) the child makes far fewer errors, giving more scope for disagreement and making the observers' performance more impressive. This shows that our calculation should take account of chance agreement. In (i) this is high; in (ii) it is lower and actual performance better as a result.

Situations like this are quite common, and Cohen's Kappa (Cohen, 1960) is the appropriate method for getting a measure of agreement that is corrected for chance. The formula for Kappa is:

$$K = \frac{P_o - P_c}{1 - P_c}$$

where P_o is the observed probability of agreement and P_c is the chance probability of agreement. Kappa is frequently used in situations where observers are asked to use more than two categories. Consider the following example, where two observers watch a child playing with other children. Time sampling is used, and the observers classify the child's play into four categories on 100 occasions.

Table 13.2 Data for two observers watching a child's play

First observer	Second observer				
	Solitary	Playing alone	Associative play	Cooperative play	Total
1. Solitary	**22**	11	–	–	33
2. Playing alone	9	**14**	4	–	27
3. Associative play	–	2	**10**	9	21
4. Cooperative play	–	–	10	**9**	19
Total	31	27	24	18	100

Observed agreement is found by adding the agreed scores on the diagonal (in bold). This is 55; so the probability of agreement (as I have cunningly decided to have 100 scores) is $P_o = 0.55$. This is not too good. We can see that the child is a bit of a loner (that's probably why we are observing him) and that the observers have some difficulty deciding whether he is playing alone or just being solitary. They have even more trouble with associative (passively joining in) and cooperative (actively joining in) play. We find the chance probability of agreement for each category by multiplying the probabilities that each observer will choose that category. So, for solitary play, it is 0.33×0.31 (the probability that the first and second observer will choose solitary play). We then add these together. So:

$$P_c = (0.33 \times 0.31) + (0.27 \times 0.27) + (0.21 \times 0.24) + (0.19 \times 0.18) = 0.26$$

Putting these values in the formula, we get:

$$K = \frac{P_o - P_c}{1 - P_c} = \frac{0.55 - 0.26}{1 - 0.26} = 0.39$$

As expected, the true level of agreement is lower than the observed. And it's pretty low. Significance is not the issue here. As with the use of correlation to assess reliability, we want as high a level as possible. Fleiss (1981) suggested that values of Kappa between 0.40 and 0.60 are fair, those between 0.60 and 0.75 are good and above 0.75 is excellent. So our observers did not do too well. With a Kappa of 0.39, we would probably want to revise our behavioural codes and/or retrain our observers. The data give us an indication of where the problems are. Observers had little difficulty deciding whether the child was alone or with a group (1 and 2 versus 3 and 4). It was what he was doing when alone or with the group that was difficult.

Exercise 13.1

A researcher asks a series of stroke patients whether they have been seen by their local SLT department. Their responses are compared with the department's own records. The resulting data are:

	Client reports having SLT	Client reports no SLT	Totals
Seen by SLT dept.	26	16	42
Not seen by SLT dept.	6	39	45
Totals	32	55	87

Work out the level of agreement between the clients' reports and departmental records.

Various amended versions of Kappa are available. Details may be found in Bakeman and Gottman (1997). There are methods for calculating agreement between several observers. There is also a weighted version of the formula for occasions when some decisions are more important than others. Suppose we want to assess how reliable decisions are about clients with dysphagia. We devise a scale and ask clinicians to use it to score videofluoroscopy results. Here we may decide that distinguishing aspiration is paramount and weight this distinction highly. Failure to agree will result in a low value of Kappa; failure to agree on less-crucial aspects of a swallow will have a less dramatic effect. Here the weights are used to reflect clinical priorities.

The fact that the researcher selects the behaviours to be observed and that the observers are reliable in observing them goes some way towards convincing us that the data are also valid. It is not sufficient, however. Failure to train the observers properly may mean that they agree but do not identify the appropriate behaviours. Such problems can be checked by comparing their data with video recordings and overcome by further training to improve their ability. Validity may also be threatened if the behaviours selected for observation are inappropriate for the purposes of the research. This is a matter for the researcher. Any doubts should be removed by observing the participants prior to the research to ensure that the most appropriate measures are being taken. Finally there is the usual concern that the presence of observers may influence the subjects' behaviour and invalidate any conclusions drawn. Again, this is a matter to be addressed in the experimental design either by using covert methods or by extensively habituating the subjects to the presence of the observer.

Participant observation

Participant observation is used to study more dynamic social situations than those studied in structured observation. The observer may expect to move from scene to scene and witness unexpected behaviours whose explanation will be an important part of the research. The study of social groups necessarily involves interactions between the individuals within them, and these add to the unpredictability of the behaviours observed. Observers are unlikely to be totally naive about the institutions they observe. Thus, in Sanger et al. (2000) and Brooks and Brown (2002) the authors no doubt began with some knowledge of and preconceptions about institutions for young offenders and about the NHS. The spirit of participant observation, however, is to question and go beyond what may be stereotyped views. Participation rather than passive observation is valuable, as Denscombe (1998) pointed out, in giving observers a sense of the meaning of the actions they observe.

Participant observation may be done covertly. Studies like those above where researchers join secretive groups or restricted organizations demand this. In contrast traditional studies such as those in social anthropology, where observers live with a social group, are unlikely to allow this to occur. Modern research is conducted with greater time pressures and seldom allows for such extensive fieldwork. Nevertheless, the researcher is likely to enter the group as an outsider and may need to participate in it for lengthy periods. Gaining access might itself be difficult, and it is common for researchers to do so through contacts with one or more persons in the organization they are to observe. These act as sponsors who can introduce and vouch for the researcher and assist access and reduce the suspicions of those to be observed. This and the need to obtain informed consent from participants make covert observation difficult. Often it is better to be completely up front with other participants and explain the purposes of the research and any possible benefits it may have. This overt approach means that researchers must judge when their presence is no longer influencing the behaviour they wish to observe. This judgement is a subjective one. The only rule is that longer periods are more likely to be successful than shorter ones.

Participant observers face the difficult task of recording their data as they observe. It might be possible to develop a shorthand so that salient features can be immediately recorded. Generally, however, writing notes during observation is not recommended and, in cases where covert observation is used, may be impossible. It both diverts the observer from the action and serves to remind others that their actions are under scrutiny. Notes must be made as soon as possible afterwards to avoid any loss of information, and it is normally recommended that the observer transcribe the data and make some attempt to identify themes within it at the end of each session of observation.

As wide a range of activities and people as possible should be observed. Observation should be conducted at different times of the day and in different locations. Both formal and informal activities should be sampled. Although use of more than one observer is helpful and provides a means of assessing the reliability of the data, the need for prolonged and discreet participation means that a single observer or, at most, a few observers are generally used.

Many of the procedures for collecting and transcribing the data are similar to those described for interviews. The analysis of the data is likely to begin as they are collected. In practice this is making a virtue out of necessity. Observers in research studies are no different from observers in everyday life. They try to understand and interpret the behaviours they see as they proceed. Any other approach would result in a mass of uninterpretable data at the end of the study. Better, then, that we formalize the process so that it is open to critical inspection. This approach is consistent with the grounded theory described in the previous chapter. Observers build theories of the behaviours as they observe them, seeking continually to test and elaborate upon their existing knowledge. As a result observation will progress from the general to the specific. Themes will emerge and can be tested through theoretical sampling. Here, the researcher deliberately observes particular situations or particular people in situations as a test of hypotheses formed during observation. The aim, as in interviewing, is theoretical saturation. Observation ends when the researcher can find no new or disconfirming behaviours and can present a comprehensive account of the observed behaviour. In practice time constraints may limit this process. Nevertheless, readers of the research should feel that they understand and can predict the ways in which the social group or organization operates.

As with interviews the aim is to develop a general account of the behaviour, which is supported by a wide variety of specific examples. These examples are an important part of the research for the reader. They add vividness and credibility to the theoretical explanation. Other checks on the validity of the account are necessary, however. Researchers have frequently sought support for their interpretations via triangulation. Studies frequently combine observation with interviews (see Westby, 1997; McAllister and Silverman, 1999; Briggs et al., 2003). Interviews may be conducted with the people who have been observed, thus providing an opportunity for respondent validation of the interpretation of the observational data. In studies of clients with communication problems, interviews with relatives and other care staff provide an alternative source of data and a means of validation.

Chapter 14
Efficacy: are we going about it in the right way?

Introduction

Legend has it that, in times past, a superior race of SLTs roamed the earth. They were confident, well-dressed ladies who believed all was well with the world and that language disorders were no match for the force of their personality. Evolution caught up with them. Evidence-based healthcare proved a hostile environment for this life form, and their descendants are an altogether more timid species.

In this book we have often discussed experiments that compare treated and untreated clients. By now you should be able to design an experiment like this yourself. Evidence-based practice requires a strategy and must answer questions that assist clinicians. In this chapter I will argue that much of the efficacy research in SLT has lacked a strategy and has asked inappropriate questions. The result has been some spectacular own goals (in the form of non-significant results) and not very much help for clinicians wondering about how to treat their clients. In the next section I will summarize one version (there are others but they are fairly similar) of what the strategy should be. First, let's consider two ways in which we could investigate the efficacy of therapy for children with language disorders.

The first approach begins by recognizing that this is a rather vague problem. Children with language disorders were not all created equal, and their different difficulties require different therapies. As a result we are going to have to answer the question a little bit at a time. We will need to subdivide children into groups who have similar disorders and investigate the effects of therapy on each of them. We will need to define clearly who the groups are and describe the therapy in detail (so that other clinicians can replicate it and know which children to treat). This is not an easy task, and we will need to draw upon theoretical accounts of language disorders as well as the clinical experience of the children. Having selected the children, we must randomly assign them to treated and untreated groups, select assessments that can detect change in the treated areas and arrange for these assessments to be carried out by clinicians who do not know which children have been treated. Ideally we will want several SLTs to give the therapy to avoid the possibility that the results are due to the skills of one or a few clinicians.

The second approach is more pragmatic. It recognizes that children are already out there receiving therapy and that a lot of bother can be avoided by assessing what happens to them. By persuading clinicians to assign children randomly to therapy or no therapy groups, it turns clinical practice into an experiment and avoids much of the inconvenience of the first approach. The children are those referred for therapy; clinicians decide what therapy is appropriate for them, and, by including many clinics, we can study a lot of children treated by a large sample of therapists giving greater generality to our results.

Let's call these two approaches 'studies of therapy' and 'studies of therapy provision'. The contrast between them is an interesting one. They address different questions. Studies of therapy test specific therapies. Studies of therapy provision evaluate a service for a client group. They are not in competition; ideally we want to know both that individual therapies work and that the service is efficient. Notice, however, that the second approach can only work if one of two conditions is fulfilled. Either clinicians know what therapy to give to a substantial proportion of the children they treat (the service can't be efficient if they don't) or it doesn't matter what therapy the children have as long as they receive it. I am going to ignore the second possibility because I don't believe it. Nor, I think, do most therapists. Seeing a therapist probably has some general benefits, but we want more than this. (If possible, 'seeing a therapist' should be the control condition in our experiment.) This leaves the first possibility. Studies of therapy provision are a test not only of the different therapies that clinicians use but also of their ability to select an appropriate therapy for each client. To do this they will require evidence from studies of therapy. I shall argue that, for the most part, such evidence does not exist. As a result therapy provision consists of many different, mainly untested, therapies. Some may work and some may not; some may work with some clients but not others. In such circumstances it is not a surprise that studies of therapy provision produce non-significant results.

The difference between the two approaches can also be described in experimental terms. In studies of therapy the IV (the therapy) is clearly defined, and we can select a DV (an assessment) that is sensitive to the predicted changes in language. By being fussy about which children we include, we can define the population to which the result may be generalized. So we can make clear recommendations about what therapy to offer and who to give it to. In contrast, studies of therapy provision are in danger of losing all control over their IV. Not only do therapists use different therapies, but we (as researchers) don't know what they use. Our IV becomes 'what therapists do with children'. A non-significant (or even a significant) result will not tell us which therapies worked and which did not, nor will it tell us which children benefited and which did not. That clinicians use different therapies and have different therapy aims also makes it difficult to select a DV. Any assessment that we choose is likely to be more sensitive to some therapy outcomes than to others.

The two types of study use the same design and are analysed in the same way (a two-factor mixed ANOVA). This similarity may be obscured because studies of therapy provision often call themselves randomized control trials (RCTs) whereas studies of therapy rarely bother to do so. There is nothing wrong with this. RCTs are the best way to investigate the effectiveness of health interventions. Studies of therapy provision are entitled to use the name. Nevertheless, RCTs are a victim of their own success. A mystique has arisen around them that tends to obscure critical appraisal of individual studies. Merely being an RCT is no guarantee that a study has asked sensible questions or obtained useful answers. It's easy to feel that the SLT has been taken for a ride here. Medical journals demand RCTs and medical opinion (see, for example, Allen, 1990; Pearson, 1995) has urged SLTs to use them. Currently studies of therapy provision are unlikely to generate positive results. Medical journals then publish the non-significant findings ensuring a maximum of bad publicity and a minimum of useful information (or encouragement) for therapists.

You may know that a study of therapy provision for young children has already taken place and that it produced mainly negative results. The purpose of the discussion above was to convince you that this outcome was predictable. We will take a more detailed look at this study shortly. First, however, let's look at a model of how efficacy research develops.

A standard model of efficacy research

Robey and Schultz (1998) outlined what they referred to as the 'standard protocol' for research on the efficacy of clinical interventions. They were particularly interested in research on aphasia, but their model applies to other areas of SLT. They argued that SLT must conform and relinquish its 'idiosyncratic approaches to clinical-outcome research'.

They began with the distinction between efficacy and effectiveness. Efficacy research tests therapy under optimal conditions; effectiveness research tests it under clinical conditions. Optimal conditions include trained therapists, more-intensive therapy and restricting entry to clients who meet certain criteria. Therapy and its assessment may be conducted in a more formal and structured way than in a clinic. Effectiveness studies accept that such circumstances do not apply in clinical situations. They evaluate what actually happens, not what might happen. Both forms of study may use RCTs and are then referred to as explanatory and pragmatic trials respectively. Bigger treatment effects are expected in efficacy studies, which should be conducted prior to effectiveness studies. The latter are used to find out if effects under optimal conditions transfer to the rough and ready of clinical life. (In SLT, efficacy is often used loosely to refer to both types of study. I will use efficacy research as a general term and efficacy and effectiveness to indicate the two types of study).

This distinction between efficacy and effectiveness studies overlaps with the one I have made between studies of therapy and therapy provision. In SLT, studies of therapy are normally efficacy studies. If these are successful, the next step is to conduct effectiveness studies of the same therapy. This rarely happens. Most effectiveness studies in SLT take the form described above. They are studies of the effectiveness of therapy provision not of the effectiveness of individual therapies.

Robey and Schultz (1998) outlined a 5-phase model of efficacy research. Phase 1 tries to detect the presence of a therapeutic effect by using small group and single case studies. The aim is to show that a treatment may be beneficial and deserves investigation. In phase 2 we decide which clients are suitable for the therapy and define exclusion criteria to select them. Outcome measures are selected or developed and the duration of therapy and its method of delivery determined. In phase 3 large-scale efficacy studies are carried out to provide stronger evidence that a treatment works. In phase 4 effectiveness studies are conducted to discover whether treatment works in a clinical environment. Efficacy studies continue with subpopulations to define more precisely those clients who benefit from the therapy. Variations in the treatment and its delivery are explored with the aim of maximizing its effects. Meta-analyses of previous studies may be conducted. Effectiveness studies continue in phase 5 to determine the cost-effectiveness of the treatment and to assess consumer satisfaction and quality-of-life issues.

The timing of efficacy and effectiveness studies is fundamental to the model. Efficacy research comes first. If a therapy works under optimal conditions, the natural sequence is to test it under clinical conditions. If it doesn't work, there is no logical case for doing this. Research with different client groups is at different stages of this model. Some areas have followed its sequence of phases; others have not; few have reached the later phases of the model. In many areas researchers have been too impatient. Effectiveness studies (phase 4), usually of therapy provision, have been conducted without testing for efficacy (phase 3), without determining for whom therapies are appropriate (phase 2) and sometimes with little evidence of a potential beneficial effect (phase 1).

So SLT for children with language disorders doesn't work

Glogowska et al. (2000) conducted a multi-centre RCT of therapy for pre-school children with language disorders. Children were randomly assigned to a treated or a 'watchful waiting' (untreated) group. Clinicians selected therapies in accordance with their normal practice. Few differences were found between the groups, and the study concluded that there was 'little evidence for the effectiveness of SLT'.

The study included a large number of children treated by 21 therapists in 16 community clinics. This suggests that the therapy was representative of typical practice and that the results hold for other children, clinics and clinicians. RCTs of therapy cannot achieve the ideal of double blinding, but efforts were made to ensure that the clinicians assessing the children did not know the group to which they were assigned. Studies like this are not difficult to design, but carrying them out requires more stamina than most us are likely to possess. Of course, if you have followed the argument above and, like me, expected a non-significant result, you may be critical of the study not because it is badly designed or because the result is wrong but because it was a waste of taxpayers' money! In fairness, however, the authors concluded that clinicians should 'reconsider the appropriateness, timing, nature and intensity of such therapy in pre-school children'.

Concern about this study has centred on the finding that the mean treatment time for a child was only 6 hours per year (Law and Conti Ramsden, 2000). Let's try to put this in perspective. Consider a family in Bristol (where the study was carried out). Four-year-old Gary seems like a sharp enough kid, but he doesn't talk much, and Mum has him referred for SLT. In contrast Dad is really impressed by his new company car, which is going a treat. Now which will get more attention in the coming year? Sadly the car will spend more time being serviced than Gary will spend receiving SLT. Now I am not a clinician; so I can't judge whether this is deliberate policy or the result of a shortage of resources. I hope there are no SLTs who think that language impairments can be sorted out in 6 hours per year. Perhaps, if people are shocked by these findings, things will change. Nevertheless, the assumption that things will improve merely by increasing the amount of therapy that children receive seems a dangerous one to me. We also need to look at the sorts of therapy that are being used.

Two curious aspects of this study deserve to be mentioned. Some attempt was made to divide the children into subgroups. Test scores were used to divide them into three groups, and members of each were randomly assigned to treatment or no treatment. Children who were more than 1.2 standard deviations below the mean on language comprehension were placed in a general language group. An expressive language group scored above this score on comprehension but below it on expressive language, and a phonology group scored above it on both comprehension and expression but had an error rate of above 40% on a test word production. A z-score of -1.2 equates to a percentile score of 11.5%. So any child in the bottom 11.5% of the population on comprehension might be placed in the general language group and further children were put in the expression and phonology groups. Even this did not exhaust all the referrals. Other children were referred; some were treated but did not qualify for the study, while some were not treated. Clearly referrals had a wide range of abilities. The percentage of the population from which they came is hard to estimate but is much greater than estimates for the prevalence of language impairment (7.4% – Tomblin et al., 1997). Given the apparent shortage of resources, more therapy might have been offered to a smaller number of more severely affected children. Although the study itself excluded some referrals, its entry criteria remained generous. Again, a more selective policy might have produced better results. The mean of 6 hours treatment conceals a large range (0–15 hours of therapy); so some children received no or very little therapy. It's possible that clinicians, invited by the authors to pursue their normal practice, decided that some children did not need therapy. This would increase the likelihood of a non-significant result.

A more serious problem concerns the measures of comprehension, expression and phonology used as outcome measures in the study. Power calculations (see Chapter 8) were used to calculate a sample size required for a medium-effect size and 80% power. This is important in view of the negative result in the study. It had an 80% chance of detecting a significant result; so we can be more confident that the non-significant result is true. But did it have an 80% chance? The children were assessed on each outcome measure, but not all of them had a problem in each area. For example, children in the expressive language and phonology groups were above the cut-off point on comprehension, and clinicians were unlikely to treat it. Figures in Roulestone et al. (2001) showed that in most cases clinicians correctly identified the children's main problem areas and treated them accordingly. So the number of children actually treated in each of the areas assessed by the outcome measures is much less than the total number of children in the study.

Both these points may have prejudiced the study in favour of a non-significant result. Nevertheless, I don't want to argue that the result was incorrect. I will stick with my view that it was no surprise and that it was due to a combination of too little evidence on which to base therapy decisions and too little time to give therapy.

Do we know what therapy to give?

Children with language problems are the largest group of clients treated by SLTs. So my suggestion that studies of therapy provision won't get significant results because clinicians don't know which therapies to use is a controversial one. So let's have some evidence before we go on.

First, some anecdotal evidence. I know we shouldn't be relying on anecdotes, but this is quite a striking one. Each year, when we talk about efficacy in lectures, I ask students if they know what treatment to give clients in their clinical placements. They admit that they don't (but they are learning their trade after all). Next I ask if they think their clinical supervisors – all experienced clinicians – know what treatment to give. As shows of hands go this is impressive. It's immediate and unanimous and the answer is 'no'. OK, so the devil in me just can't resist asking these questions. But I do have a serious purpose. I want to show that studies of therapy provision are unlikely to get significant results if clinicians are uncertain about what treatment to give to at least some of the clients in their case-loads. The answer seems to reveal something more serious than uncertainty.

This does not mean (I am trying to get back onside here) either that SLT is ineffective or that clinicians do not help clients. Most therapists believe that they are benefiting many of their clients. They recognize, of course, that this judgement is subjective and know that some clients have a habit of improving on their own. But they are also entitled to point out that therapy offers a wider range of 'benefits' than are normally assessed in research studies and that clients may improve in different and subtle ways.

Studies of therapy provision are very demanding tests of the effectiveness of therapy. To work, they require that efficacy studies have shown which therapies work and that their results have been disseminated (by publication and debate) to clinicians. My anecdote suggests this is not the case. This is not surprising. For a start, the research literature on children is not very extensive. Law et al. (1998) conducted a review of the evidence. Studies in the literature were grouped into RCTs (10), which provide the strongest evidence, quasi-experimental studies (12), and single case studies (26). The 10 RCTs cover a period of 30 years and include a total of 257 children. By way of contrast Smith and Glass (1977), who conducted a famous review of psychotherapy outcome studies, included 375 studies with over 25,000 subjects. Now this is a bit over the top (and they didn't stop there by the way), but by any standard the number of studies in an area as important as child language is small.

It is doubtful whether this evidence has had much impact on clinical practice. For example, only two RCTs examined the effects of therapy on comprehension, and one found a non-significant result. A worrying aspect of the RCTs is that six did not report using blind assessments (and you would if you had gone to the trouble of arranging it). There is evidence (see below) that non-blind assessment influences the outcomes of therapy studies, particularly when face-to-face assessments are used.

Six of the studies examined the effects of training parents to help their children, and some compared this with therapy by clinicians. Three (Fey et al., 1993; Giralometto et al., 1995, 1996) used focused stimulation where parents make frequent use of preselected target forms in talking to their children in naturalistic contexts. Fey et al. used it to improve grammar, and Giralometto et al. used it to increase spoken vocabulary. The results are impressive. Fey et al. found that treatment either by clinicians or parents was significantly better than untreated controls. Giralometto et al. found that parents modified their speech after the intervention and that children used more target words, increased their vocabulary and used more words in interactions. Both used blind assessments. The treatment is described and is replicable and is also flexible as different targets may be used to meet the needs of individual children.

This is a good example of the progress of efficacy research. The results are encouraging but questions remain. Some are theoretical.

For instance, Matheney and Panagos (1978) found that therapy for grammar improved articulation (and vice versa). This result was not replicated in Fey et al. (1994). Issues like this are best addressed by efficacy studies where greater experimental control is possible. Others are practical. Therapists had to train the parents and plan and monitor the treatment, which lasted for several months. The parents were not a random sample. In Fey et al. (1993) they responded to advertisements, and in Giralometto et al. they were described as 'middle class' with an above-average number of years in education. The therapy is demanding; so parental motivation and education may be important for its success. Treatment and training was given by a small number of therapists, who were probably highly committed and expert in the methods used. These conditions might be difficult to meet in routine clinical work and with a wider selection of parents and children. Effectiveness studies are needed to determine whether the therapy works under these more demanding conditions. The important point is that neither sort of question is answered by a study of therapy provision.

Have we not been here before?

Yes, we have. In the early 1980s several RCTs examined the effectiveness of therapy provision for people with aphasia. Three studies were conducted in the UK. Two compared clients treated by therapists and by volunteers (Meikle et al., 1979; David et al., 1982), and one compared therapy with no therapy (Lincoln et al., 1984). All reported negative results and were published in medical journals so that doctors could get a less-than-favourable view of SLT!

These studies were similar in design to the study by Glogowska et al. (2000) described above. Therapists gave the therapy they considered most appropriate to the treated group, and their progress was compared to the volunteer or no-treatment group. The negative findings showed that existing practice in the area was ineffective. These studies came in for some criticism (Pring, 1983; Howard, 1986). The case against them was similar to that above. People with aphasia vary, and it is improbable that all or even a majority will respond to any one therapy. Therapists know this and use different therapies with different clients but with little evidence to guide their selection. Studies of therapy provision are, therefore, studies of a well-intentioned lottery in which different, unproven treatments are offered to clients with different language disorders. Robertson (1994) made a similar point. Discussing the study by David et al., he wrote that it had been 'misinterpreted by influential people as showing speech therapy to be worthless'. For it to be effective 'it must be intensive, long lasting, and soundly theoretically based, none of which applied in the evaluation study in question'.

The case against using RCTs to examine therapy provision for people with dysphasia was largely misunderstood. Critics advocated the study of therapy for individual clients (Howard, 1986; Pring, 1986; Franklin, 1997), and the argument was diverted to a dispute about whether single case or group studies offered the best means of researching therapy. Robey and Schultz (1998) argued, correctly, that single case studies can never test efficacy as they do not represent any population to which a result may be generalized. They said their model resolved the dispute between single-case and RCT approaches to efficacy by putting each in its rightful place in the development of efficacy research. They are right. Single case studies can't replace RCTs, but they can tell us more about which therapies to use. We need them because, in many areas of SLT, we are at phase 1 of Robey and Schultz's model not phases 3 or 4, where efficacy and effectiveness are tested. We look at single case studies in the next chapter.

Statistical analysis of treatment studies

As I keep pointing out, studies that compare treated and untreated clients over time (whether called RCTs or not) are just two-factor mixed ANOVAs. The crucial result in the analysis is the interaction. It shows that treated clients improved significantly more over time than untreated ones. In Chapter 7 I showed how similar data could give either a significant or a non-significant interaction. Of course, the data were only superficially similar (the means were the same). In the non-significant version, I moved the scores of the treated group around so that their responses were more variable. You may think this was just a complicated way of explaining the obvious. If we give clients therapy and some progress but others don't, we can't claim that it is effective for the whole group. That ANOVA will not give a significant result just shows that there is less difference between common sense and statistics than you may have thought.

So, if we want significant results, we should avoid giving clients the opportunity to behave inconsistently. Unfortunately studies of therapy provision are an open invitation to do so. First, we take a heterogeneous group of clients. Then we tell therapists to select therapies. We use a measure of improvement that may not be sensitive to the goals of all the therapies offered. Finally we give varying amounts of therapy (but usually not much) so that, even if it is effective, clients improve by different amounts.

In fairness it should be said that some studies of therapy provision for aphasia have been more successful than those above. In most, however, steps were taken to obtain a more homogenous sample of clients. Wertz et al. (1986), for instance, screened 1,816 clients but only allowed 121 to enter their study, and Brindley et al. (1989) treated mainly young clients with relatively good levels of comprehension. The probable effect was to select groups with a good prognosis for therapy thus reducing their variability of response. Others (Basso et al., 1979; Poeck et al., 1989; Denes et al., 1996) implicitly recognized the problem that some clients might not respond to therapy (or get the right therapy) by analysing them on a case-by-case basis and showing that more treated than untreated clients improved. In addition most of these studies offered a lot of therapy over lengthy periods of time (Basso and Caporali, 2001; Brindley et al., 1989; Denes et al., 1996; Poeck et al., 1989). Poeck et al. found that about two-thirds of treated clients improved after receiving 9 hours of therapy per week for 6 to 8 weeks, and Denes et al. found that daily therapy was better than therapy three times per week (itself substantially more than standard practice). If nothing else this probably makes responses to therapy more consistent by giving those who are slow to respond a better chance to do so.

These studies are good news. Clinicians may take heart from them, although they should heed the strong message that improvement may require a lot of therapy. In most cases, however, they offer little information about different types of therapy or the response of different clients to them. Clients with, for example, high-level syntactic deficits or with fluent neologistic speech differ dramatically and need different therapies. Successful studies of therapy provision are welcome, but, after the dust has settled, we remain no wiser about how to treat these different clients. This sort of information is only available from studies of specific therapies with groups of clients with similar disorders.

RCTs in SLT and medicine

There is no question that RCTs have been successful in medicine, particularly in drug trials. This success contrasts with their uncertain history in therapy studies and has made SLT look a bit amateurish as a result. Actually the story is not as simple as this, and it's time we had a closer look.

As experiments RCTs have two great virtues – random assignment and concealment. In drug trials doctors determine if a patient is suitable for a trial. Whether they receive the drug or not is decided independently. This achieves random assignment and means that neither doctor nor patient knows who is treated. The result is a double-blind trial. Doctors can't selectively offer encouragement or advice to treated patients, and any bias in their assessment is also controlled. Use of a placebo controls for any non-specific effects of treatment. In SLT we can randomly assign but are unlikely to conceal from clients (or therapists) who is being treated. Therapy involves a social interaction and encouragement. These general effects, available to treated clients, are confounding variables. Further problems arise if those assessing the clients know who has been treated.

The advantages of drug trials do not end here. Their very nature defines the IV, DV and treated population. The IV (the drug) is precise and clearly distinguishes the treated and untreated groups (as long as they go on taking the tablets). Research should already have linked the action of the drug with a particular medical problem. Detection of the problem in patients defines the population, and changes in symptoms act as the DV (although measures such as quality of life, return to work etc. may also be used). This is very different from studies of therapy provision, where, as I keep saying, the IV is vague, the DV may be insensitive to some of the treatment goals and the clients are a mixed bunch.

In other areas of medical research RCTs are less successful. Not all, indeed not many, medical interventions are as readily assessed as drug trials. Robertson (1994) wrote that '95% of non pharmacological health technologies practiced in the UK are unevaluated' and suggested that 'treatments are offered and operations performed largely on the basis of past practice, received wisdom and good old clinical judgment'. In these areas researchers may encounter similar problems to those in SLT research. For instance, there is increasing interest in the effectiveness of primary care (Mant, 1997; Thomas, 2000). So how will RCTs fare in the exciting world of low back pain, tummy aches and unwanted pregnancies? The initial signs are not good. To assess their success I compared the number of significant findings in 25 consecutive trials in primary care with those in 25 trials in other areas of medical intervention reported in the *British Medical Journal*. As research methods go, this isn't very objective. It's not helped by the difficulty of deciding if outcomes were significant. Studies often use several DVs, and in many cases some are significant and others not which gives a positive but not entirely convincing outcome. These problems aside, however, the results were as shown in Table 14.1.

You probably don't need to do a chi square on these data to convince yourself that there is a difference. To give a few examples:

Table 14.1 Results of RCTs in primary-care and non-primary-care settings

	Trials in primary care	Trials not in primary care
Significant outcomes	10	21
Non-significant outcomes	15	4

leaflets about minor illnesses failed to convince patients not to consult their GPs, psychological therapy for depression had no greater effect than usual GP care and prevention strategies failed to reduce unwanted pregnancies in adolescents. In many of the studies the IV and DV were fairly well defined. It looks to me as if the variable nature of the caseload is the problem. So further research will be needed to discover more about the patients and why some respond to treatment and others don't. The situation is summed up by Croft (1996) when he asked, 'is the controlled trial, so well suited to the simplicity of the pharmaceutical intervention, really the best way to sort out the complex problem of back pain?' Both primary care and SLT are full of such complex problems.

Meta-analysis and systematic reviews

An irritating aspect of research is that similar studies often report inconsistent results. It's common to read a paper with significant results only to find other researchers criticizing it or reporting failures to replicate it. One response to this has been a scholarly review by an expert in the area. These can account for conflicting results by finding differences or weaknesses in the methodologies used or the subjects tested or by proposing new theories that explain contradictions in the evidence. They are influenced by the views of their authors, however, and in efficacy research are considered too subjective. Here more objective approaches, such as meta-analysis and systematic reviews, are used.

Glass (1976) distinguished three forms of data analysis. Primary analysis evaluates an experimental hypothesis and is planned before doing the research. Secondary analysis consists of looking for further information in the data. It is done after seeing the results so we must be more cautious about drawing conclusions from it. Meta-analysis is used to combine the results of studies. It does this by obtaining an effect size (d) for each study. The effect size is calculated from:

$$d = \frac{\bar{x}_e - \bar{x}_c}{s_p}$$

This is the difference in the means of the experimental and control groups divided by the pooled standard deviation (some textbooks use the control-group standard deviation). This is the formula we used in Chapter 8 to do power calculations. It gives us a standardized difference between treated and untreated groups in a study.

Strictly meta-analysis is the statistical technique, and studies that use it are systematic reviews. The terms are used more or less interchangeably, however. The term 'systematic review' is particularly used to describe meta-analyses of studies of medical interventions.

Meta-analysis can do three things for us. First, it can give us a better indication of the efficacy of therapy by getting the mean effect size across studies. Second, we can compare the effect sizes of groups of studies. This allows us to compare the effects of different types of therapy. Third we can use it to highlight the effects of methodological failings in studies. This last point needs a little explanation. Meta-analysis avoids bias by including all published studies (and unpublished ones if found). However, some studies really are poor and deserve to be excluded. There are two ways around this problem. Some meta-analyses (such as those for the Cochrane Collaboration; www.cochrane.co.uk) exclude studies with obvious failings, such as non-random assignment or non-blind assessments. The other approach is to include all the studies and compare the effect sizes obtained by good and poor studies. This approach particularly appeals to those interested in research methods. Poor studies often produce larger effect sizes, and showing this reveals the extent to which methodological weaknesses influence research findings.

Meta-analysis and psychotherapy (and some lessons for SLT)

Although meta-analysis is now widely used, its spiritual home is in psychotherapy. The efficacy of psychotherapy has been studied with great relish (not to say obsessiveness). There are countless studies and many meta-analyses. It's worth looking at what has gone on, as research on psychotherapy and SLT share many problems. Outcomes are difficult to measure; different therapies are used, and the clients may share broad diagnostic labels (for example depression, phobia) but differ in their individual problems and responses to therapy.

Meta-analyses of psychotherapy outcome studies (Smith and Glass, 1977; Shapiro and Shapiro, 1982, 1983; Wampold et al., 1997; Westen and Morrison, 2001) have found fairly large mean effect sizes (between 0.60 and 1.00) for the treatment of various types of psychological problem. These effect sizes are for comparison of treatment and no treatment. Comparisons of alternative treatments often give much smaller effect sizes. Differences between therapy and no therapy include specific effects of treatment and general benefits of having therapy. Comparisons of therapies eliminate the latter. With this removed, and given that both therapies may be beneficial to some extent, differences may be small and difficult to detect. A long-standing controversy in psychotherapy concerns whether they exist at all or whether all therapies (or all those worth investigating) contain some helpful ingredients. The hypothesis of no difference is known as the Dodo-bird verdict because Rosenzweig (1938), who initiated the debate, compared the situation to an incident in *Alice in Wonderland*, where, after a stewards' enquiry, the Dodo bird declares that, 'Everybody has won and all must have prizes.' Studies disagree on this. Shapiro and Shapiro found that about 9% of the variance in effect size was due to different treatments. They described this as a modest difference. Kazdin and Bass (1989) said differences are real but that studies have insufficient power (too few subjects) to detect them. In contrast Wampold et al. (1997) and Luborsky et al. (2002) support the verdict. Clinician- and parent-administered therapies have been compared in SLT. Often no difference is found. Whether the Dodo-bird verdict applies is unclear. It may not matter. Small advantages for clinicians may not be clinically significant when set against the savings in resources if parents can successfully deliver therapy.

Studies of psychotherapy have shown that methodology can influence effect size. Shapiro and Shapiro (1982, 1983) found that effect sizes were related to the assessment used and to the person who carried it out. Assessments vary in their reactivity (the extent to which they can be influenced by those using them). In psychotherapy, measures such as self and therapist ratings are reactive; physiological measures are not. Larger effect sizes are found when reactive measures are used, especially when they are used by clinicians who know whether clients have been treated or not. This is unlikely to be peculiar to psychotherapy. Most assessments in SLT are reactive, and arranging for blind assessment is inconvenient.

Researchers in psychotherapy have allegiances to particular therapy approaches (such as cognitive, behavioural, dynamic and so forth). Luborsky et al. (1999) showed that studies comparing different approaches were influenced by the researchers' allegiances. Sixty-nine per cent of the variance in outcomes was explained by this. In SLT theoretical divisions are less prominent, and studies usually compare therapy with no therapy. Nevertheless, we should be wary of situations, common in SLT, where therapists both propose a therapy and evaluate it. Here their allegiance may bias the results, particularly when they conduct and assess the therapy themselves.

Meta-analysis and SLT

The use of meta-analysis is increasingly popular in SLT (see Robey and Dalebout, 1998, for a review of the methods). An early example was an analysis of therapy studies for dysfluency by Andrews et al. (1980). They found that the effect size for treated clients (1.30) was substantially larger than for untreated clients (0.22). They also compared effect sizes for different therapies, finding prolonged speech, with an effect size of 1.65, most effective. Their study revealed several problems with such reviews. Like other subsequent reviews, they found that many, particularly older, papers could not be included because they did not give the data needed to calculate effect sizes. The finding in favour of prolonged speech should remind us that meta-analysis is only a statistical technique. Some therapists think prolonged speech is worse than being dysfluent and are unlikely to be convinced by its good showing. Only a few studies of attitude change were found. A large effect size from a few studies may be misleading if these are type-one errors and other non-significant outcomes are in researchers' 'file draws'. An indication that this is the case occurs when an apparently popular treatment approach has produced few studies. Andrews et al. (1983) used a method suggested by Rosenthal (1979) to estimate how many non-significant results needed to exist in file draws to override its effect size in the meta-analysis. Only six were needed; so they concluded that these probably existed and that attitude change was not effective.

Meta-analyses of efficacy research in SLT will include both studies of therapy provision and studies of therapy. The former may contribute small effect sizes to the overall mean, and the latter will include studies of different therapy methods. The mean effect size may be misleading and will not be attributable to any particular form of therapy. As with studies of therapy provision the result, positive or negative, will be of little use to practising clinicians who want guidance on what therapy to use. For the same reasons it is unlikely that meta-analyses can compare types of therapy, because many studies either fail to describe the therapy in enough detail or because the therapies used are so variable as to defy classification into groups for comparison. Andrews et al. (1980) was unusual here. In dysfluency there are distinct treatment approaches, and studies can be more easily classified.

Systematic reviews, usually for the Cochrane Collaboration, have suffered because so few studies meet the entry criteria. Greener et al. (2002) found 60 efficacy studies on aphasia therapy, but only 12 were suitable for review. Greener and Langhorne (2002) said the effectiveness of therapy cannot be confirmed or refuted by these studies, nor can clinical recommendations be made. Deane et al. (2002a) and Sellars et al. (2002) found no studies that qualified in reviews of therapy for swallowing in Parkinson's disease and dysarthria in non-progressive brain damage respectively, and Deane et al. (2002b) found only three studies of therapy for dysarthria in Parkinson's disease that qualified. These results are depressing but unsurprising. Many reviews are of areas where researchers are still trying to identify and evaluate therapies. In such cases meta-analyses, although fashionable, are probably premature.

Some meta-analyses of SLT have obtained more positive findings. Whurr et al. (1992) and Robey (1994, 1998) got mean effect sizes close to 0.60 for comparisons of treated and untreated clients with aphasia. This is a respectable result (a medium effect size according to Cohen, 1988) and Robey (1994) said it showed a 'clear superiority in performance of persons receiving treatment by a speech-language pathologist'. The review of studies of children with language problems by Law et al. (1998) gives mean effect sizes for changes in articulation and expressive and receptive language. These are positive, but their interpretation is hindered by the few studies available and by the variation in the effect sizes in individual studies. The latter is to be expected if, as described above, studies use different methods with different samples of children. A second review by Law et al. (2003) included more studies. It obtained significant effect sizes for studies targeting phonology, expressive syntax and vocabulary but not for those targeting receptive language. It again commented on the 'large degree of heterogeneity' in the results of these studies. While the review compared effect sizes for different groups of children and for procedural aspects of the treatment delivery (such as clinicians versus parents), it could not do so for the types of therapy offered. This reflects the fact that research has not developed to a point where clearly identifiable and theoretically based therapies exist. As a result the research evidence is fragmentary and includes many investigations of individual, perhaps idiosyncratic, therapies. A similar position is seen in the meta-analyses of aphasia therapy. Here studies could not be classified into meaningful subgroups. Whurr et al. (1992) described the majority as 'language stimulation' and Robey (1998) referred to the largest category as 'unspecified' therapies. Even positive results in these studies may be of little value to clinicians. Just as studies of therapy provision aggregate the effects of different therapists using different therapies, so meta-analyses aggregate the results of studies of different therapies. Neither can help much with the selection of therapy for individual clients.

A greater concern is whether the mean effect sizes in these meta-analyses are accurate. The figures are presented, explicitly or implicitly, as a measure of the effect of treatment on people with dysphasia or children with language problems. There are several reasons why they may be misleading. Studies may get large effect sizes by selectively treating clients who satisfy particular entry criteria. They may do so because either the therapy is expected to work with a particular type of client or to exclude some clients who are poor candidates for therapy. In either case the effect size will be a misleading estimate of the effect of therapy for all clients.

Other problems arise when basic methodological requirements such as random assignment and blind assessment are not met. Whurr et al. (1992) compared effect sizes of studies that did and did not use random assignment (random = 0.27, non-random = 1.13). Clearly the latter substantially increases the mean effect size. Many studies do not report using blind assessment, suggesting that it was not used. Of the 33 studies in the review by Law et al. (2003), 17 did not report doing so. To these problems must be added the potentially distorting effects of using reactive assessments. In their review Whurr et al. (1992) said that 'it appears that the more psychometrically rigorous the instrument the more conservative the effect size'. SLT may be particularly vulnerable to the affects of these factors. Many studies are conducted by practitioners with limited resources and within clinical environments. They may propose therapies to which they have some allegiance and may both conduct and assess the therapy themselves using reactive assessments. Such studies are invariably well motivated but are likely to exaggerate treatment effects. An example is the study by Ward (1999) that produced very large effects, described by Yoder (1999) as: 'larger than any I have seen in the communication disorders literature'. This is a particularly notable example, but it is unlikely to be the only case where effect sizes have been exaggerated by problems in the research design.

Conclusion

This chapter is by no means a comprehensive review of the efficacy literature in SLT. Most attention has been given to just two areas — developmental language disorders and acquired aphasia. Designing good efficacy studies in these and other areas is not easy. Good and poor research exists in all areas; so it is important that you can judge the merits of individual studies. Nevertheless, the focus of the chapter has been less on individual studies than on the shortcomings of the general research strategy. The model of efficacy research by Robey and Schultz illustrates the problem. Efficacy research is needed to show which therapies work, to define their operation and to identify clients who can benefit. When studies of therapy provision are conducted in areas where this information is unavailable, the results are likely to be negative. Clinicians are not only short of time but short of information. With no agreement on the best therapeutic approach, these studies are, inevitably, an assessment of all therapies and no therapies. Ironically, when significant results are obtained, they are of little value to clinicians. In research when you ask a silly question you find out very little at all.

In the current situation, the use of meta-analysis and the results of systematic reviews are also likely to be of little value. The shortage of research and the difficulties of conducting studies of the necessary quality mean that there may be few studies that qualify for inclusion. That many studies either fail to describe the therapies used or study therapy provision rather than individual therapies means that meta-analyses can tell us little about the effects of different approaches to therapy.

As usual more research is needed. In most areas the need is for efficacy not effectiveness studies. Ideally they should be theoretically based and should assess well-defined therapies, which can be replicated by other researchers. Replications are important to counter biases that exist when researchers assess their own favoured therapies. They can also be used to further investigate a therapy by showing that it does or does not work in different situations and with other clients.

Throughout this chapter I have assumed that clients, even those who appear superficially similar, require different therapies and that a large part of a clinician's skill is in deciding which approach to use. I also dismissed the view that the content of therapy was less important than general factors such as 'force of personality'. I may be wrong. Perhaps therapies are much the same, and benefits are more the result of the attention of a therapist than the content of the therapy. Non-significant results in studies of therapy provision suggest (unintentionally) that this is not the case. This issue is about the nature of SLT and not one for research-methods textbooks. It is important, nevertheless, and one that will shape the future of the profession.

Chapter 15
Single cases and specific therapies

Introduction

This chapter looks at two methods of investigating specific therapies. First, we look at single case studies. Single case studies are used in phase 1 of Robey and Schultz's (1998) model described in the previous chapter. They are used to assess whether a potential treatment has an effect that justifies further investigation. They also allow individual clients to be studied in more detail. Their problems can be analysed in depth, and therapies can be designed to meet their needs. Here the study can both show that a treatment works and give a clearer indication of why it works.

The second part of the chapter looks at research on specific therapies. Though they may use similar experimental designs, there is a clear contrast between these studies and those of therapy provision described in the previous chapter. They examine or contrast specific therapies that are expected to help particular groups of clients. The therapy aims can usually be stated clearly. In experimental terms they have clear independent and dependent variables, and the population tested is well defined. In most cases these are efficacy studies. Research is at phases 2 and 3 of Robey and Schwartz's model – in some areas effectiveness studies are needed or have begun to take place.

Single case studies

Single case studies come in different forms. They may be used to study a client's present condition or their change over time. They may be descriptive or experimental. We will concentrate on experimental studies of change during therapy. Single case studies have the advantage that they can be combined with clinical work with relatively little extra effort. They have two big problems, however. First, we cannot generalize their results to other clients, however similar they may be. A single client is not a random sample of any population; so a single case study cannot test the efficacy of a treatment with other clients. A second problem is that single case studies are not easy to design. In particular you may be wondering how we can have a control condition.

Single case studies have been used widely to study therapy for dysphasia, and accounts of their design concentrate on this area (Coltheart, 1983; Pring, 1986; Seron, 1997; Franklin, 1997). There are three ways to create a control condition in a single case study. We can use untreated items as a control for treated items or an untreated area as a control for a treated area or monitor a treated area during periods of no treatment and treatment so that it acts as its own control. In practice, designs often combine elements of each of these, but we will begin by looking at them separately.

Using other items as controls

Using untreated items as controls does not sound like a very promising approach. Normally we hope that effects of therapy will generalize to untreated items; so this design seems like an admission of defeat before we start. It has limited applications but is worth describing because it is quite a strong design (as single case studies go) and is easy to use.

Suppose we want to treat word finding in a client with aphasia. We randomly assign 20 pictures to two groups and ask the client to name them. We then treat one group and reassess the naming process. The design looks like Table 15.1.

Table 15.1 Basic design for a single case study of word-finding in dysphasia

	First assessment		Second assessment
20 pictures	a	treat	b
20 pictures	c	controls	d

The assessment is the number of pictures correctly named out of 20. We can compare a versus b and c versus d with a McNemar test. If therapy has worked, the former should be significant and the latter not. This is unconvincing, however. The problem is one we have met before. We need to show that treated pictures improve more than untreated ones. A better approach is to assess the pictures and then put correct and incorrect ones randomly into two groups so that an equal number is right at the beginning. Here $a = c$, and so we can compare b and d directly with a chi-square test. This tells us if $b > d$

even when $d > c$ (because of general improvement or because of generalization of the therapy effect). The design can be extended to more sets of words, further therapy and follow-up assessments, as shown in Table 15.2. Here $a = d = g$. We can assess the effects of treatment by comparing b versus e and f versus i using chi square as before. We can also compare a versus c (McNemar) to look at the maintenance of the treatment effect.

Table 15.2 Extending the design to further sets of pictures

Initial assessment			Assess 1		Assess 2
a	20 pict.	treat	b	no treatment	c
d	20 pict.	control	e	treat	f
g	20 pict.	control	h	control	i

Designs of this kind have been used to assess naming therapy in aphasia (see Marshall et al., 1990; Eales and Pring, 1998) and to assess treatment for writing in people with jargon aphasia (see Robson et al., 1998; Jackson-Waite et al., 2003). In each case they could be used because untreated items were expected to show little or no benefit from the treatment.

Improvement in these designs might result from practice or repeated exposure to the items. The client will regularly see the treated but not the untreated items. There is nothing wrong with practice, of course; but it would be nice to show that it is not the whole treatment. We could control for this by having the client do repeated naming attempts of control pictures so that they are equally exposed. It's also a good idea to have several pictures of each item so that more than one can be used in therapy and different pictures used in the assessment. This prevents a picture-specific learning effect (see Jackson-Waite et al., 2003).

The effects of therapy are particularly clear where a client's initial scores are zero (see Robson et al., 1998). It is tempting to create this situation by treating only items failed on the first assessment. This might not be a smart move, however. Naming in dysphasia, for example, fluctuates from day to day. If we use only failed items, some will be named at the next assessment whether treated or not. Although treated items should still benefit more, the results will wrongly suggest that generalization has occurred. It is better to start clients at their normal level of performance by including some items that they named correctly at the pre-therapy assessment.

Time-series designs

Before describing the other designs, it's worth considering how single case studies have been used in other areas of research. They are widely used in behavioural clinical psychology. This is not surprising. Clients are treated individually, and their problems and treatments vary, and so group studies are often inappropriate. The designs are described below. The treatments are interventions to reinforce or discourage target behaviours. In the figures I have assumed that treatment is reinforcing a particular behaviour, and the graphs show the number of times that it occurs. Large and rapid effects are often seen and are easily assessed. The designs are called 'time-series designs' because the general procedure is to compare progress over periods without treatment (A phase) and with treatment (B phase). A further feature of the designs is that they use repeated assessments within each phase (as shown in the figures) so that fluctuations in the target behaviour can be monitored.

The simplest is the 'AB design', where no treatment is compared with subsequent treatment. This design has been called 'pre-experimental'. The problem is that there is only one transition from no therapy to therapy. If change occurs, it may be difficult to convince ourselves that it is due to therapy and not to other events occurring at the same time. The ABA and ABAB designs are stronger because they have more transitions. By moving between no treatment and treatment more than once, they make it very unlikely that other events can be causing the changes that are observed. This general design may be almost indefinitely extended. For instance, we might use an ABACA(BC)A design. Here two treatments, B and C, are compared individually with no treatment; then their combined effect is examined.

Sadly the methodological requirements of these designs and our expectations of therapy are seriously at odds. The ABA design is only fully successful if performance declines in the second A phase (see Figure 15.1). We normally hope that this does not happen and may not consider therapy to be successful if it does. The ABAB design is slightly preferable as it finishes on a treatment phase.

The A phase in these designs acts as a baseline to assess change without therapy. It may show fluctuations across assessments but should not show consistent improvement. Baselines are also important in multiple baseline designs. These come in different forms. In the 'multiple baselines across situations' design (Figure 15.2) behaviour is monitored in two situations without intervention. Treatment is introduced in one but not the other; when improvement is seen,

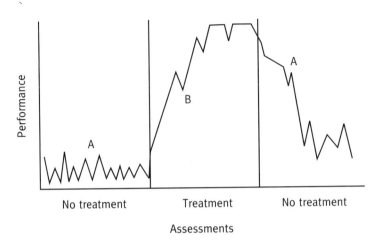

Figure 15.1 The ABA design.

treatment is transferred to the other situation. We might, for instance, reinforce a behaviour in a child first in the classroom then in the playground.

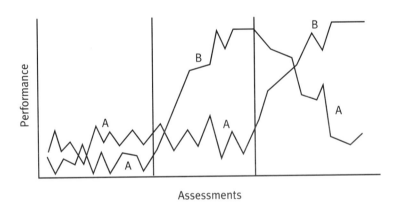

Figure 15.2 The multiple baseline design.

The design can also be used across behaviours or subjects. In the former the same treatment is given for different behaviours at different times. In the latter the same treatment is given to different people at different times. In each design it is crucial that baselines are established for each behaviour to show that it is stable. Treatment is introduced at different times and must work on each occasion to show unambiguously that it is the cause of the change in behaviour.

Other designs have been used. In the changing criteria design, shown in Figure 15.3, a criterion for success is set and treatment given until performance reaches it. Treatment is then withdrawn for a period and behaviour monitored to see if the change is maintained. If it is, a new criterion is set and treatment reintroduced. The base 10 method, described by LaPointe (1977), is similar to this design. In it clinicians set a criterion and monitor progress towards it during therapy. Once achieved, performance is monitored without therapy to ensure that gains are maintained and a new target is set.

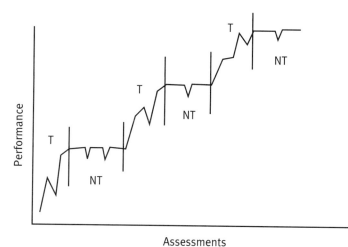

Figure 15.3 The changing criteria design.

You may already have decided that these designs are not going to get us very far. They are well adapted to behaviour modification and are convincing when treatment or its withdrawal causes rapid changes. In SLT, changes are often slower and harder to achieve. The need for treatment effects to reverse is particularly problematic. If this does not occur, the ABA design has no advantage over the AB design. A further problem is that reinforcement doesn't behave like the treatments to which we are accustomed. It is specific in some ways but general in others. It can be specific to situations as in the multiple baselines across situations design (language therapy is expected to generalize to other situations). However, the same treatment can change different behaviours, as in the 'multiple baselines across behaviours' design. A final problem is the need for repeated assessments to monitor change. It may be inconvenient and time-consuming. We look at this later. These problems suggest that only the AB design may be used in SLT. Despite the reservations about its use, Morley (1994) noted that it is widely used in clinical practice and fits the natural requirements of client and therapist.

Using another task as a control or the treated task as its own control

We can now go back and look at the other designs. Single case studies are often used to test specific therapies for particular language-processing deficits. Here, an unrelated language deficit may act as a control. If this does not improve during therapy, we can reasonably claim that the change in the treated area was not due to general recovery. The control task must not benefit from the therapy but must be one where the client wants to improve and is motivated to do so. Choosing such a task may be easier said than done. Treated and control tasks should be at similar levels of difficulty and performance. Using a control that is more difficult is silly. The difference in difficulty may mean that general recovery will lead to an improvement in the easier treated task but not in the control, making it appear as if treatment has worked. Equally the control should not be at such a low or high level of performance before therapy that it is unlikely or unable to improve under any circumstances. Another concern is that the assessments of the treated and control tasks are equally sensitive to change. Misleading results may be obtained if the assessment of the treated task is more able to detect change than that used for the control task.

A tempting solution might be to select several control tasks. If only the treated task improves, this looks convincing (surely at least one of the controls must have met the criteria above). Of course, things may not turn out like this. Some controls may improve, leaving us uncertain about the effects of therapy. A more exciting, but risky, approach is to assess several untreated tasks and to predict which will improve (owing to generalization) and which will not. A successful result here is impressive and convincing.

An alternative is to follow treatment of the first area by treatment of the control. Here we show that the control does not improve when not treated but does when treated. This shows that the control was appropriate because it can be successfully treated. It also allows us to check on maintenance of the gains in the first area. In effect the control becomes an AB design and the treated task a BA design. This has been called a 'crossover treatment' design (Coltheart, 1983). Notice that it is important that both areas improve when treated. If the second does respond to therapy, it was a suitable control for the first area. If it does not, the effects of both forms of treatment must be in doubt.

We can use the treated task as its own control in the AB design. Here we show that no change occurs without therapy, then show progress when therapy is given. A potential problem is what to do in the initial A phase. If we are testing the effect of a specific therapy, we might want the client to receive some form of general therapy or language stimulation during this period. This is better than no therapy as it controls for the general effects of receiving attention. An alternative is to offer therapy for another area of language during this baseline period. This turns the design into a crossover treatment design again.

Both these designs now look like variations on the time-series designs described above. In time-series designs, repeated assessments in each phase are used to give feedback to the clinician and to demonstrate change with therapy. In SLT, however, they may be too time-consuming to collect, and the repetition of the assessment may, in itself, cause changes in performance due to familiarity. Consequently this approach may only be used when circumstances allow. The therapy used by Matthews et al. (1997) required that repeated videos be made of a child interacting with his parents, and these were used to assess his or her progress.

A simpler alternative is to assess the client at the beginning and end of each phase of the design. This can be misleading, however. Suppose we assess a client before and after therapy and find an improved performance. The problem is that we don't know how much performance varies from day to day without therapy. Without knowing this, we can't tell whether the scores just represent a bad day and, later, a good day. This is a common problem in single-case designs. Using untreated items as controls is one way around it. They are similar to treated items and assessed in the same way, and so they are a good control for day-to-day fluctuations in performance.

Another alternative is to obtain two or more measures before and after therapy. If the pre-therapy (A) phase is equal in length to the treatment (B) phase and the assessments do not differ, this is fairly strong evidence that improvement is not occurring without therapy. Similarly, if the post-therapy assessments are higher but do not differ, this shows that the improvement is due to therapy and that it is maintained.

Analysing time-series data

When time-series designs are used in behaviour modification, the changes in behaviour are often dramatic and rapid. That they often reverse when treatment is removed may leave us in doubt about the long-term effects of the intervention, but it demonstrates quite convincingly that the changes were due to the treatment. In these circumstances you may think statistical analysis is unnecessary. Most practitioners in behaviour modification agree with you. Their approach (of which you might approve) is to draw a graph of the data, stand back and admire it for a bit and say that the treatment worked. This is called 'visual analysis'! It is sometimes used in SLT. Hesketh (1986) used two different therapies in a multiple-baseline design. The therapies aimed to reduce dyspraxic errors and promote use of a grammatical subject in speech. Baselines were established for each and the therapies introduced at different times. A dramatic increase in use of subjects left little doubt about the success of that therapy. There was a decrease in dyspraxic errors, but the change was much smaller and visual analysis less satisfactory. Single case studies of children who are dysfluent have used a similar approach. Here assessments taken during baseline are used to show a consistently high level of dysfluency and those taken after therapy to demonstrate maintenance. Graphs provide convincing evidence of treatment effects.

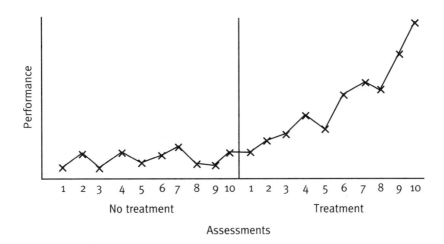

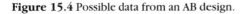

Figure 15.4 Possible data from an AB design.

Visual analysis has a further advantage. It's not at all clear what statistical tests we could use on such data. Consider the data in Figure 15.4. They look fairly convincing, but not everyone will be happy with visual analysis (they might argue that the gradually accelerating pattern of improvement is due to repeated testing). So what statistical test can we use? We might compare the assessments in the different phases of the design with a t-test. Alternatively we might get regression lines for the baseline and treatment and compare their slopes to show that a change in the trend of the data has occurred.

Unfortunately we are not going to get away with either. Data from a person over time are not subject to random variation like data from different people. Despite the variability we often see in clients, their scores are not independent, and the score on one day is a fairly good predictor of the next. Their variance will be small (an extreme example is a client who scores 0 throughout the baseline), and using them to estimate random error will lead to misleading results.

This problem is called serial dependency. Statistical methods have been developed for dealing with it in areas such as economic forecasting. There data are often a sequence of scores over time (for example unemployment figures, share prices and so forth). Changes in government policy or events can influence this data in much the same way as introducing or withdrawing therapy. Interrupted time-series analysis (ITSA) can analyse this sort of data. It is unlikely that we will want to use ITSA, however: it's complex and needs lots of data. You may also feel that it has not been a huge success in its present use!

Other methods have been proposed. Tryon (1982) suggested a simple method, called the C coefficient, for analysing time-series data when relatively few scores are available. The calculations, although not complicated, are laborious. Tryon gave worked examples of it (but see Blumberg, 1984, for some objections and corrections to the formulae) and it has been used in SLT (see Jeffries and Pring, 1987; Matthews et al., 1997; Forman et al., 2002).

Another possibility is to use non-parametric tests. These do not need estimates of error variability. Some simple method can be used to amplify visual analysis. In Figure 15.4 we might split the baseline into two halves. Then we can find two points by obtaining the median values (on the x and y axes) for the first five and the second five scores. A line through these points shows the trend in the baseline data. By continuing it into the treatment phase, we can see how many scores are above the trend (a sign test could be used to see if the number is significant). An even simpler approach may be to establish a stable baseline and then to merely assess how many assessments in the treatment phase are higher than the highest baseline assessment. Lincoln et al. (1997) used a method similar to this to assess the use of cognitive-behaviour therapy to alleviate depression after stroke in a series of single case studies.

Alternatively we might use non-parametric tests of trend. Pring (1986) described the Mann test, which can be used to assess trends in data when only a few scores are available. A more sophisticated non-parametric test of trend is Page's L. It is normally used to assess whether a trend exists in a group of subjects over time but can be used to assess responses to a group of stimuli by a single subject. An example may be found in Parkin et al. (1998), who used errorless learning to teach proper names to a client with a profound anomia after herpes simplex encephalitis.

Examples of single case studies

So far single case research has been presented as a choice between a series of well-organized designs. In fact, practice is often very far from this. Researchers must often adapt and combine different designs to meet the requirements of the research they want to do. An example is provided by a study of a client with word meaning deafness by Francis et al. (2001). In word meaning deafness clients fail to access the meanings of spoken words despite having adequate semantic information about them. They can distinguish between spoken words and non-words, repeat words and may (as a special party trick) write them down, read them and then understand them. Francis et al. compared two approaches to therapy. One used only written words; the other, written and spoken words (they referred to these as implicit and explicit therapies for their presumed or actual activation of the auditory forms of the words). Three groups of words were used, one for each treatment and a third as controls. A baseline consisting of three successive assessments showed that there was no improvement without therapy. The implicit and explicit therapies were then introduced in turn. This is described as an ABACA design; it might also be called a 'multiple baseline across treatments'. Each treatment led to significant gains when compared with untreated words. Neither was well maintained, however, although an advantage was reported here for the explicit therapy. The design is convincing because the baseline shows that there was no change without therapy and because the improvement in each set of treated words occurred at the times when treatment was introduced.

Single case studies are often successful when used to assess therapy for specific skills. Typically, as in studies of word-finding, the changes are clear and improvement is limited to the treated items, making the studies easier to control. They have been used to assess more general communication skills, however. Hopper et al. (2002) investigated the effects of coaching on the conversations of two clients with dysphasia and their spouses. Data were collected during 10 therapy sessions and coaching introduced at different points for each dyad. The design, therefore, combined two AB designs to create a multiple baseline across subjects. Performance was somewhat variable, although the means for each dyad were higher in the B phase than the A phase. More convincing changes were seen when a post-therapy conversation was compared with one taken prior to treatment.

The selection of controls becomes difficult when more-sophisticated language skills are treated. Here we meet the dilemma described above. Suppose that we treat the sentence production skills of a client with dysphasia. It seems both desirable and likely that improvement will generalize to untreated sentences. Here we might need to use an unrelated language control task. The more complex the treated task, however, the more difficult it is to determine which language skills might or might not benefit from the therapy. Marshall et al. (1997) studied a client with dysphasia who had problems assigning the thematic roles of verbs. Three argument verbs were treated. They and other untreated three argument verbs improved, but verbs from other classes did not. The latter, and the fact that the client was many years post-onset, demonstrate that therapy was effective and that it generalizes to other similar verbs.

In some cases studies of the efficacy of therapy merge with theoretical studies of language processing. Marshall et al. (1998) studied a client with a selective deficit in accessing verb phonology. They hypothesized that poor access to verb phonology led to problems in sentence production and that therapy for the former would also improve the latter. This prediction was fulfilled. Controls consisted of untreated verbs and tasks that required the production of abstract words. The former showed some improvement, suggesting that generalization was occurring; the latter did not change.

The single-case approach is being used increasingly to study treatment in areas other than dysphasia. Frazier-Norbury and Chiat (2000) treated written-word recognition in a boy with language problems. The client had poor phonological but good semantic and visual memory skills, and the treatment was designed to build on these strengths. Various semantic tasks were used in which written words appeared. Treated words improved more than sets of untreated words that either appeared or did not appear in treatment. The former set of untreated words were included to control for exposure during treatment and improved more than words that did not appear. The TROG (Bishop, 1983) and an assessment of number skills, used to control for general improvement with age, showed no change.

Crosbie and Dodd (2001) reported on the use of auditory discrimination therapy with a 7-year-old girl with severe language problems. Detection of minimal pairs was used as a measure of her auditory discrimination. A baseline was established before treatment, and improvement to within normal limits was found after treatment and 12 months later. General language assessments and reading age did not change with therapy. More surprisingly there was no change in lexical decision. These tasks act as controls and show that the therapy had a highly specific effect. Clinically, however, the results are rather disappointing. They suggest that the failure of auditory discrimination has had a lasting effect on the girl's language processing and that further therapy will be required to rectify this.

The efficacy of specific therapies: some examples

In this section I will look at efficacy research in several areas of SLT. This review is not comprehensive. I have chosen a few areas and discuss only a few studies in each. They have been selected because they appear to demonstrate positive treatments. They also illustrate some of the problems facing efficacy research in SLT.

Dysfluency

At critical points in this book I have used (fictitious) studies of treatment for dysfluency to illustrate how to do research and analyse data. Dysfluency was an obvious choice. It is common, especially in young children, and parents and children notice it, worry about it and demand that SLTs do something about it. Therapists have responded by producing a range of therapies and efficacy research. In general researchers in this area have shown good awareness of how to design efficacy studies (even if they have not always lived up to it in practice). It is accepted that studies must follow progress after therapy to assess maintenance and that assessments should be conducted in several settings to assess generalization. A series of papers have discussed the methodology of efficacy studies in dysfluency (Moscicki, 1993; Ingham and Riley, 1998; Jones et al., 2001; Thomas and Howell, 2001), and existing research has been reviewed and criticized (see Cordes, 1998; Ingham and Cordes, 1998).

Efficacy research is always more difficult when clients undergo natural recovery. Estimates of spontaneous remission in young children who are dysfluent are as high as 89% (Yairi and Ambrose, 1992). As a result clinicians must decide whether to treat or delay in the expectation of natural recovery. For researchers the situation is that described in Chapter 7. There we saw that efficacy studies can detect effects of therapy against a background of consistent recovery but struggle when clients respond inconsistently (to therapy or no therapy). Nobody has told the children about this. Spontaneous remission is seen at varying periods after onset of dysfluency; so some children will recover naturally during a study. They will have been randomly assigned, and so the effect of their recovery on the group means will be similar. However, the inconsistency of their responses will not help us get a significant interaction of groups by time of assessment. That significant results have been obtained is encouraging, therefore.

Our concern is with methodology; so we will look at just one approach and the efficacy research on it. The Lidcombe program is a behavioural treatment for stuttering in young children. Parents are trained to reward fluent speech and to point out and/or correct dysfluencies. They also rate their child's fluency daily and make recordings from which the number of dysfluencies per minute may be calculated. These provide a record of the child's speech at home and are used by clinicians to monitor and discuss therapy with parents in clinic. Measures of fluency are also taken at each clinic visit. When a child is consistently fluent at home, therapy gives way to maintenance. Parents continue monitoring speech but clinical sessions are reduced. Onslow and Packman (1998) described the programme.

The programme is an interesting example of the development of efficacy research. It was known that operant techniques could reduce dysfluency. The programme allowed parents to give and assess treatment in the child's home. The therapy was developed within clinical practice, and early data on its effectiveness came from clinical reports. Jones et al. (2000) reviewed 250 cases that were successfully treated. They found that the median treatment time was 11 sessions. The number of sessions required increased with the severity of the children's dysfluency but decreased with the time they had been dysfluent.

The use of regular assessments has allowed single case studies to be conducted. A pre-therapy baseline can be established, treatment introduced and post-therapy fluency monitored during maintenance. Single case data are presented in Onslow et al. (1990, 1994).

Robey and Schultz (1998) suggested that the initial phase of efficacy research should also investigate whether a treatment has harmful side effects. Although this may seem unlikely, behavioural treatments make some people nervous, and the programme has its critics. Woods et al. (2002) tested eight children before and after therapy and found no negative psychological impact either on the children's behaviour or the quality of their attachment with their mothers.

These data suggest that the therapy warrants further investigation in efficacy studies. A small trial of the programme was conducted by Harris et al. (2002). Children were treated for 12 sessions and compared with untreated controls. Assessments were conducted blind, and the reliability of the fluency measures was checked. Treated children improved significantly more than controls. That many children become fluent with relatively little therapy makes it easier to show an effect of treatment. If treatment is completed quickly, fewer children will show spontaneous remission and their responses will be more consistent.

These results are impressive. The next stage may be to show that the programme is superior to other types of treatment. Comparisons with other treatments may also identify the elements of the programme that are essential to the reduction in dysfluency. Such comparisons have not been undertaken to date. As usual it will be harder to produce results in these studies. If treatments are all effective to some degree, the relatively small differences between them are difficult to detect. A related question concerns whether the success of the programme is directly due to its operant nature or whether it works by inadvertently changing other variables that improve fluency. For example, it has been suggested that fluency may be increased by modifying interactions between children and parents or by changing the child's rate of speech. Bonelli et al. (2000) and Onslow et al. (2002) (see Exercise 5.8) found that measures of these variables changed inconsistently in children treated in the Lidcombe program. This suggests that the programme affects fluency directly, and not by causing secondary changes in other variables.

Clinical case-study data have already provided some evidence of the effectiveness of the therapy. Further effectiveness studies would be welcome, however. It is important that other clinicians replicate the therapy. Since both the therapy and the target population have been described in detail, this should be readily achieved. Replications by other clinicians less familiar with the programme and working in different clinical facilities would add to the generality of the findings.

Non-organic dysphonia

Carding et al. (1999) and MacKenzie et al. (2001) have conducted controlled trials of therapy for non-organic dysphonia. Carding et al.

distinguished between indirect and direct therapy. Indirect therapy seeks to correct factors such as vocal abuse and poor vocal hygiene as well as enabling client to recognize the psychological and social factors that contribute to them. Direct therapies aim to modify faulty voice production itself. Typically clinicians use a combination of methods. In Carding et al., clients treated by a combined approach were compared with clients who received only indirect therapy and a control group who received no treatment. In MacKenzie et al. (2001), a treated group received both approaches as judged appropriate by a clinician and were compared with an untreated group. Both studies obtained significant results, and Carding and Hillman (2001) argued that they show that RCTs can be used successfully to investigate complex behavioural interventions such as those used within SLT. This claim is at odds with studies in other areas of SLT and with the discussion in Chapter 14 of the reasons for their failure. So why are RCTs of voice therapy more successful than those in other areas?

As we saw in the last chapter significant results are obtained when a client group responds consistently to therapy. Consistency is more likely when the clients have similar symptoms and when broad agreement exists on the appropriate therapy. Use of a DV that is sensitive to the aims of this agreed therapy is also important. This may be more likely in dysphonia than some of the other areas we have discussed (I am sticking my neck out a bit here). Clients vary in the causes of their vocal abuse, but its symptoms are fairly consistent. Clinicians cannot change the causes; they can help clients do so by increasing their awareness of them and of their effects on voice (the indirect approach). Alternatively they can treat faulty voice production directly. Carding et al.'s results are interesting here. The combined approach was superior and produced positive and consistent results. The indirect approach produced equally good results in some clients but poor results in others. The authors suggested that the good responses in this group occurred when clients identified lifestyle causes of abuse and took responsibility for changing them.

Other factors may have contributed to the consistency of response. Both studies excluded some clients. Motivation and regular attendance were required. Professional voice users and clients with a history of dysphonia or excessive smoking or drinking, or with psychiatric or psychosomatic conditions, were excluded. Exclusion criteria play an important role in efficacy research. They remove atypical clients who might be expected, prior to the research, to not respond or to respond inconsistently to the treatment. They must be used carefully, however. Clear definitions of the criteria are needed to prevent researchers excluding clients who are merely eccentric or undesirable! Exclusion criteria serve to define the population to which the research findings may be generalized. Hence, it is equally important that consumers of the research can apply the criteria to recognize those clients to whom the results do and do not apply.

It is difficult to know whether these are efficacy or effectiveness studies. Both describe the therapies used in some detail and argue that they reflect those in current clinical use. The clients (some exclusion criteria apart) are probably typical of the many (MacKenzie et al. suggested 40,000 per annum) who seek voice therapy. In both studies, however, therapy is conducted by a single clinician. This is in contrast with those studies of therapy provision, previously described, whose strength is that they sample the therapy offered by a large number of clinicians. Use of a single experienced clinician may have contributed to the positive outcome in these studies. The therapy used will have been more consistent than would be the case if a number of clinicians were involved and may have led to a more uniform response by clients. It also means that we cannot be sure that other clinicians would achieve similar results. Carding et al. pointed out that a similar study that samples therapy by a number of clinicians is needed. They also said that the clients excluded in their study would form part of a normal clinical caseload. In both regards the studies may be deemed to examine efficacy rather than effectiveness. Nevertheless, it seems unnecessary for an effectiveness study to include clients who, by common consent, have a poor prognosis for therapy. A more appropriate approach may be to examine the effectiveness of therapy for different groups of clients separately. This approach is more informative than sampling all the clients and risking the possibility of finding non-significant results.

These studies are unusual in their use of a range of DVs. Both used self-ratings of their voices by clients, blind ratings by expert listeners and acoustic analysis of the clients' voices. MacKenzie et al. (2001) also assessed quality of life and used the hospital anxiety and depression scale (HADS) (Zigmond and Snaith, 1983) and a blind clinical interview to assess clients' psychological health. Use of several DVs is particularly useful when treatment has a number of objectives. Here ratings of voice examine its perceived normality, while acoustic measures provide an objective measure of the changes that have occurred. It is acknowledged that voice disorders frequently involve psychological factors and that they affect quality of life; so measures of these give a broader indication of the success of therapy.

In both studies the rating measures offer the clearest evidence of success. Carding et al. found that combined therapy led to significantly greater improvement than indirect therapy, which in turn was significantly better than no therapy. MacKenzie et al. found a significant improvement in self-ratings at post-therapy and follow-up assessments. Ratings by listeners showed a similar pattern but were only significant at follow-up. Although the clients' views are obviously important, self-ratings are, in some ways, the least satisfactory of the measures used. They are reactive measures and may lack validity if clients let other factors influence their judgements.

Despite the claims by both studies to have shown significant effects of therapy, changes were largely restricted to the perceptual measures. The acoustic measures were surprisingly poor at detecting change. Of greater concern is that no changes were found on the HADS, the clinical interview or in quality of life. Wilson et al.(2002) showed that the quality of life of clients with dysphonia was significantly worse than controls. This demonstrates, as expected, that dysphonia effects quality of life and leads to the expectation that it may improve with voice therapy. Using the same measure (the SF-36), MacKenzie et al. found that only one subscale had improved significantly after therapy and none had at follow-up. These non-significant results indicate that clients still have psychological problems and that their quality of life is poor. Further research is needed here. Changes in these areas may only occur after more prolonged experience of improved voice use. Alternatively it may be that their failure to change threatens the long-term improvement in voice seen in the client and listener ratings.

Children with phonological problems

Children with functional phonological problems are common and conspicuous by their disordered speech production (the 'functional' indicates that there is no known cause). Gierut (1998) states that about 10% of children are affected and that they dominate the case-loads of SLTs working in schools. Many of these children have a more general deficit in phonology. Their knowledge of the sounds of words is poor. This may affect their language generally and may lead to problems in reading and spelling (see Larrivee and Catts, 1999).

Parents of the children are concerned about their speech (and would be more so if they knew about reading and spelling too). It's likely (and who could blame them?) that they think this is exactly what speech therapists were invented for. 'And she calls herself a speech therapist', I can hear them saying. All in all, this looks like quite a stern test of competence for the profession. Happily there is a lot of research in the area, and the results, while not entirely consistent, are fairly positive.

Gierut (1998) referred to disorders of articulation as phonetic, and those affecting the stored phonological representations of words as phonemic. In contrast Almost and Rosenbaum (1998) referred to the former as phonetic, phonemic or articulatory and to the latter as linguistic. This inconsistent terminology is confusing, and those of us who already have problems with the 'ph' words can become very puzzled indeed. Gierut also used the terms 'competence' (the underlying knowledge of phonology) and 'performance' (the ability to produce it correctly in speech). These terms have not been widely used (in this context) but are less confusing, and I will adopt them here.

The term 'functional phonological disorder' is misleading. The children are referred to SLT because of their speech. They may or may not have a more general problem with phonology. As so often happens clients with a shared diagnosis differ in important respects. This suggests, as Hesketh et al. (2000) pointed out, that they may need different therapies. To put it crudely, it's a choice between attacking the mouth or the mind! Those with problems in performance may only need articulation therapy. Those with competence problems may require a different approach. Training in phonological awareness helps children with reading problems, and it is plausible that it might also improve speech. This possibility is reflected in a shift in the forms of treatment used. Gierut (1998) suggested that a traditional reliance on articulation has given way to a greater dependence on phonology.

While trying to understand phonological disorders, I have asked quite a lot of clinicians what therapy they use. The answer is fairly unanimous. They use both articulatory and phonological tasks. This eclectic approach is a sensible response to the uncertainty about which treatment to use and to the fact that many children have problems in both performance and competence. Some researchers have assessed this approach. Lancaster (1991) asked clinicians to use a range of tasks in therapy. Auditory discrimination, minimal contrast therapy, auditory bombardment, exercises from Metaphon, cued articulation and other forms of articulation work and motor-skills training were all used. Children were treated by different clinicians and blind assessment was used. Treated children improved significantly more than children whose treatment was delayed. A further group of children who were treated by their parents also improved significantly. A similar approach was taken by Almost and Rosenbaum (1998). Therapy was given twice weekly for 4 months. Single word production and the percentage of consonants correct in conversational speech were assessed. The treated group made significantly greater progress. The untreated group was then treated and substantially caught up with the treated group.

The eclectic approach takes a pragmatic view. If we hit them with everything we have (mouth and mind), something is going to work. The evidence above suggests that it does. In contrast Metaphon is more structured and more exclusively phonological. The therapy is described in Howell and Dean (1991) and Dean et al. (1995). It has 2 phases. Phase 1 differs from other phonological approaches. Child-friendly activities (involving cats' tails and trumpet blasts) are used to alert the child to the contrastive nature of first non-speech and then speech sounds and to develop a shared non-technical vocabulary for their description. In phase 2 the metaphonological knowledge gained is transferred to communicative settings.

Dean et al. (1995) described a series of single case studies in which two treated phonological processes are compared with a control untreated process. Thirteen children were treated. Five behaved themselves, progressing in the treated but not the untreated processes; four showed generalization from treated to untreated, and four showed inconsistent outcomes. These results are encouraging but show a high degree of variability in response to therapy. Initial data from a group study (Reid et al., 1996) confirmed this variability. The study used a rather eccentric design. One treated group received 6 weeks of phase 1 of the therapy; another received both phases over a 10-week period. Each had a control group who were monitored for similar periods. The results, admittedly for only a few children, show a confusing picture. There was evidence of maturational change in the control groups and the treated children responded very inconsistently.

Hesketh et al. (2000) directly compared groups of children who received articulatory or phonological therapy with a control group. The treated groups improved more than controls but did not differ from one another on phonological awareness or the percentage of consonants correct (but the articulatory group did better on a probe assessment which assessed the specific processes treated in each child). The control group in the study had normal speech. This avoided the need to delay treatment for some children but was, in other respects, an unfortunate choice. Treated children were shown to be catching up with, rather than progressing more rapidly than, controls. The evidence for maturational change in Reid et al. (1996) and the possibility that this may be greater in children with disordered speech offers an alternative explanation of the results. However, a follow-up assessment showed that improvement only occurred when the treatment was given.

The lack of difference in the therapies could be explained if some children need articulatory and others need phonological therapy. Then each group would include children who did or did not benefit from the therapy they received. Hesketh et al. had this sorted, however. Data were presented for children with good and poor phonological awareness in each group. Those with poor awareness should benefit from phonological therapy; those with good awareness may only need articulation therapy. This pattern was not found. Children with good awareness made more progress in both groups.

Very positive results in favour of phonological awareness therapy were obtained by Gillon (2000), who also compared phonological and articulatory therapy. Children receiving the former fared significantly better on measures of phonological awareness and reading and did as well in speech production. These results are impressive and are further supported by the finding that the phonological awareness group were significantly more advanced at a follow-up 11 months later (Gillon, 2002). This suggests that phonological awareness is not only to be preferred because of its effects on speech but because it benefits the children's literacy. The contrast with the findings in Hesketh et al. (2000) is puzzling, however. Gillon treated older children (5-7 years) than the Hesketh study (3.5-5). She also gave more therapy (20 hours versus 10 sessions). Twenty hours of individual therapy is likely to be more than is available in many clinics. Denne et al. (submitted) failed to replicate Gillon's finding in a study that compared phonological awareness therapy with no therapy. Children in this study were offered 12 hours of group therapy. Phonological awareness improved but neither reading nor speech did.

Given these inconsistent findings, you might wonder why I chose this area to illustrate efficacy research. You should know by now that research is rarely without contradictions and disagreements. Researchers would no doubt say that there are important problems remaining to be sorted out. There are; but there is good evidence that clinicians are treating many children with disordered speech effectively. So let's take a pat on the back when it's due.

The Lee Silverman Voice Treatment (LSVT)

I have always found SLTs to be optimistic people. So it is a shock to read the gloomy views once expressed about therapy for people with Parkinson's disease (PD). It was commonly believed that, because the illness is progressive, SLT would be an unending commitment (Allan, 1970) and that improvements in clinic would rapidly disappear (Sarno, 1968).

Two factors have changed this perception. First, pharmacological interventions have been shown to moderate many of the symptoms of PD. Second, more-optimistic findings are available on the effects of SLT. Paradoxically the former make it more imperative that SLT services are available (they seldom are). Schultz and Grant (2000) wrote that drug treatments improve many abilities but have uncertain effects on communication. Here, then, is a situation where pharmacology and SLT complement one another and where improvements in communication can enhance quality of life. Studies of the efficacy of SLT are conducted on clients on optimal drug regimes. This is important methodologically (because changes in medication during treatment may obscure research findings) and is the logical sequence to follow clinically.

Current approaches to therapy with clients with PD focus on voice and on vocal loudness in particular. Robertson and Thomson (1984) showed that intensive therapy, which included efforts to increase the volume of speech, was successful, and the effects were maintained 3 months later. Johnson and Pring (1990) also focused on vocal loudness and found positive short-term effects with a less-intensive therapy regime.

The LSVT focuses on increasing vocal loudness through increased respiratory and laryngeal effort. It uses an intensive therapy regime of 4 sessions per week for 4 weeks. Clients have a poor awareness of their speech. They seem unaware of its poor volume and feel that they are shouting when asked to increase it. Hence, emphasis is given to calibrating speech (with a sound-level meter) to increase awareness and to motivate continuing efforts to improve its volume. The therapy programme is described in Ramig et al. (1995a).

The therapy has been extensively tested. Fox et al. (2002) reviewed the evidence. Studies have used a range of dependent variables. The most immediate have been measures of sound pressure during speech tasks. Others include the rate of speech, acoustic and videostroboscopic measures and ratings by clients and families of speech quality and intelligibility. Comparisons of treated and untreated clients (see Ramig et al., 2001) show large gains by the treated clients. Other studies have compared clients receiving LSVT with clients treated for respiratory effort only (see Ramig et al., 1995b). This comparison is more exacting because respiratory effort is part of the LSVT. Results have shown that both improve but that where one has an advantage it favours LSVT. Other studies have shown that the effects of LSVT are maintained a year and 2 years (Ramig et al., 2001) after therapy.

These results are impressive. Fox et al. (2002) suggested that existing data meet the requirements of phases 1 to 3 of Robey and

Schultz's (1998) model. In other words, they show that it works under optimal conditions. The next stage is to undertake large-scale clinical trials. Such trials also have the advantage of demonstrating that the therapy is effective when offered by a larger and more varied group of clinicians. Fox et al. also suggested that studies need to examine the length and intensity of the LSVT. Its effectiveness may stem from the amount of therapy offered. We need to know if it is superior to other therapies when these are given equal time and whether it is effective at lower intensities. Finally more data are needed on the generalization of therapy effects to communication outside the clinic.

Surveys of people with PD suggest that very few actually see SLTs. Those that do make it to the clinic receive little therapy. Let's not mess about here. In the light of the evidence above, this is no longer an oversight; it's a disgrace. Nevertheless, there are aspects of the LSVT that may alarm clinicians. It is subject to copyright and should only be used by clinicians who have attended training courses. Although this is unusual, it has one advantage. Conflicting and confusing results occur when one researcher fails to replicate previous findings. This may occur if the therapy is applied inconsistently. The combination of a detailed description and training should ensure that this does not happen. A second concern may be that the therapy is not only intensive but also repetitive. It's my impression (another personal opinion coming up) that when clinicians are unsure whether a therapy is effective or not they take some comfort from the fact that it is fun (whether for the client or themselves, I am not sure)! The converse of this is that when there is evidence available that a therapy works we should roll up our sleeves and get on with it. I suspect that most effective therapies involve hard work and repetition.

Aphasia

There is no getting around the fact that aphasia is a complicated business. The following short account is not intended to do justice to the problems of assessing the efficacy of therapy for it. It would be strange not to include it, however, as the area illustrates so many of the problems with efficacy research in SLT. It may also contain some of the solutions.

Chapter 14 described the problems that arose when studies of therapy provision were conducted in the 1980s. Speech and language therapists meet people with dysphasia in hospitals where they are or have been patients. The medical influence is strong and therapists came under pressure to use RCTs to investigate their therapy despite the fact that clients required different therapies and that little information was available on what they should be. These led to non-significant results and, even when later studies obtained significant outcomes by being more selective in the clients chosen for treatment and more generous in the amounts of therapy offered, very little information was gained by clinicians. It's unclear what effect these results had on the therapy provision for people with aphasia. At best this seems very variable. Some receive extensive rehabilitation; others get little attention. In particular there is little available after the initial post-onset period. This is ironic as the only clear message from these studies was that clients could improve if given more therapy.

A welcome reaction to the failure of these early studies was the recognition of the need to use other methodologies. Two trends are apparent. One has already been described. Single case studies of individual clients offer us detailed accounts of specific deficits and of the effects of treatment upon them. This approach has been used largely, but not exclusively, to study impairments in language processing. The other approach has asked whether intervention can improve activity and participation. It has often used qualitative research methods. These approaches are sometimes portrayed as being inconsistent with one another. In fact, there is no reason why a treatment programme should not seek to achieve both.

We have seen that results of single case investigations cannot be generalized to other clients. This suggests that even successful interventions are of limited value. This need not be the case, however. Consider the study by Francis et al. (2001) described earlier. Surely a therapist treating another case of word-meaning deafness would learn from this study and would be optimistic that the approach would work? As it happens, word-meaning deafness is an unusual condition that therapists may rarely encounter. Nevertheless, studies like this have a general as well as a specific benefit for therapists. They increase our general understanding of language processing. In this case the study demonstrated that our model of auditory word recognition is broadly correct (see Franklin, 1989) and suggests that we can analyse other clients' problems in this area and identify therapies to address them.

Two areas of impairment have been studied extensively. These are word-finding (see Nickels, 2002, for a review) and mapping deficits (see Marshall, 1995, for a review). Studies in these areas have used single case studies and studies of small groups of similar clients. In neither case can we generalize the results to a larger population.

In this sense both areas are at phase 1 of Robey and Schultz's model, and there is much left to do. Their contribution is significant, however. They have not only identified therapies that work for at least some clients but have also offered theoretical accounts of why they work and a means of identifying other clients who can benefit from them. In each case the treatment is not for aphasia as such but for a particular deficit within it. From an experimental point of view this makes sense. We can study clients with the same deficit (though they may differ in other ways), apply the same therapy and select DVs that are sensitive to the treatment objectives. From a clinical point of view this approach offers the prospect that we can gradually assemble a set of treatments that benefit the different deficits that make up aphasia. This offers clinicians a means of selecting a theoretically motivated set of therapies for each client. Of course, there are problems. Progress has been slow, and clinicians may be reluctant to use therapies whose efficacy has been demonstrated with only a few clients and under experimental conditions. They may also be dubious about whether therapies for specific impairments can benefit a client's functional communication and quality of life. Researchers in this area have been slow to investigate whether clients benefit at the levels of activity and participation as a result of therapies aimed at language impairment (see Marshall, 2004).

The other approach complements the above by examining whether therapy can improve everyday life and communication in people with dysphasia. Efficacy research in communication disorders generally has had difficulty in assessing such general benefits of therapy. They are difficult to accommodate within experimental designs, and relevant DVs are hard to come by. Research into dysphasia has begun to tackle these problems using a broad range of methodologies. A first step may be to improve our knowledge of the life experience of people with dysphasia. Interviews (Parr et al., 1997), observation (Davidson et al., 2003) and quality-of-life studies (Ross and Wertz, 2003) have been used. Findings from these studies are both informative in a general sense and can help therapists identify treatment objectives and devise therapies to meet them.

Prominent among the strategies used has been the development of communication through training of carers or through the use of communication partners. Lyon et al. (1997) studied triads of clients, carers and communication partners. Their aim was both to encourage communication and to develop activities that could give the client back a sense of self, which can promote the need to engage in communication and the confidence to do so. The partner provided both respite for the carer and an external view of ways in which clients' life experiences can be expanded. The results of their study leave little doubt that the programme was successful in many diverse ways. However, as they predicted, it was difficult to show this with conventional standardized measures. Cunningham and Ward (2003) trained carers themselves to act as communication partners and reported data on four dyads. The small number of subjects prevented any clear interpretation of the results. Findings were positive but, again, suggest that it might be difficult to identify appropriate measures of improvement. These problems were not apparent in a study by Kagan et al. (2001), however. They conducted an RCT to evaluate training of conversation partners. Trained partners were compared with partners who worked with people with aphasia but had no specific training. Significant effects were found in measures of the partners' skills and in ratings of the participation of people with aphasia.

Conclusion

This book began by suggesting that SLTs need to know more about research methods. Nowhere is this need greater than in efficacy research. In the last two chapters I have argued that efficacy research in SLT has often failed to adopt a coherent strategy or to ask sensible questions. Effectiveness studies have taken place where few data on efficacy have been available and insufficient attention has been paid to the heterogeneity of the client groups chosen for study. It's hard to escape the conclusion that a little knowledge of research methods has been a dangerous thing. A shortage of research and a lack of research training have led to a profession that is uncritical of its knowledge base and unscientific in some of its practices. Research methods are not simply something to be tacked onto training as an 'extra', although they have often been treated in this way. Nor is it just a means of designing research or analysing data. It is a way of thinking about the issues that require research and of asking questions whose answers provide useful information.

Answers to exercises

Exercise 1.1

1. It is difficult to assess conversations at the best of times. There is so much going on that no single measure can capture it all. It's likely that we will have to tape or video the conversations to measure what is happening, but this may affect how and what people talk about. Children are particularly difficult. They are unlikely to be at their conversational best in a clinical situation with unfamiliar people and limited time to get over their inhibitions. It may be better if parents assess them. They know their children and see them in many different everyday settings. Giralometto (1997) described a method of getting parents to report on their children's conversational skills.

2. Dysfluency may affect a client's self-esteem, quality of life and participation in social and other activities. Being able to measure these helps us understand clients' problems and lets us find out whether therapy can improve them. Yaruss (2001) discussed the development of assessments in these areas. He pointed out that it's easier to measure the impairment of dysfluency (for example counting stammers and so forth) than to assess its effects on clients' personal and social lives. Problems of measurement may also influence choice of therapy. It's easier to obtain evidence of the effectiveness of therapies (such as slowed speech) that target impairment. Therapies with broader aims are often favoured by clinicians, but evidence for their effectiveness may be lacking due to the problem of measuring their intended outcomes.

3. Depression is common after stroke. Treatment, by counselling or by antidepressants, is important for clients and may improve their response to language therapy. Clinical psychologists have developed measures of depression (such as the Beck Depression

Inventory), but these are difficult to use with people with communication problems. You might think that clinicians would be fairly good at assessing it informally, but there is evidence that this is not the case. Stern and Bachman (1991) and Stern et al. (1997) described the use of visual analogue mood scales to assess depression. Visual analogue scales are described in Chapter 11. They are easy to use and understand and make few demands on the respondent.

4. Social behaviour is difficult to create in laboratories and is easily inhibited when other people are watching! Researchers have asked parents and teachers to complete assessments of children's social behaviour. Teachers may be a better bet here, as they are more objective and see the children in situations where they interact with their peers. The classroom is a fairly constrained setting, however. Fujiki et al. (2001) videotaped language-impaired and non-impaired children in a school playground. They classified the behaviour of the children every 5 seconds and compared the scores of the groups of children. This approach provides a naturalistic context and one where a range of child-centred behaviours may be observed.

Exercise 1.2

Common sense suggests that the ability to recognize the speech of people with cerebral palsy can be acquired through experience. However, Hunter et al. (1991) found no difference between experienced and inexperienced listeners listening to speakers they did not know. So experienced listeners may be able to recognize familiar individual speakers, not dysarthric speech itself. Recognizing individual speakers may also be helped by knowing their interests and meeting them in a familiar context that facilitates recognition. So much for common sense.

Exercise 1.3

If interest were the only factor, most people would put Freud way out in front. Piaget would be a respectable second; complicated, but kids are cute after all. Skinner would come nowhere; pigeons are definitely not cute. At the experimental level things are a little different. Psychoanalytic theory has an annoying habit of hedging its bets. More often than not a client who does x supports the theory, and a client who doesn't do x also turns out to support it. This sort of thing is useless when it comes to doing experiments. As a result the theory has become a 'religion', which some swear by and others shake their heads over. Behaviourism makes testable predictions and has had some success in clinical applications. Its bad reputation comes from overambition – you can only find out so much about people by messing about with pigeons! Piaget is somewhere in the middle: his theories are revered and have inspired much that has happened since in developmental psychology; however, his experimental methods were not exactly rigorous and later research has modified many of his ideas.

Exercise 1.4

1. Many children with language impairments have word-finding problems. We can show this by asking them to name pictures. Naming may be helped by cues giving information about the item or the first sound of its name. Suppose we give the child a sentence to be completed by the picture name. We can now compare naming of the pictures with their naming with a sentence cue. The number of pictures named provides an easy and exact measure of their success. We could put the children randomly into two groups. One names without cues; the other gets the sentences. Alternatively we might have the same children do both so that we can directly compare their success with and without sentences. This needs fewer children and has other advantages that we discuss in Chapter 2. However, performance might be affected by naming the items twice. Suppose they name first and then name with a sentence cue. They might be better with the latter because it is their second naming opportunity. We can overcome this by having half the children do naming then cued naming and half do the reverse. In this way any carryover from one naming to the other should affect both sorts of naming equally.

2. Here we don't have the choice we had in 1. We must put the children into treated and untreated groups. We do this by randomly assigning them so that the effects of other variables that influence their fluency are, on average, equal in the two groups. The groups then differ only because one receives therapy. Notice that our design means some children don't receive therapy – a necessity that, quite rightly, upsets many clinicians. We will assess the subjects before and after therapy (and the untreated group at the same times) to find out how much progress they make. How we assess them is a problem. We need something that produces a numerical score. We could count the number of stammers saying/reading a set passage or ask listeners to rate their fluency (asking them to give a numerical value on an artificial scale repre-

senting the severity of the dysfluency). Critics are bound to argue that many of the effects of therapy can't be quantified in this way. For instance, it may have other benefits, such as increasing confidence and willingness to talk and enjoy social activities. We must also be careful who carries the assessment out. Ideally they should not know which children have received therapy.

3. This is quite similar to 2. It has the advantage that we can use reaction times (RTs), which can be measured very accurately with laboratory equipment. So we test the two groups of children and compare their times. However, an important difference is that we have not put the children randomly into groups; this is determined by their language status. This often happens in SLT (and other clinical) research. As a result we are not manipulating the variable of interest, and cause-and-effect conclusions cannot be drawn – we may find that language-impaired children are slower, but we can't say that the impairment makes them slower. This is an example of a quasi-experiment. It is important to be able to spot quasi-experiments and to not draw causal conclusions from them. You may be wondering why we are so interested in RTs. Or you may know that experimental psychologists are obsessed with them. This is largely because they can be measured with great precision, in thousandths of a second (milliseconds). The argument is that things that can't be measured with precision (such as how information is processed in the brain) are reflected in RTs. There is obviously a relationship between the two, although its exact nature leaves room for much debate and disagreement.

4. This one looks easy enough until we consider what 'naturalness' is. There is no obvious measure of this and, perhaps, little agreement on what it is to sound natural. We will need to have listeners rate speakers for their naturalness. This is quite a neat solution because it kills two birds with one stone. We obtain our data, and we avoid any need to speculate about what naturalness is. It is defined for us by a cross section of listeners' opinions. We would make tapes of each speaker before and after therapy and ask listeners to rate them. It is important that all the tapes are made under the same conditions and that their content is similar. The people doing the rating should not know about the research. It would be a good idea to use people who are not SLTs to find out what they think of the speakers. They may guess that something has happened to the speakers; so we should play the tapes to them in a random order. We may even arrange things so that individual raters do not hear the same person before and after therapy. All this messing about with speakers, listeners, tapes and different orders can be trying for the experimenter and uses up a lot of nervous energy.

5. This is a tricky one. There is again the problem that we must deny some carers a potentially valuable service in order to assess its effects. Studies in this area have taken advantage of the fact that some carers are keen to have counselling and others do not want it. Thus they compare an existing service with carers who do not have counselling. This results in a quasi-experiment (see Servaes et al., 1999). The two groups may differ in other ways. Those receiving counselling may not be a random sample either, because counselling is only offered to certain carers or because it is only taken up by those who are keen to have it. Equally the comparison group that does not receive counselling may include clients who did not want it anyway, because they are old-fashioned, inhibited or just think you should pull your socks up and get on with it! Another problem is the assessment of psychological well-being. It's difficult to find an objective measure for this. We might measure mood, number of illnesses or trips to GPs. These give us a numerical score but may not be very sensitive. Alternatives such as interviewing the carers give a better picture of the situation but may be difficult to convert into quantitative data for analysis.

Exercise 2.1

1. This is a within-subjects design. The clients were assessed before and after using the computer and improved on several measures of their language. No control group was used. The IV was the time of assessment; the researchers tested before and after therapy to show a change in clients' language skills (the DV). They may have felt that a control group was unnecessary, because most clients had been dysphasic for several years and were unlikely to improve spontaneously.
2. The first experiment is a between-subjects design that compares the two groups of children. Typically developing children act as controls. The IV is the type of child and the DV their scores on the assessment. The second experiment is different. There appear to be two groups of subjects (children and teachers), but both scores belong to the children. So we can compare their scores directly using a within-subjects design. The IV is now who produced the score (children or teachers) and the DV the actual scores.
3. This is a between-subjects design; in fact, a randomized control trial (see below) was used. All clients received therapy but were also randomly assigned to groups who received either dextroamphetamine or a placebo (control group). The IV is drug versus placebo and the DV the scores on a language assessment. The group with the drug made better progress.

Exercise 2.2

1. Studies comparing smokers and non-smokers (or their children) have a problem. Smokers are not a random sample of the population; so confounding variables may be present. Tomblin et al. (1998) questioned mothers of children with SLI or with normal language development to see if they smoked during pregnancy and/or during the child's early life. Studies like this are called case-control studies. They compare people in the same population to try to find out why some have and others do not have a target behaviour/illness. Parents of children with SLI were more likely to be smokers. Other parental variables were related to SLI, however. One was parental education, and when this was taken into account smoking was no longer related to SLI. Tomblin et al. concluded that smoking is not a causal factor in SLI but may be an indicator of the sort of environment in which it occurs.
2. Allocation of children to language units or mainstream schools was clearly not random. Decisions were made about whether children would fare better in one or other setting. It's likely that more able children end up in mainstream schools, and this will affect their progress at 11 years of age. In the actual research Conti-Ramsden et al. (2002) matched mainstream children with a subset of the language unit children on measures of language ability when they were 7 years old. With this controlled no differences in their language abilities were found at 11.
3. This is a long-standing example of a general problem in discovering the mysteries of children's language development. We can select an IV and find groups of children who are good or poor at it, but we can't manipulate it and can't be sure if any relationship it has with language development is causal. Non-word repetition is related to language development. It has been suggested that it can be used as a swift, culture-free means of screening for language problems (Dollaghan and Campbell, 1998). It is plausible that it is the cause of other problems, but our inability to test this experimentally means there is no shortage of other explanations for the relationship (see, for example, Van der Lely and Howard, 1993). Again, this is an area where we just have to live with possible confounding variables. They are a nuisance, but the research is too important for us to give up on it just because of that.

Exercise 2.3

1. The problem here is the assumption that it is exclusion from school that causes later antisocial behaviour. It may; but it's equally – if not

more – plausible that people who are disruptive at school are just getting in some useful practice for being disruptive later in life. So the roots of the problem are probably elsewhere (some of us just can't help resenting authority). Notice that it's not going to be easy to sort this one out. We could randomly assign troublemakers to exclusion and non-exclusion groups and see how they get on. However, it's unlikely that education authorities would go along with this, and we would have to wait a long time to get the answer.

2. Again, the problem is that Ecstasy users are not a random sample of the population. It's possible that some other variable makes them both more likely to take the drug and more prone to psychiatric problems. This one is not quite so insoluble as 1, however. As usual, studies of rats randomly assigned to drug or no-drug conditions allow the effects of the drug on the brain to be studied in greater detail. Watch this space for further details.

3. The problem here is that we do not know what graduates would have earned had they not gone to university. They are generally more able than those who don't go; so it's more than likely that they would have earned more anyway. So purely as a financial inducement, this one is unconvincing. Of course, there may be other nice things about being an undergraduate.

   There is another problem in this example. it concerns where the data came from. Since it is about future income it must be from a sample who graduated sometime ago. In the intervening years the proportion of school leavers going to university has greatly increased. Is it likely that they will all earn £400,000 more? I think there will be a limited supply of these well paid jobs and some graduates will have to take jobs with poorer pay. Here government has over generalised from a sample to a bigger population (see below). As you can see government spokesman are either fibbing or poor at research methods (and I don't know which is worse).

Exercise 2.4

1. Here the difference in the means of the groups is larger than before. The clients are just as variable (I have increased each treated client by 3). Nevertheless, the greater difference in the means should increase your confidence that the groups differ.

2. Here the means are the same, but greater differences exist between individual clients. Improvement now ranges from 0 to 25. With such large individual differences around, a difference between the groups might easily occur by chance. As the figures show, the treated-group mean is due to some clients improving a

lot while others make much less progress. This should decrease your confidence that a difference exists between the groups.

3. Here the means are the same. However, I have doubled the number of subjects and kept their variability constant (by repeating the original data). Here you should be more confident of a significant result. As the number of subjects increases, the less likely it is that a difference between the groups is due to a few subjects who improve a lot (or a little).

Exercise 2.5

1. The probability of a type-one error is the same as the significance level in the experiment. The conventional level is 5%; we reject the null hypothesis if there is a less-than-5% probability that the result might have occurred by chance. This means we accept a 5% risk that the result is due to chance and, therefore, a 5% risk of a type-one error.

2. We don't! But we might begin to worry if other researchers do similar experiments and fail to get significant results. Our result may be significant at a higher level than $p < 0.05$ ($p < 0.01$ or $p < 0.001$ and so forth). This should make us sleep better because the probability of a type-one error is similarly reduced.

3. Type-one errors can happen any time. However, if 20 people do an experiment where the true result is not significant, we can expect one to get a significant result by chance.

4. Researchers know that journals are reluctant to publish non-significant results; so they don't bother sending them in. If several people do similar experiments (because theory suggests this is the experiment that needs doing), it's not impossible that a type-one error will get published while the correct results don't see the light of day (this is called the file-drawer problem). News of this sort of thing usually gets around eventually, but many researchers are concerned that it is a misleading way to conduct research.

Exercise 2.6

'Significance' is another of these words that has both a specialized meaning in statistics and an everyday meaning. Statisticians say a result is 'significant', meaning that it is statistically significant. The claim that a result is 'significant' when it's not statistically significant doesn't make much sense. Clinical significance is another matter. Results may be statistically significant but not clinically significant. Slight but consistent gains will give statistically significant results but may not be thought to be clinically significant, because the gain is too small, too short lived or because it requires an unrealistic amount of therapy to achieve it.

Exercise 2.7

1. There are two problems here. The first is selecting the pictures. Naming in dysphasia is affected by many other variables. The most obvious is word frequency, and longer words tend to be less frequent. So we must select short and long words that are equal in frequency to avoid it being a confounding variable. The second is deciding on the order of presentation. The easiest approach is to present the pictures in a random order. Then short and long names are equally likely to be affected by confounding variables, such as practice or fatigue. We also have the choice of keeping the same random order throughout or of shuffling the pictures to create a new one for each subject. If we do the former, we may decide to use the reverse random order for alternate subjects.

2. If each client names the items both as line drawings and photographs, naming of one may influence naming of the other. We could avoid this by using a between-subjects design with different subjects naming line drawings and photographs. However, naming in people with dysphasia is very variable, and so it's better to use a within-subjects design. One possibility is to test the items on different occasions. The gap in time would counteract any learning effects, and the order of presentation (as drawings or photographs) could be counterbalanced across subjects. Alternatively we could present half the items as drawings and half as photographs. Here, items can be presented in a random order and we can counterbalance their appearance as either drawings or photographs across subjects.

Exercise 2.8

Our analysis of the data involved subtracting post-therapy scores from pre-therapy scores to find out how much clients had changed (these are often called 'gain scores'). This is a clumsy way of doing things, and the alternative of comparing each group's pre- and post-therapy scores may appeal to you. However, we avoid situations (and they happen quite frequently) where the result of an experiment depends upon comparing separate statistical tests. The reason is simple. We want to show that the treated group improved more than the untreated group; this analysis does not do this. It's quite likely that both groups will improve with time. The treated group may improve slightly more and their test may be significant, while that on the untreated group is not. Obviously it would be misleading to claim that treatment has worked here (it's likely that all the children are improving regardless of treatment). So for the present we are stuck with subtracting the scores. In Chapter 7 we look at a better way of doing it.

Exercise 2.9

In almost all experiments that fail to get significant results there are subjects who behave perfectly. We are bound to wonder whether there is something different about them. There may be, and it may be a difference that we should know about. When we look at them after the experiment, it's surprisingly easy to find something that they have in common and to become excited about this. On the other hand, their good response may be a chance effect. To verify this we need to find further subjects of the same type and see if they behave in the same way when we do the experiment again.

Exercise 3.1

1. In (i) the normally developing and SLI children have similar scores on the BPVS. Their means are the same and the scores are equally spread out around the means. In (ii) the children with SLI have lower scores. The two distributions overlap; so the top scores in the SLI group and the bottom scores in the normal language group are similar. In (iii) the children with SLI again have lower scores. Here, however, their scores are much more spread out than those of the children with normal language (shortly we shall say that they have a bigger standard deviation). Clinically defined groups often have more variable (as well as lower) scores on assessments. In (iv) the distribution of children with SLI has two humps (it is bimodal). This suggests that they are made up of two subgroups of children, one with normal and one with below normal scores. This is a possible outcome as the BPVS is a test of comprehension and there is evidence that children with SLI may have either both a comprehension and an expressive problem or only an expressive problem – see Bishop (1997) for a discussion and some doubts about this distinction.

2. This is included just to show you that frequency distributions are not the exclusive preserve of the statistician, nor are they always the nice smooth shapes seen in part 1 of this exercise. These frequency distributions taken from Visispeech are the voice of a transsexual speaker before (left diagram) and after an operation (crico-thyroid approximation) to raise pitch.

Exercise 3.2

1. (a) There's a big difference in the mean improvement of the two groups. The standard deviations are similar but quite large (using the two-standard-deviation rule change in the treated-group ranges from about 4 to 28). It's likely that treatment has worked, but there will be some overlap in the improvement of treated and untreated clients. (b) Here the treated group makes stronger progress but has a large standard deviation. This is common in treatment studies and suggests that therapy has helped some clients but not others. It may not give us a significant result, of course. This is fair enough; the experiment is trying to show that therapy works generally, not that a few benefit. The latter may be interesting and may help us understand how or for whom it works, but it does not allow us to generalize the result to all similar clients. (c) Here the treated group makes strong gains, but the untreated group also does well, and both have large standard deviations. It does not look like therapy has worked here. There is not much difference between the groups, and the standard deviations show that change in both groups is very variable with a lot of overlap between the groups.

2. (a) Here the difference between the two groups is quite small, but the standard deviations are also small, showing that children in each group are tightly clustered around their respective means. (b) Here there is quite a large difference between the groups. The SLI group has a much larger standard deviation, showing that it is more variable than the normally developing group. The latter has a very small standard deviation that can be explained by the fact that there is a performance ceiling on the test. The maximum score is 20, and the majority of the group scores perfectly on the assessment. (c) The group with normal language development is, again, near ceiling on the test and so has a very small standard deviation. The group with SLI also scores highly but has a much larger standard deviation. Since they cannot score above 20, the standard deviation must be explained by a few children who score much lower than the others.

Exercise 3.3

In Exercise 2.4 we concluded that the first was more likely to get a significant result. The means of the two sets of data were the same; however, the individual scores in the second set were more variable. Standard deviations measure the variability in the scores and are bigger for the second set of data.

Exercise 3.4

We already know that $\sum x = 543$ and that the mean is 27.15. So $(\sum x)^2 = 294849$ and from the table below:

$$\sum(x - \bar{x})^2 = 468.5 \text{ and } \sum x^2 = 15211$$

Using the defining formula we get:

$$\text{Variance} = \frac{\sum(x - \bar{x})^2}{n - 1} = \frac{468.5}{19} = 24.66$$

so the standard deviation = 4.97

Using the computational formula:

$$\text{Variance} = \frac{\sum x^2 - \dfrac{(\sum x)^2}{n}}{n - 1} = \frac{15211 - \dfrac{294849}{20}}{19} = 24.66$$

so the standard deviation = 4.97

Subject	Score x	$(x - \bar{x})$	$(x - \bar{x})^2$	x^2
1	17	-10.15	103.02	289
2	20	-7.15	51.12	400
3	21	-6.15	37.82	441
4	23	-4.15	17.22	529
5	25	-2.15	4.62	625
6	25	-2.15	4.62	625
7	26	-1.15	1.32	676
8	26	-1.15	1.32	676
9	26	-1.15	1.32	676
10	26	-1.15	1.32	676
11	27	-0.15	0.02	729
12	28	0.85	0.72	784
13	28	0.85	0.72	784
14	29	1.85	3.42	841
15	29	1.85	3.42	841
16	30	2.85	8.12	900
17	31	3.85	14.82	961
18	33	5.85	34.22	1089
19	35	7.85	61.62	1225
20	38	10.85	117.72	1444
Totals	543		468.5	15211

Exercise 4.1

1. Heights are the sort of naturally occurring variable that is normally distributed (it's called 'normal' because of the assumption that 'normal' variables are normally distributed; many but not all are). Of course, they won't be normal if we include children, but that isn't a problem here. The presence of a few males may be, however. The heights of males and females form two normally distributed, overlapping distributions. If we combine them (ignoring gender), the overall distribution would be close to normal. However, a few taller males among a lot of females may cause a bump at the top end of the distribution.

2. Ages won't be normally distributed. People start being SLTs at about 22, and my guess is that the distribution meanders downward from there. The size of its downward slope will depend on how quickly they become exhausted!

3. The IQ is the product of a standardized test, and the makers of the test went to great lengths to make sure that it is normally distributed. This is true of the population; however, SLTs are not a random sample of the population. Their distribution will be drawn from the top of the population distribution and may be positively skewed.

4. Shoe sizes should be normally distributed (children excepted again). You may have noticed, however, that at shoe sales all the bargains are for people with very small or very large feet. I suspect retailers don't understand the normal distribution and have overstocked at the extremes.

5. I am not sure if ability at research methods is normally distributed. However, exam marks are because examiners (even those that don't know about the normal distribution) tend to mark that way. For what it's worth, I have found that the mean mark in research methods is much the same as in other exams but the standard deviation is a lot bigger!

Exercise 4.2

1. Here we just have to put the values into the z formula: $z = \dfrac{x - \bar{x}}{s}$

(a) $z = \dfrac{x - \bar{x}}{s} = \dfrac{40 - 50}{10} = -1$ (b) $z = \dfrac{x - \bar{x}}{s} = \dfrac{70 - 50}{10} = 2$

(c) $z = \dfrac{x - \bar{x}}{s} = \dfrac{37 - 50}{10} = -1.3$ (d) $z = \dfrac{x - \bar{x}}{s} = \dfrac{61 - 50}{10} = 1.1$

2. The z-tables (see Appendix 1) give the proportion (multiply by 100 to get the percentage) of people between a score and the mean. The table is for half the distribution only, the other half being a mirror image. The table value for (a) 0.5 is 0.1915. So 19.15% of people are between $z = 0.5$ and the mean. The percentile score of this person is $50 + 19.15 = 69.15$. (b) –0.5 also gives a table value of 0.1915. Here, however, the score is below the mean, and the percentile score for this person is $50 – 19.15 = 30.85\%$. (c) 1.24 has a table value of 0.3925 or 39.25%. So the percentile score is 89.25%. (d) –1.37 has a table value of 0.4147 or 41.47%. So the percentile score is $50 – 41.47 = 8.53\%$. (e) 1.96 has a table value of 0.4750 or 47.5%. So the percentile score is 97.5%. (f) –1.96 also has a table value of 0.4750. Here the percentile score is 2.5%. You will notice that the z-scores + and – 1.96 enclose 95% of the population. The 5% not included are at the extreme ends of the normal distribution.

3. Here we need to find a z-score that corresponds to the proportion 0.2500. This cuts each half of the curve into two equal parts – the 25% near the mean and the 25% further away. This score is between 0.67 and 0.68; call it 0.675.

Exercise 5.1

1. Reaction times can be measured very precisely and are clearly equal interval data. One of their great attractions is that there is usually little doubt that we may use parametric tests to analyse them.

2. If we were being fussy, we might decide that numbers of pictures named correctly are not really equal-interval data. Is one right response exactly the equal of another? This example is here to reassure you that we don't think like this. Counts of behavioural events like the number of items answered correctly or the number of eye contacts during conversation are treated as equal-interval data.

3. Here two categories of subjects (singers and non-singers) are put into three further categories by the number of symptoms of vocal attrition that they have experienced. The data are not how many symptoms they have (although they could have been) but how many people there are in each category. These are nominal (or categorical) data. Sapir et al. (1996) found that singers had significantly more symptoms of vocal attrition.

4. The GHQ measures anxiety, stress and depression. Questionnaires like this, where responses are selected (for example: 'Have you been feeling unhappy or depressed? – not at all, no more than usual, more than usual, a lot more than usual') can be used to produce a numerical score, but these are usually treated as being ordinal data. The GHQ is widely used to assess patients with a

variety of physical and mental illnesses. A cut-off score indicates the presence of significant psychological distress. Draper et al. (1992) found similar scores for the 2 groups of carers. Overall, 46% had significant levels of distress.

Exercise 5.2

1. These are equal-interval data. There are two groups: those with and without chronic sinusitis. Cecil et al. (2001) compared their fundamental frequencies with an independent t-test. They found no difference suggesting that sinusitis need not affect voice, although they warn us about accepting the null hypothesis, as only a few subjects were tested.

2. The clients rate their well-being. Many books treat these data as non-parametric (but see Chapter 8). It is a within-subjects design; so a Wilcoxon test would be used. In fact, Hoen et al. (1997) used a related t-test. You may also notice that there is no control group. The authors acknowledge this as a problem. However, change is unlikely to be due to natural recovery, as the clients had been dysphasic for at least a year. I am being rather critical of this study, but it's difficult measuring psychological well-being, and having a control group would mean denying some clients therapy for as long as 6 months!

3. The same children did the picture naming and conversational tasks, and the number of errors made was compared with a related t-test. Results on the two tests were closely related, but the picture-naming task produced more errors.

4. Quality-of-life scales are usually done by asking clients to rate themselves. So this looks like non-parametric data, and it's a between-subjects design, which means a Mann-Whitney test. In fact, Wilson et al., 2002 used an independent t-test. They found that dysphonia had strong effects on all areas of quality of life tested by the SF-36.

5. These are nominal or categorical data. The children are placed in 2 categories, with or without HIV infection and with or without language impairment. The chi-square test would normally be used here, although in this example a Fisher's exact test was used (see Chapter 9). Coplan et al. (1998) found that significantly more children with HIV were > 2 standard deviations below the mean.

You might be wondering why parametric tests are used in examples 2 and 4 despite the data being on an ordinal scale. This goes back to the disagreement between textbooks mentioned in the chapter. Some insist that equal-interval data are necessary for parametric tests. Others don't care. Researchers are keen to use parametric tests because they are more powerful. As a result non-parametric tests are mainly used when the data are clearly non-normal or have unequal variances.

Exercise 5.3

1. (a) 1.81, (b) 2.23, (c) 2.23, (d) 2.53, (e) 2.75
2. (a) 28. (b) The result is significant for a one-tail but not for a two-tail test. So this is one of those occasions when it is important to have made a prediction and, therefore, to have decided whether to use a one- or two-tail test in advance. The children with SLI would, if anything, score worse; so a one-tail test appears to be justified here.

Exercise 5.4

In each case we have to calculate the pooled variance and substitute this and the means into the formula for the independent t-test. A one-tail test is used. For the original data:

$$s_p^2 = \frac{(n_1 - 1)s_1^2 + (n_2 - 1)s_2^2}{n_1 + n_2 - 2} = \frac{5 \times 5.40^2 + 5 \times 5.66^2}{10} = 30.59$$

$$t = \frac{(\bar{x}_1 - \bar{x}_2)}{\sqrt{\left(\frac{1}{n_1} + \frac{1}{n_2}\right)s_p^2}} = \frac{13 - 8}{\sqrt{\left(\frac{2}{6}\right) \times 30.59}} = \frac{5}{3.19} = 1.57$$

$t(10) = 1.57$, not sig.

For Exercise 2.3 (i) $s_p^2 = 30.59$ again and:

$$t = \frac{(\bar{x}_1 - \bar{x}_2)}{\sqrt{\left(\frac{1}{n_1} + \frac{1}{n_2}\right)s_p^2}} = \frac{16 - 8}{\sqrt{\left(\frac{2}{6}\right) \times 30.59}} = \frac{8}{3.19} = 2.51$$

$t(10) = 2.51$, $p < 0.05$

For Exercise 2.3 (ii) $s_p^2 = \dfrac{5 \times 9.82^2 + 5 \times 6.07^2}{10} = 66.63$

$$t = \dfrac{(\bar{x}_1 - \bar{x}_2)}{\sqrt{\left(\dfrac{1}{n_1} + \dfrac{1}{n_2}\right)s_p^2}} = \dfrac{13 - 8}{\sqrt{\left(\dfrac{2}{6}\right) \times 66.63}} = \dfrac{5}{4.71} = 1.06$$

$t(10) = 1.06$, not sig.

For Exercise 2.3 (iii) $s_p^2 = \dfrac{11 \times 5.39^2 + 11 \times 5.15^2}{22} = 27.79$

$$t = \dfrac{(\bar{x}_1 - \bar{x}_2)}{\sqrt{\left(\dfrac{1}{n_1} + \dfrac{1}{n_2}\right)s_p^2}} = \dfrac{13 - 8}{\sqrt{\left(\dfrac{2}{12}\right) \times 27.79}} = \dfrac{5}{2.15} = 2.32$$

$t(22) = 2.32$, $p < 0.05$

To obtain a significant result at $p < 0.05$ for a one-tail test and 10 d.f., t must be > 1.81. So the original data are not significant. In Exercise 2.4 part 1 the difference in the means is greater and the result is significant. In Exercise 2.3 part 2 the variability of the scores is increased and gives a lower t value and a non-significant result. In Exercise 2.3 part 3 the difference in the means now gives a significant result because twice as many subjects are used (the standard deviations change slightly as $n - 1$ is used in their calculation).

Exercise 5.5

1. The means and standard deviations are in Table 5.3. Calculate the pooled variance:

$$s_p^2 = \dfrac{(n_1 - 1)\, s_1^2 + (n_2 - 1)\, s_2^2}{n_1 + n_2 - 2} = \dfrac{9 \times 5.23^2 + 9 \times 5.89^2}{18} = 31.02$$

Then calculate the value of t:

$$t = \dfrac{(\bar{x}_1 - \bar{x}_2)}{\sqrt{\left(\dfrac{1}{n_1} + \dfrac{1}{n_2}\right)s_p^2}} = \dfrac{12 - 8.6}{\sqrt{\left(\dfrac{2}{10}\right) \times 31.02}} = \dfrac{3.4}{2.49} = 1.36$$

The table value for a one-tail test at p < 0.05 with 18 d.f. is 1.73 so this result is well short of significant. Contrast this with the strongly significant result from the related t-test. The independent t-test is non-significant because of large differences between the subjects. As a result the difference between the groups might occur by chance. The related t-test is unaffected by these as it looks at differences between the two conditions for each subject disregarding their overall level of naming.

(ii)

	Before	After	Difference (d)	d^2
Subject 1	92	104	12	144
Subject 2	124	123	-1	1
Subject 3	203	186	-17	289
Subject 4	156	162	6	36
Subject 5	132	140	8	64
Subject 6	86	91	5	25
Subject 7	141	139	-2	4
Subject 8	167	160	-7	49
Subject 9	101	115	14	196
Subject 10	97	101	4	16

$$s_d = \sqrt{\frac{\sum d^2 - \frac{(\sum d)^2}{n}}{n-1}} = \sqrt{\frac{824 - \frac{484}{10}}{9}} = 9.28$$

$$\text{and } t = \frac{\overline{d}}{s_d / \sqrt{n}} = \frac{2.2}{9.28 / \sqrt{10}} = 0.748$$

The result is not significant. This is what Goberman et al. (2002) found. It shouldn't have taken you long to realize that this would be the case. The differences between before and after states are inconsistent. Some clients increase and some decrease their fundamental frequencies. As a result d is small and s_d is large and the value of t suffers accordingly.

Exercise 5.6

The children's standardized score of 92 compares with a mean of 100 and a standard deviation of 15 for all 5-year-olds. Here we can use a z-test to see if the children differ from this mean:

$$z = \frac{\bar{x} - \mu}{\sigma/\sqrt{n}} = \frac{92 - 100}{15/\sqrt{16}} = \frac{-8}{15/4} = -2.13$$

The table value for a z-score of –2.13 is 0.4834. So a sample with a mean as low as this would occur less than 2% of the time by chance. The result is significant whether we are using a one-tail or a two-tail test (we would presumably use a one-tail test here). Note that it wouldn't be surprising if an individual child scored this low (the child would have an individual z-score of –0.533), but it is very unlikely that we would find a sample of children with a mean score this low).

Exercise 5.7

People with cleft palate			People without cleft palate		
Subject	Score	Rank	Subject	Score	Rank
1	6	6	9	8	12
2	5	3.5	10	5	3.5
3	4	1	11	6	6
4	4.5	2	12	8.5	13
5	6	6	13	9	14.5
6	9	14.5	14	7.5	11
7	7	10	15	10	17
8	6.5	8.5	16	9.5	16
			17	6.5	8.5
		$R_1 = 51.5$			$R_2 = 101.5$

$$U = n_1 n_2 + \frac{n_1(n_1+1)}{2} - R_1 = 8 \times 9 + \frac{8 \times 9}{2} - 51.5 = 56.5$$

and $U' = n_1 n_2 - U = 8 \times 9 - 56.5 = 15.5$

This result is significant for a one-tail test (table value = 18) but not for a two-tail test (table value = 15) at the p < 0.05 level. Kunkel et al. (1997) found a significant difference. They noted, however, that there was considerable overlap in the scores suggesting that the measure cannot distinguish absolutely between normal and pathological function. Nevertheless, they argued that it can be used to monitor change with therapy.

Exercise 5.8

	Pre-treatment	Post-treatment	Difference (d)	Rank
Subject 1	0.116	0.122	0.006	3
Subject 2	0.140	0.141	0.001	1
Subject 3	0.114	0.124	0.010	4
Subject 4	0.126	0.106	-0.020	7
Subject 5	0.114	0.136	0.022	8
Subject 6	0.150	0.139	-0.011	5
Subject 7	0.127	0.129	0.002	2
Subject 8	0.165	0.152	-0.013	6

The sum of the ranks of the least occurring sign is 18 (7 + 5 + 6). The table values for $p < 0.05$ are 5 (for a one-tail test) and 3 (for a two-tail test); so the result is clearly not significant. Onslow et al. (2001) failed to find significant differences on any of their measures and concluded that the Lidcombe program does not affect speech timing.

Exercise 5.9

This example illustrates how useful the sign test can be. All we know is that an event with two possible outcomes had the same outcome on 9 occasions (the equivalent of treating 9 clients who all improve). Here we use a two-tail test as there is no reason to predict the outcome. The result is significant at the 5% level. There is a possible confounding variable, however. The north dressing room is given to the team from further north in the country. So perhaps it's just a case of southern softies not having any bottle on the big day. In fact, there is some support for this hypothesis! The feng shui expert failed miserably, and the trend continued for 3 more matches. The thirteenth match was the second division play-off final between Stoke City and Brentford. Traditional practice was changed, and Stoke (the more northerly team) was given the unlucky dressing room (so disconfounding the two variables). They won 2–0.

Exercise 6.1

1. The IV is the situation in which the children were tested. It has 5 levels. Either a within- or a between-subjects design might be used. Yaruss (1997) used the former, which (because children differ widely in their fluency rates) is more likely to detect differences. This means that each child was tested quite a lot and that, order of

testing had to counterbalanced across children. The DV was the number of dysfluencies per 100 syllables.

2. This has to be a between-subjects design. The IV is the type of subjects and has 3 levels: monolinguals and 2 types of bilinguals. The DV is performance on the Boston naming test. The bilingual were proficient in both languages, although English was their second language. Both groups were found to have significantly poorer naming scores than the monolinguals. Other methodological problems in this research include ensuring that the groups are equal on other variables that might affect naming performance and the definition of bilingualism and monolingualism. See the paper for more on this.

3. The IV here is the age of the people tested. It is a between-subjects variable with 8 levels! Proverb explanations were given a score of 1 when partially correct and 2 when fully correct, and the total score was the DV. The researchers marked the answers themselves but were blind as to the age of the subjects they were marking.

4. The IV here is time (when assessments were carried out) and has 5 levels. The clients were followed throughout the training period and repeatedly assessed; so it's a within-subjects design. These clients are very variable in their use of objects; so their mean score with several objects on different occasions was used to smooth out variation in use of the objects.

5. This is also a between-subjects design. The IV is the type of child, with 4 levels (3 groups with language problems and children with no history of language problems). Educational progress (the DV) was assessed by the number and grades of GCSEs they obtained. Where more than one DV is available, it's tempting to use them. There are potential difficulties with this, however. It is confusing if one DV is significant but another is not. The significant result may be a type-one error or may occur because that measure is more sensitive. Another problem is that DVs may be related. For instance, children may obtain better grades by entering fewer exams, thus confusing the outcome.

Exercise 6.2

The Anova tables are shown below. Notice that the within-subjects design produces a highly significant result, while the same data analysed as a between-subjects design does not. This shows the advantage of using a within-subjects design. The mathematical explanation for this is seen in the tables. The sums of squares for the IV (time) and the total sums of squares (the sum of squares of all the scores) are the same in each table. The error variance is also the same (508.62 = 451.62 + 57.00). In the between-subjects design this is used in the F-ratio. In the within-subjects design it is split into error variance due to differences between subjects and error variance owing to differences in their changes over time. The former is much bigger but is irrelevant to the analysis. The consistency of the subjects over time is used in the F-ratio, and error variance due to differences between subjects is ignored.

Source of variance	Sum of squares	d.f.	Mean square	F	p
Time	70.33	2	35.17	1.45	0.2567
Within groups (error)	508.62	21	24.22		
Total	578.95	23			

Source of variance	Sum of squares	d.f.	Mean square	F	p
Time	70.33	2	35.17	8.64	0.0036
Subjects (error)	451.62	7	64.52		
Subjects × time (error)	57.00	14	4.07		
Total	578.95	23			

Exercise 6.3

Suppose there are 3 routes to work. Routes are the IV with 3 levels. To find out which is faster you must randomly select a route each day. You will need strict rules about timing the journey, starting and stopping the stopwatch at the same point each day. Suppose you collect 10 times for each journey. The mean times will differ, and the individual times will vary. So, is one route faster than the others? ANOVA will find out. This is an odd ANOVA. The data are different journey times rather than scores from different people. This doesn't matter; we often use ANOVA (and other tests) like this. It is a between-subjects design. If we produce a significant result, we will need to compare pairs of means to find out which are different. Our hypothesis asks whether any route is faster (it does not predict which), and so we use an unplanned comparison.

Exercise 6.4

1. No prediction was made about the levels of dysfluency in the various situations; so an unplanned comparison was used. The Tukey test found that play under pressure elicited more dysfluencies than each of the other conditions.

2. In this study it might be argued that a planned comparison was justified on theoretical grounds. The expectation was that bilingual subjects would perform less well than monolinguals. However, a Tukey test was used to carry out an unplanned comparison.

3. Proverb explanation was expected to improve with age before declining in old age. An unplanned comparison found that young adolescents were significantly poorer than all other groups, and older adolescents were significantly poorer than 20-, 30-, 40- and 50-year-olds but not 60- and 70-year-olds. The 70-year-olds were significantly poorer than those in their 20s and 40s. The results are broadly consistent with the hypothesis, but notice the potential for confusing findings when comparing so many groups. Comparisons across different ages also face the problem that language use changes with time so that differences may occur because age groups differ in their familiarity with the materials tested.

4. Improvement was expected over time and a significant result was obtained. A Newman-Keuls unplanned comparison was used to look at differences between all the assessments. This showed that almost all the improvement occurred in the first 2 5-week periods.

5. The authors wanted to know whether the groups of children with language problems differed from controls and whether they differed from one another; so a Scheffé test was used to compare all the groups. This showed that the group with persisting problems and general delay entered significantly fewer examinations than the recovered or control groups. Examination results showed a different pattern, with controls doing better than all the other groups. So children classified as recovered continue to experience educational disadvantage.

Notice that unplanned comparisons were used in all the above. You may think predictions could have been made. In 1 it might have been expected that play under pressure would differ from the other conditions, and in 3 a general expectation about the results was stated yet an unplanned comparison was used. As the number of conditions increases it becomes more difficult to be explicit about where differences will be and the option of comparing all conditions with an unplanned comparison becomes more attractive.

Exercise 6.5

									n	R	R^2/n
MS+	Scores	257	156	248	243				4		
	Ranks	6	1	4	2					13	42.25
MS−	Scores	270	276	298	281	259			5		
	Ranks	9	11	16	12	7				55	605
controls	Scores	261	253	247	291	286	287	273	7		
	Ranks	8	5	3	15	13	14	10		68	660.57

$$\sum \frac{R^2}{n} = 1307.82$$

$$H = \frac{12}{N(N+1)} \sum \frac{R^2}{n} - 3(N+1) = \frac{12}{16 \times 17} \times 1307.82 - 3 \times 17 = 6.70$$

With $k - 1 = 2$ d.f. this value is significant at the $p < 0.05$ level. The data suggest the difference is due to the MS+ group, but to check this Laakso et al. (2000) compared the conditions with Mann-Whitney tests. Although the result is significant, you may feel unconvinced. Normally we fail to get significance with small numbers of subjects and need more. Here, you feel it would be nice to have more to see if the result is still significant. In fairness Laakso et al. called this a pilot study, and the groups were found not to differ on a test designed for people with aphasia. It won't help your confidence, however, to hear that 2 control subjects who scored poorly on the test were omitted from the data!

Exercise 7.1

Figure 7.1 shows the expected outcome of our dysfluency experiment. The figures in this exercise show some less likely outcomes (but you never know). In (i) neither group has improved but the treated group have lower scores. This should give us a main effect of 'type of subject' but not of time. There is no interaction because both types of subject behave similarly over the course of the experiment. In (ii) both treated and untreated subjects improve. There will be a main effect of time but not of type of subject. Again, there is no interaction as both types of subject behave in the same way. In (iii) the treated group has improved and the untreated group has deteriorated. There is a very pronounced crossover in the graph, which should produce a significant interaction. This is a fairly unlikely outcome, but I have included it to illustrate an important point. There is unlikely to be either a main effect of type of subject or of time. The mean performance of the subjects is the same (despite the difference in their performance over time), and the mean of all the subjects is the same at the 2 assessments. So a significant interaction occurs despite there being no significant main effects. The fact that the groups started at different levels, as they did in (i), should tell you that something is wrong here. After all, the groups were supposed to be randomly assigned. In (iv) the outcome is similar to Figure 7.1 except that the untreated group has deteriorated slightly. The interaction should be strongly significant. It's hard to tell whether there will be significant main effects, however.

Exercise 7.2

1. The variables here are the ages of the children with 3 levels (1.5, 2.5 and 3.5 years) and the person to whom they are talking, which has 2 levels (Mum or Dad). You would expect the former to be a between-subjects variable and the latter a within-subjects variable and the ANOVA to be a two-factor mixed design. In fact, McLaughlin et al. (1983) followed the same children across time (so the research took a while!); so it's a two-factor within-subjects ANOVA.

2. Here the subjects must be different people. There are 3 groups, so type of subject is a between-subjects variable with 3 levels. Each child would be asked to do both the naming and the naming-with-a-cue conditions, however, so this is a within-subjects variable with 2 levels, and the ANOVA is a two-factor mixed design.

3. Here the groups of people with dysphasia are a between-subject variable with 3 levels – no treatment, computer (reading), and computer (non-verbal). The time of assessment is a within-subjects variable with 3 levels (before treatment and at 13 and 26 weeks). So the ANOVA is a two-factor mixed design.

4. The trick in this one is realizing that the listeners (not the single speaker) are the subjects. Whether the listeners are experienced or not is a between-subjects variable with 2 levels. There are 2 within-subjects variables. These are whether they hear single words or 5- or 10-word sentences (3 levels) and whether they are produced with the valve or with finger occlusion (3 levels). So it's a three-factor mixed ANOVA.

5. Here there is a single between-subjects variable with 2 levels (children and adults). In (i) they see 4 types of symbol. You may think that this is a single within-subjects variable with 4 levels, but you would be wrong. The researcher is obviously interested in both

complexity and translucency (and whether they interact), and so they are separate within-subjects variables each with 2 levels. In (ii) an extra within-subjects variable, time of test, with 4 levels, is added. So three- and four-factor mixed ANOVAs will be used.

Exercise 8.1

This seems worth doing. It's not much work, and we may find something useful in all those clinical records. There are problems, however. First, we can't draw cause-and-effect conclusions because the variables have not been manipulated. Suppose children who respond well had more therapy. We can't be sure that therapy caused the improvement. Perhaps they had hyperactive parents who took them down to the clinic, nagged the therapist and then gave the kids a hard time at home, the latter being the real cause of improvement (not a very convincing explanation, but – and this is the point – the experiment can't rule it out).

Then there is the problem discussed in this chapter. Because we have done many tests, the chance of a type-one error has increased. Suppose we find that 1 variable is significant. Can we assume this tells us something about children who do and do not improve? Unfortunately, this is just the sort of situation where the result may be a type-one error. We can overcome this by using a higher significance level, but this may then lose our significant result.

Exercise 8.2

This just goes to show that type-one errors are not limited to research methods. If we are looking for evidence of 'intelligent design' and have all the fruits of the world to choose from, then we are likely to find some that fit the bill. This overlooks the fact that some don't (what about coconuts and pineapples?) not to mention those that look well designed but then poison us. It's just like doing a lot of statistical tests and then selecting just those that are significant to support our case.

Exercise 8.3

For a one-tail test at $p < 0.05$, 80% power requires $\delta = 2.50$:

$$\delta = d\sqrt{\frac{n}{2}} \qquad 2.50 = 0.92\sqrt{\frac{n}{2}} \qquad \frac{n}{2} = \left(\frac{2.50}{0.92}\right)^2 \qquad n = 15$$

Exercise 8.4

The way to conduct experiments is to use the effect size to calculate the number of subjects required to stand a good chance (perhaps 80%) of obtaining a significant result. If we don't, or are unable to do this, we might be tempted to analyse the data every so often as we go along. The data are tested more than once, and the chance of a type-one error is increased. The use of a power analysis removes this problem as we only test the data when we reach the required number of subjects. Recognizing that researchers can't resist temptation, Arnold and Harvey (1998) have described a process of 'data monitoring' that allows for repeated analyses by correcting for the increased type-one error rate. A further problem is that effect sizes are, like all statistics, estimates of true values. Jones et al. (2002) suggested we discontinue a clinical trial where the effect size is greater than expected. Here a significant result may be obtained with fewer than the calculated number of subjects and, since the trial involves withholding treatment, it is unethical to continue it unnecessarily.

Exercise 8.5

$$F = \frac{11.63}{2.02} = 5.76$$

The variances of the two groups are 2.02 and 11.63. So:
    Each variance is for 10 subjects; so the degrees of freedom are (9, 9) and the table value for $p < 0.05$ is 3.18. So the 2 variances differ significantly. So it looks like treatment has had a variable effect improving some children but having little or no effect on others.

Exercise 9.1

The expected frequencies are shown in brackets in the first table. The calculations are shown in the table below it.

	Qualitative methods	Quantitative methods	
Female authors	13 (7.83)	5 (10.17)	18
Male authors	17 (22.17)	34 (28.83)	51
Totals	30	39	69

O	E	$(O-E)$	$(O-E)$	$\dfrac{(O-E)^2}{E}$
13	7.83	5.17	26.73	3.41
5	10.17	-5.17	26.73	2.63
17	22.17	-5.17	26.73	1.21
34	28.83	5.17	26.73	0.93
				$\sum \dfrac{(O-E)^2}{E} = 8.18$

With 1 d.f. this is significant at the $p < .01$ level.

As you will shortly discover, we must be careful drawing conclusions from the results of chi-square tests, which are normally used in situations, as here, where confounding variables may be at work. In this example there is a further danger of overgeneralizing from these casually acquired data. The results appear to show a gender difference in writing about research. Perhaps males get a kick out of mathematical formulae and females prefer the more rambling style of qualitative research (well thats my experience of them - the books I mean).

Exercise 9.2

The data, with the expected frequencies in brackets, were:

	Regular words	Exception words	
Correct	24 (20)	16 (20)	40
Incorrect	6 (10)	14 (10)	20
	30	30	60

The calculations are as follows:

O	E	$(O-E)$	$(O-E)$	$\dfrac{(O-E)^2}{E}$
24	20	4	16	0.8
16	20	-4	16	0.8
6	10	-4	16	1.6
14	10	4	16	1.6
				$\sum \dfrac{(O-E)^2}{E} = 4.8$

Chi square = 4.8, which is significant at the $p < 0.05$ level. So the above scores show that the subject was reading non-lexically and is likely to be a surface dyslexic.

Exercise 9.3

1. The first test compares the correct responses with errors. The expected frequencies are 8 and 32 (because there are 4 opportunities to make an error by chance). With d.f. = 1 the calculated value is easily significant at the $p < 0.01$ level.

	Correct	All errors
Observed score	17	23
Expected score	8	32

O	E	$(O-E)$	$(O-E)$	$\dfrac{(O-E)^2}{E}$
17	8	9	81	10.1
23	32	-9	81	2.5
				$\sum \dfrac{(O-E)^2}{E} = 12.6$

There are 2 possibilities of a semantic error and 2 of a non-semantic error; so we expect the 23 errors to divide equally between them. So the expected score is 11.5.

	Semantic errors	Other errors
Observed score	15	8
Expected score	11.5	11.5

O	E	$(O-E)$	$(O-E)$	$\dfrac{(O-E)^2}{E}$
15	11.5	3.5	12.25	1.06
8	11.5	-3.5	12.25	1.06
				$\sum \dfrac{(O-E)^2}{E} = 2.12$

This result is not significant, and so there are not more semantic errors than expected by chance. Had we not analysed the data it's likely we would have concluded that there were; so perhaps we should analyse this sort of data more often.

2. Using a one-sample chi square with 6 d.f. we get a value of 13.8, which is higher than the table value of 12.59 at the $p < 0.05$ level. So the distribution is uneven, with Monday looking like the

favourite day for meeting your maker. As usual with such data we need to be careful about drawing conclusions. Nevertheless, you may agree with Evans et al. (2000) that it has quite a lot to do with the Scottish fondness for getting legless at the weekend. They go to some length to rule out confounding variables. The trend is not seen in those with a previous history of coronary heart disease (who may have mended their ways) or those dying in hospital (who can't get a drink). Nor is it seen among other causes of death (so it's not because people die at the weekend and are not found till Monday). The trend is particularly strong among men under 50. Finally there is evidence of a similar trend in Russia, another country with an understandable desire to drown its sorrows at the weekend.

Exercise 10.1

1. As Yaruss et al. (2002) pointed out, it is not surprising that strong positive correlations were found between satisfaction with therapy and perceptions of the competence of therapists. Respondents were asked to rate their best and worst experiences of therapy and of the clinicians involved. The correlations were 0.67 and 0.72 respectively. These researchers believed competence causes satisfaction and argue, for increasing it by further training. They were probably right, but it's possible that perceived competence is the result of satisfaction.

2. A significant negative correlation was found between time of starting the programme and PPVT scores (−0.46). This supports the case for early intervention and for more thorough screening for these children. A significant positive correlation of 0.65 was found between PPVT scores and family involvement. Again, we need to be careful about these results as uncontrolled variables were present.

3. A significant correlation was found between improvement in language and change in CBF in the left (0.56) but not the right hemisphere. The result looks dodgy to me. The correlation for the right hemisphere was 0.42, which is just below significant; so the trend in each hemisphere is the same, with the right just failing to be significant (see Exercise 2.7). In a second study with clients 7 years after onset, CBF in the right but not the left hemisphere was related to good recovery. Mimura et al. (1998) argued that initial recovery was in the left hemisphere but that long-term recovery was due to gradual compensation by the right hemisphere.

Exercise 10.2

The table below allows us to obtain the necessary values to calculate r.

	Rated severity (x)	ALS (y)	PRS	xy	x^2	y^2
Client 1	4	8	3	12	16	9
Client 2	2	5	3	6	4	9
Client 3	8	6	8	64	64	64
Client 4	3	2	7	21	9	49
Client 5	4	6	7	28	16	49
Client 6	9	7	8	72	81	64
Client 7	8	9	6	48	64	36
Client 8	3	6	4	12	9	16
Client 9	9	10	8	72	81	64
Client 10	5	8	7	35	25	49
	55	67	61	370	369	409

$$r = \frac{n\sum xy - (\sum x)(\sum y)}{\sqrt{(n\sum x^2 - (\sum x)^2)(n\sum y^2 - (\sum y)^2)}} = \frac{10\times370 - 55\times61}{(10\times369 - 55^2)(10\times409 - 61^2)}$$

$$r = \frac{3700 - 3355}{\sqrt{(3690 - 3025)(4090 - 3721)}} = \frac{345}{\sqrt{665 \times 369}} = 0.696$$

With 10 subjects (d.f. = 8) r is significant at $p < 0.05$ for either a one- or a two-tail test.

Exercise 10.3

It's perfectly possible, although sometimes confusing, to compare both the means of sets of scores to see if they are correlated. Both may be significant, each may be significant but not the other, or neither may be significant. Suppose parents give higher scores than teachers, indicating that they feel their children have better language skills. The scores may still be correlated showing that parents and teachers agree on the relative levels of skill of different children. If the correlation is significant but the t-test is not, this suggests that there is good agreement on both the level and relative skills of the children. If neither test is significant, there is no agreement between them at all.

Exercise 10.4

The value of b can be worked out using the values calculated in Exercise 10.2 to obtain the correlation coefficient.

$$b = \frac{n\sum xy - (\sum x)(\sum y)}{n\sum x^2 - (\sum x)^2} = \frac{10 \times 403 - 55 \times 67}{10 \times 369 - 3025} = \frac{345}{665} = 0.52$$

We can then work out a by substituting the means of x and y into the regression equation:

$$y = a + bx$$

$$6.7 = a + 0.52 \times 5.5 \quad \text{So } a = 6.7 - 2.86 = 3.84$$

and the regression equation is $y = 3.84 + 0.52x$

Exercise 10.5

1. This example illustrates some of the difficulties of interpreting multiple regression. As usual, correlation does not indicate causality. It's not surprising that length of time in present job or age predict satisfaction since clinicians are more likely to stay in their current job if satisfied with it and more likely to stay in the profession if they enjoy the work. So the former may be less a cause of satisfaction than an indication that some jobs are better than others and that, once therapists get one, they stay with it. Age and length of time in a job are also likely to be correlated with one another. This leaves size of caseload looking like the most important variable.

2. A way of examining this would be to study people at school learning a language. Sanz (2000) studied Spanish/Catalan- and Spanish-only speaking people learning English. Of course, they were not randomly assigned; so the 2 groups differed on other variables. Sanz tackled this problem using hierarchical multiple regression. She first controlled other variables that might affect their ability to learn English by entering them in the regression equation. Then their language status was entered. This contributed a further significant proportion of the variance of their ability in English.

Exercise 11.1

1. Fimian et al. (1991) developed a test of occupational stress among therapists. They had worked on measures of stress in teachers and so had experience of the sort of items needed. They reviewed

the literature and consulted a number of clinicians. As a result they obtained 67 items, which were reduced to 49 by eliminating redundant and similar items. Factor analysis led to the test being divided into 6 sections – 4 about sources of stress and 2 about reactions to it. Cronbach's alpha showed that items in each section were consistent, and only 1 further item was removed.

2. Wilson et al. (1991) developed a tinnitus-reaction questionnaire. They selected items by consulting the literature on the symptoms of tinnitus and through interviews with sufferers conducted during earlier research by one of the authors. Twenty-eight items were found. Cronbach's alpha was used to examine their consistency. As this was very high all were retained.

3. Many general measures of QOL exist. In creating client-specific measures researchers must choose whether to use or adapt these or to start afresh. Cella et al. (1996) started with a 28-item assessment for patients with cancer. They added 60 more items generated from interviews with clients and clinicians and after a survey of the literature. After factor analysis (see text) the measure was reduced to 44 items in 6 subscales.

4. Tests of functional communication have been developed in different ways. Items in the Communicative Effectiveness Index (CETI) (Lomas et al., 1989) were generated by people with aphasia and their families. The ASHA Functional Assessment of Communication Skills for Adults (FACS) (Frattali et al., 1995) used a panel of clinicians, and the Communication Activities of Daily Living (CADL 2) (Holland et al., 1998) used interviews with family members and observation of people with aphasia.

Exercise 11.2

1. A test of language in dementia must distinguish between people with early dementia and normal elderly people and should detect differences in language at different stages of dementia. The Arizona Battery for Communication Disorders of Dementia (ABCD) (Bayles and Tomoeda, 1993) is such a measure. During its development, it was shown to distinguish mild dementia readily from normal elderly language. Scores were also correlated with scores on other tests of general cognitive decline. Its use with people in the UK has been investigated by Armstrong et al. (1996).

2. Tests that can predict the later language of preverbal children or children with slow language development would allow us to identify and give early treatment to children at risk. One measure that

claims to do this is the Communication and Symbolic Behaviour Scales Developmental Profile (CSBS DP). Parents complete a short checklist and a questionnaire, and clinicians score a sample of behaviour. The measure was investigated by Wetherby et al. (2002). They looked at the concurrent validity of the parental measures by correlating them with the behaviour sample. Then they looked at its predictive validity by obtaining language scores for the children at 2 years of age.

3. Glogowska et al. (2001) developed a questionnaire for parents of children taking part in a study of therapy effectiveness. Factor analysis revealed three factors – practical help from SLTs, help with emotional responses to their child's problems and perceptions of the effectiveness of therapy. Assessing the validity of such a measure will be difficult as no similar measures are available. Construct validity was used. The measure was part of a larger questionnaire to assess parents' views of the speech and language therapy service they received. The authors showed that the 3 scales were correlated with parents' perceptions of the quality of the service, although not always significantly, but were not related to the type of language problem experienced by their children.

Exercise 13.1

The level of observed agreement is 65/87. So $P_o = 0.75$. This is quite a high level but has not been corrected for chance. P_c in this case is 0.51. So:

$$K = \frac{P_o - P_c}{1 - P_c} = \frac{0.75 - 0.51}{1 - 0.51} = 0.49$$

which is only at a 'fair' level of agreement. Luther et al. (1998), who carried out a research project similar to this, found a Kappa value of 0.48. Agreement for other rehabilitation services was also quite poor, with only occupational therapy making it into the 'good' range. They concluded that client reports were quite inaccurate and that care should be taken when using them as a guide to service provision.

Appendices

Appendix 1: the normal distribution (z-scores)

z	0	1	2	3	4	5	6	7	8	9
0.0	0.0000	0.0040	0.0080	0.0120	0.0160	0.0199	0.0239	0.0279	0.0319	0.0359
0.1	0.0389	0.0438	0.0478	0.0517	0.0557	0.0596	0.0636	0.0675	0.0714	0.0754
0.2	0.0793	0.0832	0.0871	0.0910	0.0948	0.0987	0.1026	0.1064	0.1134	0.1141
0.3	0.1179	0.1217	0.1255	0.1293	0.1331	0.1368	0.1406	0.1443	0.1480	0.1517
0.4	0.1554	0.1591	0.1628	0.1664	0.1700	0.1736	0.1772	0.1808	0.1844	0.1879
0.5	0.1915	0.1950	0.1985	0.2019	0.2054	0.2088	0.2123	0.2157	0.2190	0.2224
0.6	0.2258	0.2291	0.2324	0.2357	0.2389	0.2422	0.2454	0.2486	0.2518	0.2549
0.7	0.2580	0.2612	0.2642	0.2673	0.2704	0.2734	0.2764	0.2794	0.2823	0.2852
0.8	0.2881	0.2910	0.2939	0.2967	0.2996	0.3023	0.3051	0.3078	0.3106	0.3133
0.9	0.3159	0.3186	0.3212	0.3238	0.3264	0.3289	0.3315	0.3340	0.3365	0.3389
1.0	0.3413	0.3438	0.3461	0.3485	0.3508	0.3531	0.3554	0.3577	0.3599	0.3621
1.1	0.3643	0.3665	0.3686	0.3708	0.3729	0.3749	0.3770	0.3790	0.3810	0.3830
1.2	0.3849	0.3869	0.3888	0.3907	0.3925	0.3944	0.3962	0.3980	0.3997	0.4015
1.3	0.4032	0.4049	0.4066	0.4082	0.4099	0.4115	0.4131	0.4147	0.4162	0.4177
1.4	0.4192	0.4207	0.4222	0.4236	0.4251	0.4265	0.4279	0.4292	0.4306	0.4319
1.5	0.4332	0.4345	0.4357	0.4370	0.4382	0.4394	0.4406	0.4418	0.4429	0.4441
1.6	0.4452	0.4463	0.4474	0.4484	0.4495	0.4505	0.4515	0.4525	0.4535	0.4545
1.7	0.4554	0.4564	0.4573	0.4582	0.4591	0.4599	0.4608	0.4616	0.4625	0.4633
1.8	0.4641	0.4649	0.4656	0.4664	0.4671	0.4678	0.4686	0.4693	0.4699	0.4706
1.9	0.4713	0.4719	0.4726	0.4732	0.4738	0.4744	0.4750	0.4756	0.4761	0.4767
2.0	0.4772	0.4778	0.4783	0.4788	0.4793	0.4798	0.4803	0.4808	0.4812	0.4817
2.1	0.4821	0.4826	0.4830	0.4834	0.4838	0.4842	0.4846	0.4850	0.4854	0.4857
2.2	0.4861	0.4864	0.4868	0.4871	0.4875	0.4878	0.4881	0.4884	0.4887	0.4890
2.3	0.4893	0.4869	0.4898	0.4901	0.4904	0.4906	0.4909	0.4911	0.4913	0.4916
2.4	0.4918	0.4920	0.4922	0.4925	0.4927	0.4929	0.4931	0.4932	0.4934	0.4936
2.5	0.4938	0.4940	0.4941	0.4943	0.4945	0.4946	0.4948	0.4949	0.4951	0.4952
2.6	0.4953	0.4955	0.4956	0.4957	0.4959	0.4960	0.4961	0.4962	0.4963	0.4964
2.7	0.4965	0.4966	0.4967	0.4968	0.4969	0.4970	0.4971	0.4972	0.4973	0.4974
2.8	0.4974	0.4975	0.4976	0.4977	0.4977	0.4978	0.4979	0.4979	0.4980	0.4981
2.9	0.4981	0.4982	0.4982	0.4983	0.4984	0.4984	0.4985	0.4985	0.4986	0.4986
30.0	0.4987	0.4987	0.4987	0.4988	0.4988	0.4989	0.4989	0.4989	0.4990	0.4990
3.1	0.4990	0.4991	0.4991	0.4991	0.4992	0.4992	0.4992	0.4992	0.4993	0.4993
3.2	0.4993	0.4993	0.4994	0.4994	0.4994	0.4994	0.4994	0.4995	0.4995	0.4995
3.3	0.4995	0.4995	0.4995	0.4996	0.4996	0.4996	0.4996	0.4996	0.4996	0.4997
3.4	0.4997	0.4997	0.4997	0.4997	0.4997	0.4997	0.4997	0.4997	0.4997	0.4998
3.5	0.4998	0.4998	0.4998	0.4998	0.4998	0.4998	0.4998	0.4998	0.4998	0.4998
3.6	0.4998	0.4998	0.4999	0.4999	0.4999	0.4999	0.4999	0.4999	0.4999	0.4999
3.7	0.4999	0.4999	0.4999	0.4999	0.4999	0.4999	0.4999	0.4999	0.4999	0.4999
3.8	0.4999	0.4999	0.4999	0.4999	0.4999	0.4999	0.4999	0.4999	0.4999	0.4999
3.9	0.5000	0.5000	0.5000	0.5000	0.5000	0.5000	0.5000	0.5000	0.5000	0.5000

The table gives the proportion (multiply by 100 to find the percentage) of the curve between the mean and the z-score. Column 1 gives the value of z to one decimal place. Row 1 allows the value for a second decimal place to be obtained.

Appendix 2: the t-distribution

One-tail test	0.05	0.025	0.01	0.005
Two-tail test	0.10	0.05	0.025	0.01
d.f.				
1	6.31	12.71	31.82	63.66
2	2.92	4.30	6.97	9.93
3	2.35	3.18	4.54	5.84
4	2.13	2.78	3.75	4.61
5	2.01	2.57	3.37	4.03
6	1.94	2.45	3.14	3.71
7	1.90	2.37	3.00	3.50
8	1.86	2.31	2.90	3.36
9	1.83	2.26	2.82	3.25
10	1.81	2.23	2.76	3.17
11	1.80	2.20	2.72	3.11
12	1.78	2.18	2.68	3.06
13	1.77	2.16	2.65	3.01
14	1.76	2.15	2.62	2.98
15	1.75	2.13	2.60	2.95
16	1.75	2.12	2.58	2.92
17	1.74	2.11	2.57	2.90
18	1.73	2.10	2.55	2.88
19	1.73	2.09	2.54	2.86
20	1.73	2.09	2.53	2.85
21	1.72	2.08	2.52	2.83
22	1.72	2.07	2.51	2.82
23	1.71	2.07	2.50	2.81
24	1.71	2.06	2.49	2.80
25	1.71	2.06	2.49	2.79
26	1.71	2.06	2.48	2.78
27	1.70	2.05	2.47	2.77
28	1.70	2.05	2.47	2.76
29	1.70	2.05	2.46	2.76
30	1.70	2.04	2.46	2.75
60	1.67	2.00	2.39	2.66
120	1.66	1.98	2.36	2.62

Critical values of t for one- and two-tail tests. The value of t must be greater than or equal to the table value.

Appendix 3: the Mann-Whitney test

One-tail test: 0.05 level of significance

	$n_1 =$											
$n_2 =$	1	2	3	4	5	6	7	8	9	10	11	12
1	-	-	-	-	-	-	-	-	-	-	-	-
2	-	-	-	-	0	0	0	1	1	1	1	2
3	-	-	0	0	1	2	2	3	3	4	5	5
4	-	-	0	1	2	3	4	5	6	7	8	9
5	-	0	1	2	4	5	6	8	9	11	12	13
6	-	0	2	3	5	7	8	10	12	14	16	17
7	-	0	2	4	6	8	11	13	15	17	19	21
8	-	1	3	5	8	10	13	15	18	20	23	26
9	-	1	3	6	9	12	15	18	21	24	27	30
10	-	1	4	7	11	14	17	20	24	27	31	34
11	-	1	5	8	12	16	19	23	27	31	34	38
12	-	2	5	9	13	17	21	26	30	34	38	42

One-tail test: 0.01 level of significance

	$n_1 =$											
$n_2 =$	1	2	3	4	5	6	7	8	9	10	11	12
1	-	-	-	-	-	-	-	-	-	-	-	-
2	-	-	-	-	-	-	-	-	-	-	-	-
3	-	-	-	-	-	-	0	0	1	1	1	2
4	-	-	-	-	0	1	1	2	3	3	4	5
5	-	-	-	0	1	2	3	4	5	6	7	8
6	-	-	-	1	2	3	4	6	7	8	9	11
7	-	-	0	1	3	4	6	7	9	11	12	14
8	-	-	0	2	4	6	7	9	11	13	15	17
9	-	-	1	3	5	7	9	11	14	16	18	21
10	-	-	1	3	6	8	11	13	16	19	22	24
11	-	-	1	4	7	9	12	15	18	22	25	28
12	-	-	2	5	8	11	14	17	21	24	28	31

Two-tail test: 0.05 level of significance

$n_2 =$	$n_1 =$											
	1	2	3	4	5	6	7	8	9	10	11	12
1	–	–	–	–	–	–	–	–	–	–	–	–
2	–	–	–	–	–	–	–	0	0	0	0	1
3	–	–	–	–	0	1	1	2	2	3	3	4
4	–	–	–	0	1	2	3	4	4	5	6	7
5	–	–	0	1	2	3	5	6	7	8	9	11
6	–	–	1	2	3	5	6	8	10	11	13	14
7	–	–	1	3	5	6	8	10	12	14	16	18
8	–	0	2	4	6	8	10	13	15	17	19	22
9	–	0	2	4	7	10	12	15	17	20	23	26
10	–	0	3	5	8	11	14	17	20	23	26	29
11	–	0	3	6	9	13	16	19	23	26	30	33
12	–	1	4	7	11	14	18	22	26	29	33	37

Two-tail test: 0.01 level of significance

$n_2 =$	$n_1 =$											
	1	2	3	4	5	6	7	8	9	10	11	12
1	–	–	–	–	–	–	–	–	–	–	–	–
2	–	–	–	–	–	–	–	–	–	–	–	–
3	–	–	–	–	–	–	–	–	0	0	0	1
4	–	–	–	–	–	0	0	1	1	2	2	3
5	–	–	–	–	0	1	1	2	3	4	5	6
6	–	–	–	0	1	2	3	4	5	6	7	9
7	–	–	–	0	1	3	4	6	7	9	10	12
8	–	–	–	1	2	4	6	7	9	11	13	15
9	–	–	0	1	3	5	7	9	11	13	16	18
10	–	–	0	2	4	6	9	11	13	16	18	21
11	–	–	0	2	5	7	10	13	16	18	21	24
12	–	–	1	3	6	9	12	15	18	21	24	27

Appendix 4: table of critical values for the Wilcoxon test

	One-tail test		Two-tail test	
n	$p < 0.05$	$p < 0.01$	$p < 0.05$	$p < 0.01$
5	0	–	–	–
6	2	–	0	–
7	3	0	2	–
8	5	1	3	0
9	8	3	5	1
10	10	5	8	3
11	13	7	10	5
12	17	9	13	7
13	21	12	17	9
14	25	15	21	12
15	30	19	25	15
16	35	23	29	19
17	41	27	34	23
18	47	32	40	27
19	53	37	46	32
20	60	43	52	37
21	67	49	58	42
22	75	55	65	48
23	83	62	73	54
24	91	69	81	61
25	100	76	89	68

W must be less than or equal to the table value.

Appendix 5: the sign test

n	One-tail test		Two-tail test	
	$p < 0.05$	$p < 0.01$	$p < 0.05$	$p < 0.01$
5	0	–	–	–
6	0	–	0	–
7	0	0	0	–
8	1	0	0	0
9	1	0	1	0
10	1	0	1	0
11	2	1	1	0
12	2	1	2	1
13	3	1	2	1
14	3	2	2	1
15	3	2	3	2
16	4	2	3	2
17	4	3	4	2
18	5	3	4	3
19	5	4	4	3
20	5	4	5	3
21	6	4	5	4
22	6	5	5	4
23	7	5	6	4
24	7	5	6	5
25	7	6	7	5

Appendix 6: critical values of the F-distribution

Critical values of the F-distribution at the p < 0.05 level of significance

	df_1									
df_2	1	2	3	4	5	6	7	8	9	10
2	18.51	19.00	19.16	19.25	19.30	19.33	19.35	19.37	19.38	19.40
3	10.13	9.55	9.28	9.12	9.01	8.94	8.89	8.85	8.81	8.79
4	7.71	6.94	6.59	6.39	6.26	6.16	6.09	6.04	6.00	5.96
5	6.61	5.79	5.41	5.19	5.05	4.95	4.88	4.82	4.77	4.74
6	5.99	5.14	4.76	4.53	4.39	4.28	4.21	4.15	4.10	4.06
7	5.59	4.74	4.35	4.12	3.97	3.87	3.79	3.73	3.68	3.64
8	5.32	4.46	4.07	3.84	3.69	3.58	3.50	3.44	3.39	3.35
9	5.12	4.26	3.86	3.63	3.48	3.37	3.29	3.23	3.18	3.14
10	4.96	4.10	3.71	3.48	3.33	3.22	3.14	3.07	3.02	2.98
11	4.84	3.98	3.59	3.36	3.20	3.09	3.01	2.95	2.90	2.85
12	4.75	3.89	3.49	3.26	3.11	3.00	2.91	2.85	2.80	2.75
13	4.67	3.81	3.41	3.18	3.03	2.92	2.83	2.77	2.71	2.67
14	4.60	3.74	3.34	3.11	2.96	2.85	2.76	2.70	2.65	2.60
15	4.54	3.68	3.29	3.06	2.90	2.79	2.71	2.64	2.59	2.54
16	4.49	3.63	3.24	3.01	2.85	2.74	2.66	2.59	2.54	2.49
17	4.45	3.59	3.20	2.96	2.81	2.70	2.61	2.55	2.49	2.45
18	4.41	3.55	3.16	2.93	2.77	2.66	2.58	2.51	2.46	2.41
19	4.38	3.52	3.13	2.90	2.74	2.63	2.54	2.48	2.42	2.38
20	4.35	3.49	3.10	2.87	2.71	2.60	2.51	2.45	2.39	2.35
25	4.24	3.39	2.99	2.76	2.60	2.49	2.40	2.34	2.28	2.24
30	4.17	3.32	2.92	2.69	2.53	2.42	2.33	2.27	2.21	2.16
40	4.08	3.23	2.84	2.61	2.45	2.34	2.25	2.18	2.12	2.08
60	4.00	3.15	2.76	2.53	2.37	2.25	2.17	2.10	2.04	1.99
120	3.92	3.07	2.68	2.45	2.29	2.18	2.09	2.02	1.96	1.91

Critical values of the F-distribution at the p < 0.01 level of significance.

	df_1									
df_2	1	2	3	4	5	6	7	8	9	10
2	98.50	99.00	99.17	99.25	99.30	99.33	99.36	99.37	99.39	99.40
3	34.12	30.82	29.46	28.71	28.24	27.91	27.67	27.49	27.34	27.23
4	21.20	18.00	16.69	15.98	15.52	15.21	14.98	14.80	14.66	14.55
5	16.26	13.27	12.06	11.39	10.97	10.67	10.46	10.29	10.16	10.05
6	13.74	10.92	9.78	9.15	8.75	8.47	8.26	8.10	7.98	7.87
7	12.25	9.55	8.45	7.85	7.46	7.19	6.99	6.84	6.72	6.62
8	11.26	8.65	7.59	7.01	6.63	6.37	6.18	6.03	5.91	5.81
9	10.56	8.02	6.99	6.42	6.06	5.80	5.61	5.47	5.35	5.26
10	10.04	7.56	6.55	5.99	5.64	5.39	5.20	5.06	4.94	4.85
11	9.65	7.21	6.22	5.67	5.32	5.07	4.89	4.74	4.63	4.54
12	9.33	6.93	5.95	5.41	5.06	4.82	4.64	4.50	4.39	4.30
13	9.07	6.70	5.74	5.21	4.86	4.62	4.44	4.30	4.19	4.10
14	8.86	6.51	5.56	5.04	4.70	4.46	4.28	4.14	4.03	3.94
15	8.68	6.36	5.42	4.89	4.56	4.32	4.14	4.00	3.89	3.80
16	8.53	6.23	5.29	4.77	4.44	4.20	4.03	3.89	3.78	3.69
17	8.40	6.11	5.18	4.67	4.34	4.10	3.93	3.79	3.68	3.59
18	8.29	6.01	5.09	4.58	4.25	4.01	3.84	3.71	3.60	3.51
19	8.18	5.93	5.01	4.50	4.17	3.94	3.77	3.63	3.52	3.43
20	8.10	5.85	4.94	4.43	4.10	3.87	3.70	3.56	3.46	3.37
25	7.77	5.57	4.68	4.18	3.86	3.63	3.46	3.32	3.22	3.13
30	7.56	5.39	4.51	4.02	3.70	3.47	3.30	3.17	3.07	2.98
40	7.31	5.18	4.31	3.83	3.51	3.29	3.12	2.99	2.89	2.80
60	7.08	4.98	4.13	3.65	3.34	3.12	2.95	2.82	2.72	2.63
120	6.85	4.79	3.95	3.48	3.17	2.96	2.79	2.66	2.56	2.47

Appendix 7: power

δ	One-tail test		Two-tail test	
	$p < 0.05$	$p < 0.01$	$p < 0.05$	$p < 0.01$
1.00	0.26	0.09	0.17	0.06
1.10	0.29	0.11	0.20	0.07
1.20	0.33	0.13	0.22	0.08
1.30	0.37	0.15	0.26	0.10
1.40	0.40	0.18	0.29	0.12
1.50	0.44	0.20	0.32	0.14
1.60	0.48	0.23	0.36	0.17
1.70	0.52	0.27	0.40	0.19
1.80	0.56	0.30	0.44	0.22
1.90	0.60	0.34	0.48	0.25
2.00	0.64	0.37	0.52	0.28
2.10	0.68	0.41	0.56	0.32
2.20	0.71	0.45	0.60	0.35
2.30	0.74	0.49	0.63	0.39
2.40	0.78	0.53	0.67	0.43
2.50	0.80	0.57	0.71	0.47
2.60	0.83	0.61	0.74	0.51
2.70	0.85	0.65	0.77	0.55
2.80	0.88	0.68	0.80	0.59
2.90	0.90	0.72	0.83	0.63
3.00	0.91	0.75	0.85	0.66
3.10	0.93	0.78	0.87	0.70
3.20	0.94	0.81	0.89	0.73
3.30	0.95	0.84	0.91	0.77
3.40	0.96	0.86	0.93	0.80
3.50	0.97	0.88	0.94	0.82
3.60	0.98	0.90	0.95	0.85
3.70	0.98	0.92	0.96	0.87
3.80	0.98	0.93	0.97	0.89
3.90	0.99	0.94	0.97	0.91
4.00	0.99	0.95	0.98	0.92
4.10	0.99	0.96	0.98	0.94
4.20	–	0.97	0.99	0.95
4.30	–	0.98	0.99	0.96
4.40	–	0.98	0.99	0.97
4.50	–	0.99	0.99	0.97
4.60	–	0.99	–	0.98
4.70	–	0.99	–	0.98
4.80	–	0.99	–	0.99
4.90	–	–	–	0.99
5.00	–	–	–	0.99

From Statistical Methods for Psychology (with InfoTrac) 4th edition by Howell© 1997. Reprinted with permission of Brooks/Cole, a division of Thomson Learning: www.thomsonrights.com. Fax 800 730–2215.

Appendix 8: critical values of chi square

The actual value must be greater than or equal to the table value.

Degrees of freedom	$p < 0.05$	$p < 0.01$
1	3.84	6.64
2	5.99	9.21
3	7.82	11.34
4	9.49	13.28
5	11.07	15.09
6	12.59	16.81
7	14.07	18.48
8	15.51	20.09
9	16.92	21.67
10	18.31	23.21

Appendix 9: critical values for the Pearson product-moment correlation coefficient

Degrees of freedom	One-tail test		Two-tail test	
	$p < 0.05$	$p < 0.01$	$p < 0.05$	$p < 0.01$
5	0.670	0.833	0.754	0.874
6	0.621	0.789	0.707	0.834
7	0.582	0.750	0.666	0.798
8	0.549	0.715	0.632	0.765
9	0.521	0.685	0.602	0.735
10	0.497	0.658	0.576	0.708
11	0.476	0.634	0.553	0.683
12	0.458	0.612	0.532	0.661
13	0.441	0.592	0.514	0.641
14	0.426	0.574	0.497	0.623
15	0.412	0.558	0.482	0.605
16	0.400	0.542	0.468	0.590
17	0.389	0.528	0.455	0.575
18	0.378	0.515	0.444	0.561
19	0.369	0.503	0.433	0.549
20	0.360	0.492	0.423	0.537
25	0.323	0.445	0.381	0.487
30	0.296	0.409	0.349	0.449
40	0.257	0.357	0.304	0.393
60	0.211	0.295	0.250	0.325
80	0.183	0.256	0.217	0.283
100	0.164	0.230	0.195	0.254

r must be larger than or equal to the table value.

Appendix 10: critical values for the Spearmen rank-order correlation coefficient

Degrees of freedom	One-tail test		Two-tail test	
	$p < 0.05$	$p < 0.01$	$p < 0.05$	$p < 0.01$
5	0.900	1.000	1.000	–
6	0.829	0.943	0.886	1.000
7	0.714	0.893	0.786	0.929
8	0.643	0.833	0.738	0.881
9	0.600	0.783	0.700	0.833
10	0.564	0.745	0.648	0.794
11	0.536	0.709	0.618	0.755
12	0.503	0.671	0.587	0.727
13	0.484	0.648	0.560	0.703
14	0.464	0.622	0.538	0.675
15	0.443	0.604	0.521	0.654
16	0.429	0.582	0.503	0.635
17	0.414	0.566	0.485	0.615
18	0.401	0.550	0.472	0.600
19	0.391	0.535	0.460	0.584
20	0.380	0.520	0.447	0.570
25	0.337	0.466	0.398	0.511
30	0.306	0.425	0.362	0.467
40	0.264	0.368	0.313	0.405
60	0.214	0.300	0.255	0.331
80	0.185	0.260	0.220	0.287
100	0.165	0.233	0.197	0.257

r must be larger than or equal to the table value.

References

Adams A-M, Gathercole SE (1995) Phonological working memory and speech production in preschool children. Journal of Speech and Hearing Research 38: 403-13.

Adams A-M, Gathercole SE (1996) Phonological working memory and spoken language development in young children. Quarterly Journal of Experimental Psychology 49A: 216-33.

Aftonomos LB, Steele RD, Wertz RT (1997) Promoting recovery in chronic aphasia with interactive technology. Archives of Physical Medicine and Rehabilitation 78: 841-6.

Allan CM (1970) Treatment of non-fluent speech resulting from neurological disease – treatment of dysarthria. British Journal of Disorders of Communication 5: 3-5.

Allen CMC (1990) Trials and tribulations in speech therapy. British Medical Journal 301: 302-3.

Almost D, Rosenbaum P (1998) Effectiveness of speech intervention for phonological disorders: a randomized control trial. Developmental Medicine and Child Neurology 40: 319-25.

Andrews G, Craig A, Feyer AM, Hoddinott S, Howie P, Neilson M (1983) Stuttering: a review of research findings and theories circa 1982. Journal of Speech and Hearing Disorder 48: 226-46.

Andrews G, Guitar G, Howie P (1980) Meta-analysis of the effects of stuttering treatment. Journal of Speech and Hearing Disorders 45: 287-307.

Armstrong L, Bayles KA, Borthwick SE, Tomoeda CK (1996) Use of the Arizona Battery for Communication Disorders of Dementia in the UK. European Journal of Disorders of Communication 31: 171-80.

Arndt J, Healy EC (2001) Concomitant disorders in school-age children who stutter. Language, Speech and Hearing Services in Schools 32: 68-78.

Arnold DH, Harvey EA (1998) Data monitoring: a hypothesis-testing approach for treatment outcome research. Journal of Consulting and Clinical Psychology 66: 1030-5.

Bakeman R, Gottman JM (1997) Observing Interaction: An Introduction to Sequential Analysis. Cambridge: Cambridge University Press.

Banat D, Summers S, Pring T (2002) An investigation into carers' perceptions of the verbal comprehension ability of adults with severe learning disabilities. British Journal of Learning Disabilities 30: 78-81.

Basso A, Capitani E, Vignolo LA (1979) Influence of rehabilitation on language skills in aphasic patients: a controlled study. Archives of Neurology 36: 190-6.

Basso A, Caporali A (2001) Aphasia therapy or the importance of being earnest. Aphasiology 15: 307-32.

Bayles KA, Tomoeda CK (1993) Arizona Battery for Communication Disorders of Dementia. Tucson, AZ: Canyonlands Publishing.

Best W, Melvin D, Williams S (1993) The effectiveness of communication groups in day nurseries. European Journal of Disorders of Communication 28: 187-212.

Bishop DVM (1983) Test for the reception of grammar. 2nd edn. Privately published.

Bishop DVM (1997) Uncommon Understanding Development and Disorders of Language Comprehension in Children. Hove: Psychology Press.

Bishop DVM (2002) The role of genes in the etiology of specific language impairment. Journal of Communication Disorders 35: 311-28.

Blood GW, Ridenour JS, Thomas EA, Qualls CD, Hammer CS (2002) Predicting job satisfaction among speech-language pathologists working in public schools. Language Speech and Hearing Services in Schools 33: 282-90.

Blood GW, Simpson KC, Raimondi SC, Dineen M, Kauffman SM, and Stagaard KA (1994) Social support in laryngeal cancer survivors: voice and adjustment issues. American Journal of Speech Language Pathology 3: 37-44.

Blood IM, Wertz H, Blood GW, Bennett S, Simpson KC (1997) The effects of life stressors and daily stressors on stuttering. Journal of Speech, Language and Hearing Research 40: 134-43.

Blumberg CJ (1984) Comments on 'a simplified time series analysis for evaluating treatment interventions'. Journal of Applied Behavioural Analysis 17: 539-42.

Bonelli P, Dixon M, Bernstein-Ratner N, Onslow M (2000) Child and parent speech and language following the Lidcombe programme of early stuttering intervention. Clinical Linguistics and Phonetics 14: 427-46.

Booth T, Booth W (2002) Men in the lives of mothers with intellectual disabilities. Journal of Applied Research in Intellectual Disabilities 187-99.

Botting N, Conti Ramsden G (2000) Social and behavioural difficulties in children with language impairment. Child Language Teaching and Therapy 16: 105-20.

Bowling A (1997) Research Methods in Health. Buckingham: Open University Press.

Boyd S, Hewlett N (2001) The gender imbalance among speech and language therapists and students. International Journal of Language and Communication Disorders 36: 167-72.

Bradley L, Bryant P (1983) Categorising sounds and learning to read: a causal connection. Nature 301: 419-21.

Brantley PJ, Waggoner CD, Jones GN, Rappaport NB (1987) A daily stress inventory: development, reliability and validity. Journal of Behavioural Medicine 10: 61-74.

Briggs K, Askham J, Norman I, Redfern S (2003) Accomplishing care at home for people with dementia: using observational methodology. Qualitative Health Research 13: 268-80.

Brindley P, Copeland M, Demain C, Martyn P (1989) A comparison of ten chronic Broca's aphasics following intensive and non-intensive periods of therapy. Aphasiology 3: 695-707.

Brooks I, Brown RB (2002) The role of ritualistic ceremony in removing barriers between subcultures in the National Health Service. Journal of Advanced Nursing 38: 341-52.

Brown M, Perry A, Cheesman T, Pring T (2000) Pitch change in male-to-female transsexuals: has phonosurgery a role to play? International Journal of Language and Communication Disorders 35: 129–36.

Bryman A (2001) Social Research Methods. Oxford: Oxford University Press.

Bryman A, Burgess RG (1994) Reflections on qualitative data analysis. In Bryman A, Burgess RG (eds) Analysing Qualitative Data. London: Routledge.

Campbell TF, Needleman HL, Riess J, Tobin M (2000) Bone lead levels and language processing performance. Developmental Neuropsychology 18: 171–86.

Cannito MP, Burch AR, Watts C, Rappold PW, Sherrard K (1997) Dysfluency in spasmodic dysphonia: a multivariate analysis. Journal of Speech, Language and Hearing Research 40: 627–41.

Carding P, Hillman R (2001) More randomised controlled studies in speech and language therapy: complex behavioural interventions can be evaluated. British Medical Journal 323: 645–7.

Carding P, Horsley IA, Docherty GJ (1999) A study of the effectiveness of voice therapy in the treatment of 45 patients with non-organic dysphonia. Journal of Voice 13: 72–104.

Catts HW, Fey ME, Zhang X, Tomblin JB (2001) Estimating the risk of future reading difficulties in kindergarten children: a research model and its clinical implementation. Language, Speech and Hearing Services in Schools 32: 38–50.

Cecil M, Tyndall L, Haydon R (2001) The relationship between dysphonia and sinusitis: a pilot study. Journal of Voice 15: 270–7.

Cella D, Dineen K, Arnason B, Reder A, Webster K, Karabatsos G, Chang C, Lloyd S, Mo F, Stewart J, Stefoski D (1996) Validation of the functional assessment of multiple sclerosis quality of life instrument. Neurology 47: 129–39.

Chadwick DD, Jolliffe J, Goldbart J (2002) Carer knowledge of dysphagia management strategies. International Journal of Language and Communication Disorders 37: 345–57.

Clark HH (1973) The language as fixed effect fallacy: a critique of language statistics in psychological research. Journal of Verbal Learning and Verbal Behaviour 15: 257–61.

Clark-Carter D (1997) Doing Quantitative Psychological Research: From Design to Report. Hove: Psychology Press.

Cohen J (1960) Coefficient of agreement for nominal scales. Educational and Pschological Measurement 20: 37–46.

Cohen J (1988) Statistical power analysis for the behavioural sciences. 2nd edn. New York: Academic Press.

Coltheart M (1983) Aphasia therapy research: a single case study approach. In Code C, Muller DJ (eds) Aphasia Therapy. London: Arnold.

Conti-Ramsden G, Botting N, Knox E, Simkin Z (2002) Different school placements following language unit attendance: which factors effect language outcome? International Journal of Language and Communication Disorders 37: 185–95.

Coplan J, Contello KA, Cunningham CK, Weiner LB, Dye TD, Roberge L, Wojtowycz MA, Kirkwood K (1998) Early language development in children exposed to or infected with human immunodeficiency virus. Pediatrics 102: e8.

Cordes A (1998) Current status of the stuttering treatment literature. In Cordes AK, Ingham RJ (eds) Treatment Efficacy for Stuttering: A Search for Empirical Bases. San Diego: Singular.

Cossu G, Rossini F, Marshall JC (1993) When reading is acquired but phonemic awareness is not: a study of literacy in Down's syndrome. Cognition 46: 129–38.

Crichton-Smith I (2002) Communicating in the real world: accounts from people who stammer. Journal of Fluency Disorders 27: 333–52.

Croft P (1996) Review of MW van Tulder, BW Koes and LM Bouter (eds) 'Low back pain in primary care: effectiveness of diagnostic and therapeutic interventions.' British Medical Journal 313: 122.

Cronbach LJ (1951) Coefficient alpha and the internal consistency of tests. Psychometrika 16: 297–334.

Crosbie S, Dodd B (2001) Training auditory discrimination: a single case study. Child Language Teaching and Therapy 17: 173–94.

Culton GL, Gershwin JM (1998) Current trends in laryngectomy rehabilitation: a survey of speech language pathologists. Otolaryngology – Head and Neck Surgery 118: 458–63.

Cunningham R, Ward CD (2003) Evaluation of a training programme to facilitate conversation between people with aphasia and their partners. Aphasiology 17: 687–707.

Dale PS (1991) Validity of a parent report measure of vocabulary and syntax at 24 months: preschool children with language impairment. Journal of Speech and Hearing Research 34: 565–71.

Dancey CP, Reidy J (2002) Statistics without maths for psychology: using SPSS for Windows™. 2nd edn. London: Prentice Hall.

David RM, Enderby R, Bainton D (1982) Treatment of acquired aphasia: speech therapists and volunteers compared. Journal of Neurology, Neurosurgery and Psychiatry 45: 957–61.

Davidson B, Worrall L, Hickson L (2003) Identifying the communication activities of older people with aphasia: evidence from naturalistic observation. Aphasiology 17: 243–64.

Dean EC, Howell J, Waters D, Reid J (1995) Metaphon: a metalinguistic approach to the treatment of phonological disorder in children. Clinical Linguistics and Phonetics 9: 1–19.

Deane KHO, Whurr R, Clarke CE, Playford ED, Ben-Shlomo Y (2002a) Non-pharmacological Therapies for Dysphagia in Parkinson's Disease (Cochrane review). In The Cochrane Library, Issue 1. Oxford: Update software.

Deane KHO, Whurr R, Playford ED, Ben-Shlomo Y, Clarke CE (2002b) Speech and Language Therapy for Dysarthria in Parkinson's Disease: a Comparison of Techniques (Cochrane Review). In The Cochrane Library, Issue 1. Oxford: Update Software.

Deary IJ, Wilson JA, Harris MB, MacDougal G (1995) Globus pharyngis: development of a symptom assessment scale. Journal of Psychosomatic Research 39: 203–13.

Defries JC, Fulker DW (1985) Multiple regression analysis of twin data. Behaviour Genetics 15: 467–73.

Denes G, Perrazzolo C, Piani A, Piccione F (1996) Intensive versus regular speech therapy in global aphasia: a controlled study. Aphasiology 10: 385–94.

Denne M, Langdown N, Pring T, Roy P (submitted) Treating children with expressive phonological disorders: does phonological awareness therapy work in the clinic?

Denscombe M (1998) The Good Research Guide for Small Scale Social Research Projects. Buckingham: Open University Press.

De Nil LF, Brutten GJ (1991) Speech associated attitudes of stuttering and non-stuttering children. Journal of Speech and Hearing Research 34: 60–66.

Dollaghan C, Campbell TF (1998) Non-word repetition and child language impairment. Journal of Speech, Language and Hearing Research 41: 1136–46.

Dormandy K, Van der Gaag A (1989) What colour are the alligators? A critical look at methods used to assess communication skills in adults with learning difficulties. British Journal of Disorders of Communication 24: 265–79.

Draper BM, Poulos CJ, Cole AMD, Poulos RG, Ehrlich F (1992) A comparison of caregivers for elderly stroke and dementia victims. Journal of the American Geriatrics Society 40: 896–901.

DuBois E, Bernthal J (1978) A comparison of three methods for obtaining articulatory responses. Journal of Speech and Hearing Disorders 43: 295–305.

Dunn LM, Dunn LM, Whetton C, Burley J (1997) British Picture Vocabulary Scales. 2nd edn. Windsor: NFER-Nelson.

Eales C, Pring T (1998) Using individual and group therapy to remediate word-finding difficulties. Aphasiology 12: 913–18.

Eastwood J (1988) Qualitative research: an additional research methodology for speech pathology? British Journal of Disorders of Communication 23: 171–84.

Edwards S, Fletcher P, Garman M, Hughes A, Letts C, Sinka I (1997) The Reynell Developmental Language Scales III. Windsor: NFER-Nelson.

Erzberger C, Prein G (1997) Triangulation: validity and empirically based hypothesis construction. Quality and Quantity 31: 141–54.

Evans C, Chalmers J, Capewell S, Redpath A, Finlayson A, Boyd J, Pell J, McMurray J, Macintyre K, Graham L (2000) 'I don't like Mondays' – day of the week of coronary heart disease deaths in Scotland: study of routinely collected data. British Medical Journal 320: 218.

Festinger L, Reichen HW, Schacter S (1956) When Prophecy Fails. New York: Harper & Row.

Fey ME, Cleave PL, Long SH, Hughes DL (1993) Two approaches to the facilitation of grammar in children with language impairments: an experimental evaluation. Journal of Speech and Hearing Research 36: 141–57.

Fey ME, Cleave PL, Ravida AI, Long SH, Dejmal AE, Easton DL (1994) Effects of grammar facilitation on the phonological performance of children with speech and language impairments. Journal of Speech and Hearing Research 37: 594–607.

Field A (2000) Discovering Statistics using SPSS for Windows. London: Sage.

Fimian MJ, Lieberman RJ, Fastenau PS (1991) Development and validation of an instrument to measure occupational stress in speech–language pathologists. Journal of Speech and Hearing Research 34: 439–46.

Fleiss JL (1981) Statistical Methods for Rates and Proportions. New York: Wiley.

Forman D, Hall S, Oliver C (2002) Descriptive analysis of self-injurious behaviour and self-restraint. Journal of Applied Research in Intellectual Disabilities 15: 1–7.

Fox CM, Morrison CE, Ramig LO, Sapir S (2002) Current perspectives on the Lee Silverman Voice Treatment (LSVT) for individuals with idiopathic Parkinson disease. American Journal of Speech-Language Pathology 11: 111–23.

Francis DR, Riddoch MJ, Humphreys GW (2001) Cognitive rehabilitation of word meaning deafness. Aphasiology 15: 749–66.

Franklin S (1989) Dissociations in auditory word comprehension: evidence from nine fluent aphasic patients. Aphasiology 3: 189–207.

Franklin S (1997) Designing single case treatment studies for aphasic patients. Neuropsychological Rehabilitation 7: 401–18.

Frattali CM, Thompson CK, Holland AL, Wohl CB, Ferketic MM (1995) The American Speech-Hearing-Language Association Functional Assessment of Communication Skills for Adults (ASHA FACS). Rockville, MD: ASHA.

Frazier-Norbury C, Chiat S (2000) Semantic intervention to support word recognition: a single case study. Child Language Teaching and Therapy 16: 141–61.

Fujiki M, Brinton B, Isaacson T, Summer C (2001) Social behaviours of children with language impairment in the playground: a pilot study. Language, Speech and Hearing Services in Schools 32: 101–13.

Fujimoto PA, Madison CL, Larrigan LB (1991) The effects of a tracheostoma valve on the intelligibility and quality of tracheoesophageal speech. Journal of Speech and Hearing Research 34: 33–6.

Fuller DR (1997) Initial study into the effects of translucency and complexity on the learning of Blissymbols by children and adults with normal cognitive abilities. Augmentative and Alternative Communication 13: 30–9.

Gathercole SE, Baddeley AD (1990) Phonological memory deficits in language disordered children: is there a causal connection? Journal of Memory and Language 29: 336–60.

Geers AE (2002) Factors affecting the development of speech, langauge and literacy in children with early cochlear implantation. Language, Speech and Hearing Services in Schools 33: 172–83.

Gibbard D (1994) Parental based intervention with preschool language delayed children. European Journal of Disorders of Communication 29: 131–50.

Gierut JA (1998) Treatment efficacy: functional phonological disorders in children. Journal of Speech, Language and Hearing Research 41: S85–S100.

Gillon GT (2000) The efficacy of phonological awareness intervention for children with spoken language impairment. Language, Speech and Hearing Services in Schools 31: 126–41.

Gillon GT (2002) Follow-up study investigating the benefits of phonological awareness intervention for children with spoken language impairment. International Journal of Language and Communication Disorders 37: 381–400.

Giralometto L (1997) Development of a parent report measure for profiling the conversational skills of preschool children. American Journal of Speech-Language Pathology 6: 25–33.

Giralometto L, Pearce PS, Weitzman E (1995) Interactive focused stimulation for toddlers with expressive vocabulary delays. Journal of Speech and Hearing Research 39: 1274–83.

Giralometto L, Pearce PS, Weitzman E (1996) The effects of focused stimulation for promoting vocabulary in young children with delays: a pilot study. Journal of Child Communication and Development 17: 39–49.

Glaser BG, Strauss AL (1967) The Discovery of Grounded Theory: Strategies for Qualitative Research. New York: Aldine.

Glass GV (1976) Primary, secondary and meta analysis of research. The Educational Researcher 10: 3–8.

Glogowska M, Campbell R (2000) Investigating parental views of involvement in preschool speech and language therapy. International Journal of Language and Communication Disorders 35: 391–405.

Glogowska M, Campbell R, Peters TJ, Roulestone S, Enderby P (2001) Developing a scale to measure parental attitudes towards preschool speech and language therapy services. International Journal of Language and Communication Disorders 35: 391–405.

Glogowska M, Campbell R, Peters TJ, Roulestone S, Enderby P (2002) A multimethod approach to the evaluation of community preschool speech and language therapy provision. Child: Care, Health and Development 28: 507–12.

Glogowska M, Roulestone S, Enderby P, Peters T (2000) Randomised control trial of community based speech and language therapy in preschool children. British Medical Journal 321: 923–6.

Goberman A, Coelho C, Robb M (2002) Phonatory characteristics of Parkinsonian Speech before and after morning medication: the ON and OFF states. Journal of Communication Disorders 35: 217–39.

Goffman E (1961) Asylums. New York: Doubleday.

Goldberg DP, Williams P (1988) A User's Guide to the General Health Questionnaire. Windsor: NFER-Nelson.

Goodglass H, Kaplan E, Weintraub S (1983) Boston Naming Test. Philadelphia: Lea & Febiger.

Greene J, D'Oliveira M (1982) Learning to Use Statistical Tests in Psychology: A Student Guide. Milton Keynes: Open University Press.

Greener J, Enderby P, Whurr R (2002) Speech and Language Therapy for Aphasia following Stroke (Cochrane Review). In The Cochrane Library, Issue 2. Oxford: Update Software, 2000.

Greener J, Langhorne P (2002) Systematic reviews in rehabilitation for stroke: issues and approaches to addressing them. Clinical Rehabilitation 16: 69–74.

Gutierrez VF, Pena E (2001) Dynamic assessment of diverse children: a tutorial. Language Speech and Hearing Services in Schools 32: 212–24.

Hall DMB (1999) Letter to the editor. International Journal of Language and Communication Disorders 34: 445–7.

Harris V, Onslow M, Packman A, Harrison E, Menzies R (2002) An experimental investigation of the Lidcombe program on early stuttering. Journal of Fluency Disorders 27: 203–14.

Hatcher PJ, Hulme C, Ellis AW (1994) Ameliorating early reading failure by integrating the teaching of reading and phonological skills: the phonological linkage hypothesis. Child Development 65: 41–57.

Hauerwas LB, Stone CA (2000) Are parents of school age children with specific language impairments accurate estimators of their child's language skills? Child Language Teaching and Therapy 16: 73–86.

Hayhow R, Cray AM, Enderby P (2002) Stammering and therapy views of people who stammer. Journal of Fluency Disorders 27: 1–17.

Hesketh A (1986) Measuring progress in aphasia therapy: a multiple baseline study. British Journal of Disorders of Communication 21: 47–62.

Hesketh A, Adams C, Nightingale C, Hall R (2000) Phonological awareness therapy and articulatory training approaches for children with phonological disorders: a comparative outcome study. International Journal of Language and Communication Disorders 35: 337–54.

Hilari K, Wiggins RD, Roy P, Byng S, Smith SC (2003) Predictors of health related quality of life (HRQL) in people with chronic aphasia. Aphasiology 17: 365–81.

Hinton PR (1995) Statistics Explained: A Guide for Social Science Students. London: Routledge.

Hodgson R, Rollnick S (1996) More fun, less stress: how to survive in research. In Parry G, Watts FN (eds) Behavioural and Mental Health Research: A Handbook of Skills and Methods. 2nd edn. Hove: Erlbaum/Taylor & Francis.

Hodson B (1986) The Assessment of Phonological Processes – Revised. Danville, IL: Interstate Printers and Publishers.

Hoen B, Thelander M, Worsley J (1997) Improvement in psychological well-being of people with aphasia and their families: evaluation of a community-based programme. Aphasiology 11: 681–91.

Holland AL, Frattali CM, Fromm D (1998) Communication Activities of Daily Living. 2nd edn. Austin, TX: Pro Ed.

Holmes TH, Rahe RH (1967) The Social Readjustment Rating Scale. Journal of Psychosomatic Research 11: 213–18.

Hopper T, Holland A, Rewega M (2002) Conversational coaching: treatment outcomes and future directions. Aphasiology 16: 745–61.

Howard D (1986) Beyond randomised control trials: the case for effective case studies of the effects of treatment in aphasia. British Journal of Disorders of Communication 21: 89–102.

Howard D, Patterson K (1992) The Pyramids and Palm Trees Test: A Test of Semantic Access from Words and Pictures. Bury St Edmunds: Thames Valley Test Company.

Howell DC (1997) Statistical Methods for Psychology. Belmont, CA: Duxbury.

Howell J, Deane EC (1991) Teaching Phonological Disorders in Children: Metaphon – Theory to Practice. London: Whurr.

Howitt D, Cramer D (1999) A Guide to Computing Statistics with SPSS for Windows™. London: Prentice Hall.

Hunter L, Pring TR, Martin S (1991) An experimental evaluation of the use of strategies to improve the intelligibility of cerebral-palsied speech. British Journal of Disorders of Communication 26: 163–74.

Ingham JC, Riley G (1998) Guidlines for documentation of treatment efficacy for young children who stutter. Journal of Speech, Language and Hearing Research 41: 753–70.

Ingham RJ, Cordes AK (1998) On watching a discipline shoot itself in the foot: some observations on current trends in stuttering treatment research. In Healey C, Ratner N (eds) Stuttering Treatment Efficacy. New York: Lawrence Erlbaum.

ISIS-2 (Second International Study of Infarct Survival) Collaborative Group (1988) Randomised intravenous streptokinase, oral asprin, both, or neither among 17,187 cases of suspected myocardial infaction: ISIS-2. Lancet ii: 349–60.

Iversen-Thoburn SK, Hayden PA (2000) Alaryngeal speech utilization: a survey. Journal of Medical Speech Language Pathology 8: 85–99.

Jackson-Waite K, Robson J, Pring T (2003) Written communication using a Lightwriter in undifferentiated jargon aphasia: a single case study. Aphasiology 17: 767–80.

Jacoby GP, Levin L, Lee L, Creaghead NA, Kummer AW (2002) The number of individual treatment units necessary to facilitate functional communication improvements in the speech and language of young children. American Journal of Speech-Language Pathology 11: 370–80.

Jeffries K, Pring T (1987) Assessing the effects of teaching a learning disabled child. British Journal of Special Education 14: 24–26.

Johnson JA, Pring TR (1990) Speech therapy and Parkinson's disease: a review and further data. British Journal of Disorders of Communication 25: 183–94.

Jones F, Pring T, Grove N (2002) Developing communication in adults with profound and multiple learning difficulties using objects of reference. International Journal of Language and Communication Disorders 37: 173–84.

Jones M, Onslow M, Harrison E, Packman A (2000) Treating stuttering in children: Predicting treatment time in the Lidcombe program. Journal of Speech, Language and Hearing Research 43: 1440–50.

Jones M, Gebski V, Onslow M, Packman A (2001) Design of randomized control trials. Principles and methods applied to a treatment for early stuttering. Journal of Fluency Disorders 26: 247–67.

Jones M, Gebski V, Onslow M, Packman A (2002) Statistical power in stuttering research: a tutorial. Journal of Speech, Language and Hearing Research 45: 243–55.

Kaderavek JN, Sulzby E (1998) Parent–child joint book reading: an observational protocol for young children. American Journal of Speech-Language Pathology 7: 33–47.

Kagan A, Black SE, Duchan J, Simmons-Mackie N, Square P (2001) Training volunteers as conversation partners using 'Supported Conversation for Adults with Aphasia' (SCA): a controlled trial. Journal of Speech, Language and Hearing Research 44: 624–38.

Kail R (1994) A method of studying the generalized slowing hypothesis in children with specific language impairment. Journal of Speech and Hearing Research 37: 418–21.

Kalinowski J, Stuart A, Armson J (1996) Perceptions of stutterers and non-stutterers during speaking and non-speaking situations. American Journal of Speech, Language Pathology 5: 61–6.

Katz RC, Wertz RT (1997) The efficacy of computer provided reading treatment for chronic aphasia. Journal of Speech, Language and Hearing Research 40: 493–507.

Kay J, Lesser R, Coltheart M (1992) PALPA: Psycholinguistic Assessment of Language Processing in Aphasia. Hove: Lawrence Erlbaum.

Kay J, Lesser R, Coltheart M (1996) PALPA: the proof of the pudding is in the eating. Aphasiology 10: 202–15.

Kay-Raining Bird E, Cleave PL, McConnell L (2000) Reading and phonological awareness in children with Down Syndrome: a longitudinal study. American Journal of Speech-Language Pathology 9: 319–30.

Kazdin AE, Bass D (1989) Power to detect differences between alternative treatments in comparative psychotherapy outcome research. Journal of Consulting and Clinical Psychology 57: 138–47.

Keppel G (1991) Design and Analysis: A Researcher's Handbook. Englewood Cliffs, NJ: Prentice Hall.

Kersten P, Low JTS, Ashburn A, George SL, McClellan DL (2002) The unmet needs of young people who have had a stroke: results of a national UK survey. Disability and Rehabilitation 24: 860–6.

Kingston M, Huber A, Onslow M, Jones M, Packman A (2003) Predicting treatment time with the Lidcombe program: replication and meta–analysis. International Journal of Language and Communication Disorders 38: 165–78.

Kitzinger J (1995) Introducing focus groups. British Medical Journal 311: 299–302.

Knight RG, Devereux RC, Godfrey HPD (1997) Psychosocial consequences of caring for a spouse with multiple sclerosis. Journal of Clinical and Experimental Neuropsychology 19: 7-19.

Knowles W, Masidlover M (1982) The Derbyshire Language Scheme. Derby: Derbyshire County Council.

Knox M, Parmenter TR, Atkinson N, Yazbeck M (2000) Family control: the view of families who have a child with an intellectual disability. Journal of Applied Research in Intellectual Disabilities 13: 17-28.

Kuder GF, Richardson MW (1937) The theory of the estimation of test reliability. Psychometrica 2: 151-60.

Kunkel M, Wahlmann U, Wagner W (1997) Objective non-invasive evaluation of velopharyngeal function in cleft and non cleft patients. Cleft Palate - Craniofacial Journal 35: 35-9.

Laakso K, Brunnegard K, Hartelius L, Ahlsen E (2000) Assessing high level language in individuals with multiple sclerosis: a pilot study. Clinical Linguistics and Phonetics 14: 329-49.

Lahey M, Edwards J (1996) Why do children with specific language impairment name pictures more slowly than their peers? Journal of Speech and Hearing Research 39: 1081-98.

Lahey M, Edwards J (1999) Naming errors of children with specific language impairment. Journal of Speech, Language and Hearing Research 42: 195-205.

Lancaster G (1991) The effectiveness of parent administered input training for children with phonological disorders. Unpublished MSc thesis, City Iniversity.

LaPointe LL (1977) Base 10 programmed stimulation: task specification scoring and plotting performance in aphasia therapy. Journal of Speech and Hearing Disorders 42: 90-105.

Larrivee LS, Catts HW (1999) Early reading achievement in children with expressive phonological disorders. American Journal of Speech-Language Pathology 8: 118-28.

Law J, Boyle J, Harris F, Harkness A, Nye C (1998) Screening for speech and language delay: a systematic review of the literature. International Journal of Language and Communication Disorders 33 (supplement): 21-3.

Law J, Conti Ramsden G (2000) Treating children with speech and language impairments: six hours' therapy is not enough. British Medical Journal 321: 908-9.

Law J, Garrett Z, Nye C (2003) Speech and Language Therapy Interventions for Children with Primary Speech and Language Delay or Disorder. Cochrane Developmental Psychosocial and Learning Problems Group: Cochrane Database of Systematic Reviews 1.

Leach C (1979) Introduction to Statistics: A Non-parametric Approach for the Social Sciences. Chichester: Wiley.

Lincoln NB, McGuirk E, Mulley GP, Lendrem W, Jones AC, Mitchell JRA (1984) Effectiveness of speech therapy for aphasic stroke patients: a randomised control trial. The Lancet 1: 1197-200.

Lincoln NB, Flannaghan T, Sutcliffe L, Rother L (1997) Evaluation of cognitive behavioural treatment for depression after stroke: a pilot study. Clinical Rehabilitation 11: 114-22.

Lindsay G, Dockrell J, Letchford B, Mackie C (2002a) Self-esteem of children with specific speech and language difficulties. Child Language Teaching and Therapy 18: 125-43.

Lindsay G, Soloff N, Law J, Band S, Peacey N, Gascoigne M, Radford J (2002b) Speech and language therapy services to education in England and Wales. International Journal of Language and Communication Disorders 37: 173–84.

Lomas J, Pickard L, Bester S, Elbard H, Finlayson A, Zoghaib C (1989) The Communicative Effectiveness Index: Development and psychometric evaluation of a functional communication measure for adult aphasia. Journal of Speech and Hearing Disorders 54: 113–24.

Lowe M, Costello AJ (1988) Symbolic Play Test. 2nd edn. Windsor: NFER-Nelson.

Luborsky L, Diguer L, Seligman DA, Rosenthal R, Krause ED, Johnson S, Halperin G, Bishop M, Berman JS, Schweizer E (1999) The researcher's own therapy allegiances: a wild card in comparisons of treatment efficacy. Clinical Psychology: Science and Practice 6: 95–106.

Luborsky L, Rosenthal R, Diguer L, Andrusyna TP, Berman JS, Levitt JT, Seligman DA, Krause ED (2002) The Dodo-bird verdict is alive and well – mostly. Clinical Psychology: Science and Practice 9: 2–12.

Luther A, Lincoln NB, Grant F (1998) Reliability of stroke patients' reports on rehabilitation services received. Clinical Rehabilitation 12: 238–44.

Lyon JG, Cariski D, Keisler L, Rosenbek J, Levine R, Kumpula J, Ryff C, Coyne S, Blanc M (1997) Communication partners: enhancing participation in life and communication for adults with aphasia in natural settings. Aphasiology 11: 693–708.

Ma EP-M, Yiu EM-L (2001) Voice activity and participation profile: assessing the impact of voice disorders on daily activities. Journal of Speech, Language and Hearing Research 44: 511–24.

MacKenzie K, Millar A, Wilson JA, Sellars C, Deary IJ (2001) Is voice therapy an effective treatment for dysphonia? A randomised control trial. British Medical Journal 323: 658–61.

Mant D (1997) Research and Development in Primary Care. London: HMSO.

Marshall J (1995) The mapping hypothesis and aphasia therapy. Aphasiology 9: 517–39.

Marshall J (2004) Can speech and language therapy with aphasic people reduce disability and increase social participation? A review of the literature. In Halligan P, Wade D (eds) The Effectiveness of Rehabilitation for Cognitive Deficits. Oxford: Oxford University Press.

Marshall J, Chiat S, Pring T (1997) An impairment in processing verbs' thematic roles: a therapy study. Aphasiology 11: 845–54.

Marshall J, Pound C, White-Thompson M, Pring T (1990) The use of picture/word matching tasks to assist word retrieval in aphasic patients. Aphasiology 4: 167–84.

Marshall J, Pring T, Chiat S (1998) Verb retrieval and sentence production in aphasia. Brain and Language 63: 159–83.

Matheney N, Panagos JM (1978) Comparing the effects of articulation and syntax programs on syntax and articulation improvement. Language Speech and Hearing Services in Schools 9: 57–61.

Matthews S, Williams R, Pring T (1997) Parent–child interaction therapy and dysfluency: a single case study. European Journal of Disorders of Communication 32: 346–57.

Mays N, Pope C (2000) Assessing quality in qualitative research. British Medical Journal 320: 50–2.

Mazzoni M, Vista M, Geri E, Avila L, Bianchi F, Moretti P (1995) Comparison of language recovery in rehabilitated and matched non-rehabilitated aphasic patients. Aphasiology 9: 553-63.

McAllister CL, Silverman MA (1999) Community formation and community roles among persons with Alzheimer's disease: a comparative study of experiences in a residential Alzheimer's facility and a traditional nursing home. Qualitative Health Research 9: 65-85.

McGregor KK, Windsor J (1996) Effects of priming on the naming accuracy of preschoolers with word finding deficits. Journal of Speech and Hearing Research 39: 1048-58.

McLaughlin B, White D, McDevitt T, Raskin R (1983) Mothers' and fathers' speech to their young children: similar or different? Journal of Child Language 10: 245-52.

Meikle M, Weschler E, Tupper A, Benenson M, Butler J, Mulhall D, Stern G (1979) Comparative trial of volunteer and professional treatments after stroke. British Medical Journal 2: 87-9.

Michallet B, Le Dorze G, Tetreault S (2001) The needs of spouses caring for severely aphasic persons. Aphasiology 15: 731-47.

Miles S, Bernstein Ratner N (2001) Parental language input to children at stuttering onset. Journal of Speech, Language and Hearing Research 44: 1116-30.

Miller C (2001) False belief understanding in children with specific language impairment. Journal of Communication Disorders 34: 73-86.

Miller CA, Kail R, Leonard LB, Tomblin JB (2001) Speed of processing in children with specific language impairment. Journal of Speech, Language and Hearing Research 44: 416-33.

Miller JF, Sedey AL, Miolo G (1995) Validity of parent report measures of vocabulary development for children with Down syndrome. Journal of Speech and Hearing Research 38: 1037-44.

Mimura M, Kato M, Kato M, Sano Y, Kojima T, Naeser M, Kashima H (1998) Prospective and retrospective studies of recovery in aphasia: changes in cerebral blood flow and language functions. Brain 121: 2083-94.

Moeller MP (2000) Early intervention and language development in children who are deaf and hard of hearing. Pediatrics 106: e43.

Morison M, Moir J (1998) The role of computer software in the analysis of qualitative data: efficient clerk research assistant or Trojan horse? Journal of Advanced Nursing 28: 106-16.

Morley S (1994) Single case methodology in psychological therapy. In Lyndsay SJE, Powell GE (eds) A Handbook of Clinical Adult Psychology (2nd edn). London: Routledge.

Moscicki EK (1993) Fundamental methodological considerations in controlled clinical trials. Journal of Fluency Disorders 18: 183-96.

Nickels L (2002) Therapy for naming disorders: revisiting revising, and reviewing. Aphasiology 16: 935-79.

Nippold MA, Uhden LD, Scwhartz IE (1997) Proverb explanation through the lifespan: a developmental study of adolescents and adults. Journal of Speech, Language and Hearing Research 40: 245-53.

Onslow M, Andrews C, Lincoln M (1994) A control/experimental trial of an operant treatment for early stuttering. Journal of Speech and Hearing Research 26: 531-6.

Onslow M, Costa L, Rue S (1990) Direct early intervention with stuttering: some preliminary data. Journal of Speech and Hearing Disorders 55: 405-16.

Onslow M, Packman A (1998) The Lidcombe program of early stuttering intervention. In Healey C, Ratner N (eds) Stuttering Treatment Efficacy. New York: Lawrence Erlbaum.

Onslow M, Stocker S, Packman A, McLeod S (2002) Speech timing in children after the Lidcombe program of early stuttering intervention. Clinical Linguistics and Phonetics 16: 21-33.

Owen SE, McKinlay IA (1997) Motor difficulties in children with developmental disorders of speech and language. Child: Care, Health and Development 23: 315-25.

Paradice R, Adewusi A (2002) 'It's a continuous fight, isn't it?' Parents' views of educational provision for children with speech and language difficulties. Child Language Teaching and Therapy 18: 257-88.

Parkin AJ, Hunkin NM, Squires EJ (1998) Unlearning John Major: the use of errorless learning in the reaquisition of proper names following herpes simplex encephalitis. Cognitive Neuropsychology 15: 361-75.

Parkinson K, Rae JP (1996) The understanding and use of counselling by speech and language therapists at different levels of experience. European Journal of Disorders of Communication 31: 140-52.

Parr S, Byng S, Gilpin S, Ireland C (1997) Talking about Aphasia. Buckingham: Open University Press.

Pearson VAH (1995) Speech and language therapy: is it effective? Public Health 109: 143-53.

Poeck K, Huber W, Wilmes K (1989) Outcome of intensive language treatment in aphasia. Journal of Speech and Hearing Disorders 54: 471-9.

Polit DF (1996) Data Analysis and Statistics for Nursing Research. Stamford, CT: Appleton & Lange.

Pope C, Ziebland S, Mays N (2000) Analyzing qualitative data. British Medical Journal 320: 114-16.

Pound P, Gompertz P, Ebrahim S (1993) Development and results of a questionnaire to measure carer satisfaction after stroke. Journal of Epidemiology and Community Health 47: 500-5.

Pring TR (1983) Speech therapists and volunteers: some comments on recent investigations of their effectiveness in the treatment of aphasia. British Journal of Disorders of Communication 18: 65-73.

Pring TR (1986) Evaluating the effects of speech therapy for aphasics: developing the single case methodology. British Journal of Disorders of Communication 21: 103-15.

Pring TR, Hunter L (1994) Speakers and listeners: some problems of generalising from a common speech pathology research design. European Journal of Disorders of Communication 29: 51-9.

Ramig LO, Countryman S, Thompson S, Horii Y (1995b) A comparison of two forms of intensive speech treatment for Parkinson's disease. Journal of Speech and Hearing Research 38: 1232-51.

Ramig LO, Pawlas AA, Countryman S (1995a) The Lee Silverman Voice Treatment: a practical guide to treating the voice and speech disorders in Parkinson disease. Iowa City: National Center for Voice and Speech.

Ramig LO, Sapir S, Fox C, Countryman S (2001) Changes in vocal intensity following intensive voice treatment (LSVT) in individuals with Parkinson disease: a comparison with untreated patients and age matched controls. Movement Disorders 16: 79–83.

Reid J, Donaldson M, Howell J, Dean EC, Grieve R (1996) The effectiveness of therapy for child phonological disorder: the Metaphon approach. In Aldridge M (ed.) Child Language. Clevedon: Multilingual Matters.

Renfrew CE (1997) Bus Story Test: A Test of Narrative Speech. Bicester: Winslow.

Rescorla L, Roberts J, Dahlsgaard K (1997) Late talkers at 2: outcome at age 3. Journal of Speech, Language and Hearing Research 40: 556–66.

Ritchie J, Spencer L (1994) Qualitative data analysis for applied policy research. In Bryman A, Burgess RG (eds) Analysing Qualitative Data. London: Routledge.

Roberts PM, Garcia LJ, Desroches A, Hernandez D (2002) English performance of proficient bilingual adults on the Boston Naming Test. Aphasiology 16: 635–45.

Robertson I (1994) Clinical freedom and scientific fact. British Medical Journal 308: 1243.

Robertson SJ, Thomson F (1984) Speech therapy in Parkinson's disease: a study of the efficacy and long-term effects of intensive treatment. British Journal of Disorders of Human Communication 19: 213–24.

Robey RR (1994) The efficacy of treatment for aphasic persons: a meta analysis. Brain and Language 47: 582–608.

Robey RR (1998) A meta analysis of clinical outcomes in the clinical treatment of aphasia. Journal of Speech, Language and Hearing Research 41: 172–87.

Robey RR, Dalebout SD (1998) A tutorial on conducting meta analysis of clinical outcome research. Journal of Speech, Language and Hearing Research 41 1227–41.

Robey RR, Schultz MC (1998) A model for conducting clinical outcomes research: an adaptation of the standard protocol for use in aphasiology. Aphasiology 12: 787–810.

Robson C (2002) Real World Research. Oxford: Blackwell.

Robson J, Pring T, Marshall J, Morrison S, Chiat S (1998) Written communication in undifferentiated jargon aphasia: a therapy study. International Journal of Language and Communication Disorders 33: 305–28.

Rosenhan DL (1973) On being sane in insane places. Science 179: 350–8.

Rosenthal R (1979) The 'file-drawer problem' and tolerance for null results. Psychological Bulletin 86: 638–41.

Rosenthal R, Rosnow RL (1991) Essentials of Behavioural Research. New York: McGraw Hill.

Rosenzweig S (1938) Some implicit common factors in diverse methods in psychotherapy. American Journal of Orthopsychiatry 6: 412–15.

Ross KB, Wertz RT (2003) Quality of life with and without aphasia. Aphasiology 17: 355–64.

Roulestone S (2001) Consensus and variation between speech and language therapists in the assessment and selection of preschool children for intervention: a body of knowledge or idiosyncratic decisions? International Journal of Language and Communication Disorders 36: 329–48.

Roulestone S, Glogowska M, Peters T, Enderby P (2001) Day in day out: the everyday therapy of community clinics. International Journal of Language and Communication Disorders 36 (supplement): 435–40.

Rust J, Golombok S (2000) Modern Psychometrics: The Science of Psychological Assessment. London: Routledge.

Sanger DD, Creswell JW, Dworak J, Schultz L (2000) Cultural analysis of communication behaviours among juveniles in a correctional facility. Journal of Communication Disorders 33: 31-57.

Sanz C (2000) Bilingual education enhances third language acquisition: evidence from Catalonia. Applied Psycholinguistics 21: 23-44.

Sapir S, Mathers-Schmidt B, Larson GW (1996) Singers' and non singers' vocal health, vocal behaviours and attitudes towards singing: indirect findings from a questionnaire. European Journal of Disorders of Communication 31: 193-209.

Sarno MT (1968) Peech impairment in Parkinson's disease. Archives of Physical Medicine and Rehabilitation 49: 269-75.

Schmidt CL, Lawson KR (2002) Caregiving attention – focusing and children's attention sharing behaviours as predictors of later verbal IQ in very low birth weight children. Journal of Child Language 29: 3-22.

Schultz GM, Grant MK (2000) Effects of speech therapy and pharmacological and surgical treatments on voice and speech in Parkinson's disease: a review of the literature. Journal of Communication Disorders 33: 59-88.

Sellars C, Hughes T, Langhorne P (2002) Speech and language therapy for dysarthria due to non-progressive brain damage: a systematic Cochrane review. Clinical Rehabilitation 16: 61-8.

Semel E, Wiig EH, Secord WA (1987) Clinical Evaluation of Language Fundamentals – Revised. San Antonio, TX: The Psychological Corporation.

Semel E, Wiig EH, Secord WA (1995) Clinical Evaluation of Language Fundamentals. 3rd edn. Orlando: Harcourt Brace.

Seron X (1997) Effectiveness and specifity in neurosychological therapies: a cognitive point of view. Aphasiology 11: 105-23.

Servaes P, Draper B, Conroy P, Bowring G (1998) Informal carers of aphasic stroke patients: stresses and interventions. A literature review. Aphasiology 13: 889-900.

Shapiro DA, Shapiro D (1982) Meta-analysis of comparative therapy outcome studies: a replication and refinement. Psychological Bulletin 92: 581-604.

Shapiro DA, Shapiro D (1983) Comparative therapy outcome research: methodological implications of meta-analysis. Journal of Consulting and Clinical Psychology 51: 42-53.

Silverman D (1993) Interpreting qualitative data. Methods for analyzing talk text and interaction. London: Sage.

Smith ML, Glass GV (1977) Meta analysis of psychotherapy outcome studies. American Psychologist 32: 752-60.

Snowling MJ, Adams JW, Bishop DVM, Stothard SE (2001) Educational attainment of school leavers with a preschool history of speech language impairments. International Journal of Language and Communication Disorders 36: 173-83.

Spector A, Thorgrimsen L, Woods B, Royan L, Davies S, Butterworth M, Orrell M (2003) Efficacy of an evidence-based cognitive stimulatiom therapy programme for people with dementia – randomised control trial. British Journal of Psychiatry 183: 248-54.

Starkweather CW, Gottwald SR (1990) The demands and capacities model II: clinical implications. Journal of Fluency Disorders 15: 143-57.

Stern RA, Arruda JE, Hooper CR, Wolfner GD, Morey CE (1997) Visual analogue mood scales to measure internal mood state in neurologically impaired patients: description and initial validity evidence. Aphasiology 11: 59-71.

Stern RA, Bachman DL (1991) Depressive symptoms following stroke. American Journal of Psychiatry 148: 351–6.

Streiner DL, Norman GR (1995) Health Measurement Scales: A Practical Guide to Their Development and Use. 2nd edn. Oxford: Oxford University.

Tabachnick BG, Fidell LS (2001) Using Multivariate Statistics. 4th edn. Boston: Allyn & Bacon.

Thal DJ, O'Hanlon L, Clemmons M, Fralin L (1999) Validity of a parent report measure of vocabulary and syntax for preschool children with language impairment. Journal of Speech, Language and Hearing Research 42: 482–96.

Thomas C, Howell P (2001) Assessing efficacy of stuttering treatments. Journal of Fluency Disorders 26: 311–33.

Thomas P (2000) The research needs of primary care: trials must be relevant to patients. British Medical Journal 321: 2–3.

Tomblin JB, Hammer CS, Zhang X (1998) The association of parental tobacco use and SLI. International Journal of Language and Communication Disorders 33: 357–68.

Tomblin JB, Records NL, Buckwalter P, Zhang X, Smith E, O'Brien M (1997) Prevalence of specific language impairment in kindergarten children. Journal of Speech, Language and Hearing Research 40: 1245–60.

Tryon WW (1982) A simplified time series analysis for evaluating treatment interventions. Journal of Applied Behavioural Analysis 15: 423–9.

Van der Gaag A (1988) The Communication Assessment Profile (CASP). London: Speach Profiles.

Walker–Batson D, Curtis S, Natarajan R, Ford J, Dronkers N, Salmeron E, Lai J, Unwin DH (2001) A double blind placebo-controlled study of the use of amphetamine in the treatment of aphasia. Stroke 32: 2093–7.

Wampold BE, Mondin GW, Moody M, Stich F, Benson K, Ahn H (1997) A meta analysis of outcome studies comparing bona fide psychotherapies: Empirically 'All must have prizes'. Psychological Bulletin 122: 203–15.

Ward S (1999) An investigation into the effectiveness of an early intervention method for delayed language development in young children. International Journal of Language and Communication Disorders 34: 243–64.

Ware JE, Snow KK, Kosinski M, Gandek B (1993) SF-36 Health Survey: Manual and Interpretation Guide. Boston, MA: The Health Institute, New England Medical Center.

Wertz RT, Weiss DG, Aten JL, Brookshire R, Garcia-Bunuel L, Holland A, Kurtzke J, LaPointe L, Milianti F, Brannegan R, Greenbaum H, Marshall R, Vogel D, Carter J, Barnes N, Goodman R (1986) Comparison of clinic, and home deferred language treatment for aphasia: a veterans administration cooperative study. Archives of Neurology 43: 653–8.

Wertz RT (1996) The PALPA's proof is in the predicting. Aphasiology 10: 180–90.

Westby C (1997) There's more to passing than knowing the answers. Language, Speech and Hearing Services in Schools 28: 274–87.

Westen D, Morrison K (2001) A multidimensional meta analysis of treatments for depression, panic and generalized anxiety disorder: An empirical examination of the status of empirically supported therapies. Journal of Consulting and Clinical Psychology 69: 875–99.

Wetherby AM, Allen L, Cleary J, Kublin K, Goldstein H (2002) Validity and reliability of the Communication and Symbolic Behaviour Scales Developmental Profile with very young children. Journal of Speech, Language and Hearing Research 45: 1202–18.

Whurr R, Lorch MP, Nye C (1992) A meta analysis of studies between 1946 and 1988 concerned with the efficacy of speech and language therapy treatment for aphasic persons. European Journal of Disorders of Communication 27: 1–17.

Wilson JA, Deary IJ, Millar A, MacKenzie K (2002) The quality of life impact of dysphonia. Clinical Otolaryngology 27: 179–82.

Wilson PH, Henry J, Bowen M, Haralambous G (1991) Tinnitus reaction questionnaire: psychometric properties of a measure of distress associates with tinnitus. Journal of Speech and Hearing Research 34: 197–201.

Windsor J, Hwang M (1999) Testing the generalized slowing hypothesis in specific language impairment. Journal of Speech, Language and Hearing Research 42: 1205–18.

Winter K (1999) Speech and language therapy provision for bilingual children: aspects of the current service. International Journal of Language and Communication Disorders 34: 85–98.

Wolk L, Meisler AW (1998) Phonological assessment: a systematic comparison of conversation and picture naming. Journal of Communication Disorders 31: 291–313.

Woods CL, Williams DE (1976) Traits attributed to stuttering and normally fluent males. Journal of Speech and Hearing Research 19: 267–78.

Woods S, Shearsby J, Onslow M, Burnham D (2002) The psychological impact of the Lidcombe program of early stuttering intervention: eight case studies. International Journal of Language and Communication Disorders 37: 31–40.

World Health Organization (WHO) (1999) International Classification of Functioning and Disability (ICIDH-2 beta-2 version). Geneva: WHO.

Yairi E, Ambrose N (1992) A longitudinal study of stuttering children: a preliminary report. Journal of Speech and Hearing Research 35: 755–60.

Yaruss JS (1997) Clinical implications of situational variability in preschool children who stutter. Journal of Fluency Disorders 22: 187–203.

Yaruss JS (2001) Evaluating treatment outcomes for adults who stutter. Journal of Communication Disorders 34: 163–82.

Yaruss JS, Quesal RW, Reeves L, Molt LF, Kluetz B, Caruso AJ, McClure JA, Lewis F (2002) Speech treatment and support group experiences of people who participate in the National Stuttering Association. Journal of Fluency Disorders 27: 115–34.

Yoder P (1999) Letter to the editor. International Journal of Language and Communication Disorders 34: 441–3.

Yorkston KM, Beukleman DR (1980) An analysis of connected speech samples of aphasic and normal speakers. Journal of Speech and Hearing Disorders 45: 27–36.

Yorkston KM, Klasner ER, Swanson KM (2001) Communication in context: a qualitative study of the experiences of individuals with multiple sclerosis. American Journal of Speech-Language Pathology 10: 126–37.

Zigmond AS, Snaith RP (1983) The Hospital Anxiety and Depression Scale. Acta Psychiatrica Scandinavica 7: 361–70.

Index